Antibiotics and Chemotherapy

Vol. 30

Series Editors

H. Schönfeld, Grenzach; *R. W. Brockman,* Birmingham, Ala., and
F. E. Hahn, Washington, D. C.

S. Karger · Basel · München · Paris · London · New York · Sydney

Antiparasitic Chemotherapy

Antiparasitic Chemotherapy

Volume Editor
H. Schönfeld, Grenzach

19 figures, 1 color plate and 14 tables, 1981

S. Karger · Basel · München · Paris · London · New York · Sydney

Antibiotics and Chemotherapy

Vol. 27: Virus Chemotherapy. Hahn, F. E., Washington, D. C. (ed.)
VI + 306 p., 58 fig., 12 schemes, 34 tab., 1980. ISBN 3–8055–0263–X
Vol. 28: Design of Cancer Chemotherapy. Experimental and Clinical Approaches.
Mihich, E., Buffalo, N. Y. and Eckhardt, S., Budapest (eds.)
X + 194 p., 14 fig., 27 tab., 1980. ISBN 3–8055–0411–X

National Library of Medicine, Cataloging in Publication
Antiparasitic chemotherapy
Volume editor, H. Schönfeld. – Basel, New York, Karger, 1981
(Antibiotics and chemotherapy; v. 30)
1. Parasitic Diseases – drug therapy I. Schönfeld, H. (Hans) II. Series
W1 AN855G v.30/ [WC A633]
ISBN 3-8055-2160-X

Drug Dosage
The author and publisher have exerted every effort to ensure that drug selection and dosage set forth in this text are in accord with current recommendations and practice at the time of publication. However, in view of ongoing research, changes in government regulations, and the constant flow of information relating to drug therapy and drug reactions, the reader is urged to check the package insert for each drug for any change in indications and dosage and for added warnings and precautions. This is particularly important when the recommended agent is a new and/or infrequently employed drug.

Printed in Switzerland by Merkur AG, Langenthal.
ISBN 3-8055-2160-X

Contents

Introduction VII

Botero, D. (Medellin): Intestinal Parasitic Infections 1
Biagi, F. (Mexico): Amebiasis 20
Culbertson C. G. (Indianapolis, Ind.): Amebic Meningoencephalitis (with 1 color plate) 28
Gemmell, M. A.; Johnstone, P. D. (Dunedin/Mosgiel): Cestodes . . 54
Ribeiro-dos-Santos, R.; Rassi, A.; Köberle, F. (Sao Paulo/Goiás): Chagas' Disease 115
Hawking, F. (St. Albans): Chemotherapy of Filariasis 135
Meingassner, J. G.; Heyworth, P. G. (Vienna): Intestinal and Urogenital Flagellates 163
Kern, P. (Hamburg): Leishmaniasis 203
Dietrich, M.; Kern, P. (Hamburg): Malaria 224
Hughes, W. T. (Baltimore, Md.): *Pneumocystis Carinii* Pneumonitis 257
Evans, D. A. (London): African Trypanosomes 272

Introduction

In recent years, numerous publications have pointed to the particular problems of health and hygiene that have resulted from mass tourism in tropical regions as well as from the foreign travels, for political and business purposes, of inhabitants from these regions.

For the most part, these publications have concentrated on the 'major' infectious diseases, with malaria continuing to require prime attention despite intense efforts to eradicate this disease. In 'civilized' countries, other parasitic diseases tend to be regarded as insignificant and rare – so rare, in fact, that they seldom achieve mention in the colorful brochures issued by travel agencies. It is exactly these lesser known parasitoses, however, that can pose a particularly dangerous and insidious threat to human health.

The present volume of Antibiotics and Chemotherapy is intended to serve as a source of information covering important human parasitoses which have received inadequate attention. The editors are aware that a complete review of all such diseases would be beyond the scope of this series and have therefore chosen to concentrate on selected disorders of major interest.

Unfortunately, two contributions scheduled to cover schistosomiasis and distome flukes were not submitted in time. These papers will appear in forthcoming issues of the journal Chemotherapy.

In keeping with the editorial policy of Antibiotics and Chemotherapy, all contributions feature the original work of well-known experts. The editorial board respects the authority of these contributions and has not altered their contents.

H. Schönfeld, Grenzach

Antibiotics Chemother., vol. 30, pp. 1–19 (Karger, Basel 1981)

Intestinal Parasitic Infections

David Botero

School of Medicine, University of Antioquia, Medellín, Colombia

Introduction

Intestinal parasitic infections belong to the most common and widespread infections throughout the world. The prevalence in developing countries in Latin America, Asia and Africa is very high, sometimes near 100 % in the poorest communities. Fecal contamination of the soil is the main dissemination mechanism of these parasites, which invade the human host mainly through the mouth, when ingesting contaminated food or water, or directly when eating portions of soil or feces. Some intestinal parasites invade through the skin; this is facilitated by the custom of walking barefooted, mainly in rural areas. The high prevalence of intestinal parasites always runs parallel to the deficient living conditions, low family income and poor sanitation. It can be assured that the frequency of intestinal parasitism is an indicator of the level of development of the communities studied. For these reasons the control of these parasitic infections is very difficult and it is not only a public-health task, but a matter of economic development and raising of living standards [1].

In the tropical areas of the world the high prevalence of intestinal parasites has been observed for many years, and unfortunately, in rural areas the frequencies are similar to those found when the first surveys were done, 50 or 80 years ago. In the recent decades these parasites have expanded their geographical distribution, due to the frequent traveling to the temperate zone and to the increased number of visitors to the tropics. These are reasons why medical doctors and paramedical personnel, all over the world, should be acquainted with parasitic diseases [2].

Although some pathogenic intestinal parasites may not produce symptomatology at a certain time, they can cause lesions at any moment and can be responsible for symptoms of varying intensity. Because the number of affected people in the poor countries is so high, the effects on the general health of the population is considerable. These parasites are an important cause of diarrhea, some produce anemia and others may invade internal organs and become responsible for diseases that are fatal in some cases [3].

The treatment of the intestinal parasitic infections is mandatory when the patient complains of disease caused by these parasitic agents. It is frequent that a patient consulting for other disease is found to harbor intestinal parasites. This carrier state is usually treated because its elimination is a good measure to prevent dissemination to others. At the present time, when the antiparasitic drugs are more effective and less toxic, their use in mass therapy has been practiced as a public health measure, along with the traditional preventive procedures, such as sanitation, personal hygiene, use of latrines, wearing of shoes, etc. These methods of control, including the periodic treatments, are necessary in endemic areas, where reinfections are the rule for the people that live in contaminated environments [4]. Multiparasitism is more frequent than the presence of only one species of parasite, which makes proper treatment, usually by using more than one drug, necessary. Chemoprophylaxis for intestinal parasitic infections is not currently used and immunizations are nonexisting. Only under special circumstances chemoprophylaxis is recommended and effectively practised for amebiasis. This is possible because there are good nonabsorbable drugs that act by contact with the parasites in the lumen of the large intestine, where the ameba are attacked promptly after they reach the colon. This measure is not applicable to other intestinal protozoa or helminths [5].

Pathology

The different biological characteristics of the intestinal parasites, which include location in the bowel, capacity of invading, migration, blood sucking, etc., are the reasons for the variable pathology and symptomatology they can produce. The human factors responsible for the susceptibility to disease due to these agents are also important variables to be considered.

A simple biological classification of the intestinal parasites can be made in three groups: protozoa, which are microscopic unicellular organisms; nematodes or roundworms, which have a cilindrical shape, and cestodes or tapeworms, which have a flat morphology. For review of the pathology, a separate paragraph is dedicated to each one of the common parasites, within these three groups.

Intestinal Protozoa

Entamoeba histolytica. This parasite is transmitted by ingestion of mature cysts; each of them capable to produce eight trophozoites in the large intestine. The trophozoites, or motile forms, reproduce by binary fission within the lumen or the intestinal wall. These trophozoites encyst again in the intestinal lumen and are eliminated with the formed stool. Contamination of hands, food, water, etc., by these stools are the origin of new infections.

E. histolytica is the only human intestinal ameba pathogenic for man. It is fairly widespread in all countries and shows a prevalence of 20–40% in endemic areas of developing tropical countries. It has been observed that in some endemic areas approximately 75% of the persons positive for this parasite in stool examinations are asymptomatic at certain times. Of the remaining 25% symptomatic cases, about 1/4 of them are acute or dysenteric cases, while the rest are chronic cases. This last group, presenting mainly with abdominal cramps and slight diarrhea, correspond to those in which the tissue invasion by the amebic trophozoites is scanty and superficial. In the dysenteric patients the pathological findings are ulcerations of varying intensity, sometimes deep enough to cause intestinal perforation. The asymptomatic cases do not have tissue invasion and the parasites reproduce in the intestinal lumen. The extraintestinal forms of amebiasis are less frequent, hepatic abscess being the most frequent location. Cutaneous amebiasis, genital infections, ameboma and brain abscess are rare forms of this disease.

Giardia lamblia. These flagellate protozoa inhabit the duodenum and proximal part of the small intestine where they adhere to the intestinal mucosa and sometimes penetrate superficially. They are transmitted from person to person through cysts eliminated with the formed feces. In the diarrheic stools or the duodenal fluid the trophozoites are observed. These are noninfective by oral route, but multiply actively in the intestine. Some reservoirs including dogs and wild animals can harbor the parasites and occasionally be the source of infection. Giardiasis is more common in children, especially in the developing areas of the world, where fecal contamination is common. The prevalence in these areas and age groups is around 20%. Recently, an increasing frequency in persons from temperate countries traveling abroad has been observed. More than 50% of the cases, mainly adults, are asymptomatic or show slight symptomatology such as meteorism, abdominal malaise and loose stools. When frankly symptomatic, the patients complain of diarrhea, abdominal pain, steatorrhea, malabsorption syndrome and weight loss.

Balantidium coli. These ciliated Protozoa inhabit the large intestine of humans and pigs, multiply in the intestinal lumen as trophozoites and are encysted in the cecum. The cysts are eliminated with the feces and constitute the infective forms by oral ingestion. The frequency of this parasite is usually less than 1% in tropical areas. When symptoms are present they are due to the production of colonic ulcerations. The clinical picture is represented mainly by diarrhea and colicky pain, but in severe cases a dysenteric syndrome is observed, similar to the amebic dysentery.

Intestinal Nematodes

Ascaris lumbricoides (Roundworm). The roundworm is the most frequent parasitic worm throughout the world, prevalence rates being from 50 to 80% in developing countries. Infection occurs when the host is ingesting embryonated eggs. The larvae liberated in the small intestine penetrate the blood stream and reach the lungs, where they produce transient tissue damage and microscopic hemorrhage; the subsequent respiratory symptoms are rarely attributed to the parasite. These larvae travel to the epiglottis and are swallowed to become adult parasites in the small intestine. The adult worms produce periumbilical pain and occasional diarrhea. When the number of worms is high, intestinal obstruction can be seen. Impairment of nutrition is also observed in these cases, mainly in children with a low food intake. The most important complications of ascariasis are caused by migratory worms; invasion to the bile ducts, liver, appendix, peritoneal cavity, etc., cause serious disease, sometimes requiring surgical treatment.

Trichuris trichiura (Whipworm). This helminth is nearly as frequent as *A. lumbricoides*, mainly in tropical countries. The worms inhabit the large intestine, where they are partially introduced in the mucosa. Eggs are eliminated in the stools and embryonate in the soil, they are infective by mouth, but there is no pulmonary migration of the larvae; the adult worms are directly developed in the large intestine. The pathology is dependent on the worm burden, the majority of the light infections being asymptomatic. In the moderate infections the symptoms are diarrhea and colicky pain. In the intense infections, most frequently seen in children living in poor environmental conditions, a dysenteric syndrome can be observed. When malnutrition is associated, rectal prolapse can occur. Blood loss due to intestinal hemorrhage is the cause of anemia in these children.

Necator americanus and Ancylostoma duodenale (Hookworms). These parasites predominate in the rural areas of the tropical countries where the prevalence varies much depending on several epidemiological conditions. In endemic areas frequencies are from 20 to 80 %. The eggs eliminated in the stools form larvae in the soil, able to penetrate the skin, travel through the blood stream, invade the lungs and produce transient pneumonitis with high circulating eosinophilia. The initial lesions in the skin cause pruriginous lesions, called ground itch. From the lungs the larvae go to the epiglottis and are swallowed to become adult worms in the duodenum; there they attach to the mucosa by means of hooks and produce hemorrhage. The parasites ingest blood and cause chronic anemia when the intensity of the worm burden is high. Undernutrition and nutritional anemia are frequently associated and aggravate the clinical manifestations of the disease. Epigastric pain, vomiting and other symptoms of duodenitis are frequent in this disease.

Strongyloides stercoralis (Threadworm). This small helminth presents prevalence rates around 10 % in tropical countries. The parasites live within the mucosa and submucosa of the small intestine, where they produce larvae that are eliminated in the feces. After becoming infective in the soil, the larvae penetrate the skin, pass through the lungs and reach the small intestine again. Lesions and symptoms are presented in the port of entry and in the lungs similarly to the hookworms. Intestinal symptoms are those of duodenitis, such as epigastric pain, nausea etc., resembling peptic ulcer. Malabsorption syndrome is sometimes present. High eosinophilia always accompany this parasitic infection. The most important pathological effect of strongiloidiasis may occur in debilitated patients and in those receiving corticosteroids or other immunosuppressive drugs, in which autohyperinfection can produce a massive invasion of the worms to the whole intestine and other viscera, sometimes fatal. This infection is especially important to prevent in transplanted patients and in others receiving immunosuppressive treatment.

Enterobius vermicularis (Pinworm). The location of this parasite is the colonic lumen; the adult females migrate through the anus to deposit the eggs in the perianal skin. These migrations produce pruritus ani and vulvae, the main symptoms of this parasitic infection. The female genital tract, especially in children, can be invaded by the parasites. Enterobiasis is easily spread from person to person and is prevalent not only in the developing countries, but also in those with high living standards. Prevalence rates in children are from 10 to 50%.

Intestinal Cestodes

The most important human intestinal tapeworms are: (a) the long parasites, acquired by ingesting raw or undercooked meat or fish, *Taenia saginata,* or beef tapeworm, *Taenia solium,* or pork tapeworm, and *Dyphillobothrium latum,* or fish tapeworm; (b) the small or dwarf tapeworm *Hymenolepis nana,* transmitted by ingestion of eggs eliminated in the feces of the infected persons. Most cases of the four mentioned cestodiasis are asymptomatic; when symptoms occur, they are of low intensity and mainly referred to the intestinal tract.

Cysticercosis is an important disease produced when the eggs of *T. solium* reach the stomach; this is possible when the eggs are ingested or when they are regurgitated from the intestine. Hydatid disease is produced when ingesting eggs of the dog tapeworm *Echinococcus granulosus.* These last two cestodiasis are produced by larvae of the parasites that have tissue invasion different from the intestine. The treatment is by surgical procedures, but some trials with mebendazole have shown benefits for hydatic cyst, while praziquantel is promising in human cysticercosis.

Chemotherapy [6–8]

Important advance in the treatment of intestinal parasitic infections has been obtained in the last decade, although the ideal single dose of a nontoxic and wide-spectrum antiparasitic drug that at the same time is of low cost, has not been found yet. The enormous number of parasitized people in the world requires a simple treatment that may be used in mass campaings. Treatment is an important complementary control measure for the intestinal parasites, since the traditional, well-known methods of control that include sanitation, housing, water supply, personal hygiene, etc., are difficult to implant in the developing countries and sometimes impossible to obtain by the poorest infected groups. Individual treatment is necessary in most cases, especially when the parasitic infection is causing symptomatology.

The drugs of choice and the alternative treatments will be mentioned for each of the infections considered in this chapter.

Amebiasis

In cases of symptomatic intestinal amebiasis two types of drugs are always necessary, one for attacking the trophozoites in the tissues and the other against those in the lumen. In the first group, the drugs of choice are the nitroimidazole derivatives and in the second group the dichloroacetamide derivatives. Alternative treatment among the tissue amebicides is dehydroemetine. In cases of asymptomatic amebiasis the oral luminal amebicides of the dichloroacetamide group are sufficient to eliminate the infection. Hydroxyquinolines are not recommended any more due to their toxicity and low efficacy. Paromomycin is poorly tolerated, expensive and of low therapeutic value.

Giardiasis

The drugs of choice are the nitroimidazoles and the alternative treatment is based on the use of furazolidone. Quinacrine is still used in some countries, but the poor tolerability and the lower efficacy compared with the other two drugs already mentioned, makes the use of quinacrine unnecessary.

Balantidiasis, Ascariasis and Trichuriasis

The nitroimidazoles found effective for *balantidiasis* are metronidazole and nimorazole. The others have not been tried in this parasitic disease. *Ascariasis* is effectively treated with pyrantel pamoate or mebendazole. Alternative treatment are tetramisole-levamisole, the new anthelmintic flubendazole and the old anthelmintic piperazine. For *trichuriasis* the drug of choice is mebendazole or its analogue flubendazole. An alternative drug is oxantel pamoate.

Necatoriasis and Ancylostomiasis, and Strongyloidiasis

Both pyrantel pamoate and mebendazole are similarly effective against the two hookworms parasitic for man *(Ancylostoma* and *Necator).* Bephenium hydroxynaphthoate is still used in some countries as an alternative only for *Ancylostoma duodenale,* since the action against *Necator americanus* is very low. This drug is poorly tolerated and much less effective than the two other mentioned drugs. For these reasons its use is not necessary. Tetrachloroethylene is toxic and not very effective. The only drug effective for *strongyloidiasis* is thiabendazole.

Enterobiasis and Cestodiasis

Similarly good for the treatment of enterobiasis are pyrantel pamoate and mebendazole. The alternative drugs are flubendazole and piperazine. Pyrvinium pamoate is not necessary at the present time. The tapeworm infections (cestodiasis) are preferably treated with praziquantel and alternatively with niclosamide.

Description of the Drugs

The drugs for the treatment of intestinal parasites are divided into three groups, according to their benefits:

(1) Those considered drugs of choice: dichloroacetamide derivatives, nitroimidazoles, mebendazole, pyrantel pamoate, thiabendazole and praziquantel. For these drugs, except thiabendazole, a description is made under the following aspects: (a) chemical composition and mode of action; (b) toxicity, side effects and contraindications; (c) individual therapy indications and dosages; (d) uses in mass treatment, when applicable.

(2) Alternative drugs: emetine and dehydroemetine, furazolidone, flubendazole, piperazine, tetramisole-levamisole, oxantel pamoate and niclosamide. These drugs are described in a shorter manner.

(3) Drugs not necessary at the present time or contraindicated, which still are on the market and are used in some countries: hydroxyquinolines, paromomycin, quinacrine, bephenium hydroxynaphthoate, tetrachloroethylene and pyrvinium pamoate. These drugs are not described in this text.

Antiprotozoan Drugs

Oral Luminal Amebicides: Dichloroacetamide Derivatives

(a) These compounds are very slightly absorbed from the intestine and are presented as white or yellowish powders almost insoluble in water, of no special taste. Four compounds are currently in use: teclozan, dichloroacetyl-ethyl-aminoethyl-benzene (100-mg tablets); diloxanide furoate, 4-(N-methyldichloroacetamide) phenyl-2-furoate (500-mg tablets); etofamide, a derivative of clefamide, closely related in chemical structure (200-mg tablets); clefamide, N-(β-oxyethyl)-N-(p-phenoxy-)4-nitrobenzyl dichloroacetamide (250-mg tablets).

These compounds are amebicides by contact in the intestinal lumen. As all antiamebic drugs, they act against the trophozoites, since the cysts are unpenetrable by these chemicals. The amides are effective in high dilutions, over 1:80,000. The intimate mode of action against the parasites is not completely known.

(b) Experimental toxicity is low, being LD_{50} by oral route over 5,000 mg/kg. At therapeutical dosages no toxic side effects have been reported. No contraindications are known. A frequent side effect is flatulence, a symptom that disappears after the treatment is finished.

(c) Indications for these drugs are treatment of asymptomatic cyst passers and treatment of symptomatic intestinal amebiasis, in this case combined with an amebicide that acts in the tissues. The dosage for adults is 3–6 tablets per day for 5–10 days. For children lower dosages can be used in suspension form.

(d) Mass treatment for amebiasis is not commonly used. Chemoprophylaxis is effective with these drugs; it can be used in highly endemic areas, mainly for visitors; in mental institutions and in communities with very poor hygienic conditions. One tablet, 2 or 3 times per week, is sufficient for prevention.

Oral Tissue Amebicides: Nitroimidazole Derivatives

These drugs are administered by mouth only, they are absorbed from the small intestine and act against the ameba trophozoites in the intestinal wall and in other body tissues. They have very little activity against the parasites in the intestinal lumen. For this reason it is necessary to associate them with luminal amebicides. There are good number of compounds pertaining to the 5-nitroimidazole group, all with anti-protozoan activity. The drugs more commonly used will be mentioned below.

Metronidazole

(a) This was the first compound clinically used in protozoan diseases. Since 1959 it has been used for *Trichomonas vaginalis* infections with excellent results. Several years later the use was expanded to the treatment of amebiasis and giardiasis. Metronidazole (1-(2hydroxyethyl)-2-methyl-5-nitroimidazole) is a crystaline powder, soluble in water and readily absorbed from the small intestine. The plasma levels rise rapidly, reach effective concentrations in 2–3 h, and maintain these levels for 12 h after a single oral dose. It is excreted mainly through the urine, which sometimes presents a redish color; it is also eliminated through the bile in the form of a metabolite, that added to the small amount of the nonabsorbed drug, is responsible for some activity against the luminal amebic trophozoites. Other secretions presenting the metabolite are saliva, semen, vaginal secretions and milk. The drug crosses the placenta, a fact that restricts its use in pregnant women.

(b) The drug has a bitter taste and produces side effects in 15–30% of the treated cases, usually of low intensity. The most common symptoms are of the gastrointestinal tract, such as nausea, vomiting, abdominal pain, metallic taste and diarrhea. Symptoms of the nervous system are seen less frequently, such as dizziness, joint and muscle pain, headache and numbness of the extremities. The inhibition of several enzymes concerned with the metabolism of alcohol, are responsible for the frequent symptoms present when alcohol is ingested during or shortly after the treatment with metronidazole. This disulfiram-like effect is characterized by confusional state, flushing, headache, nausea, vomiting, drowsiness and fall in blood pressure. Contraindications are pregnancy during the first trimester, blood discrasias and diseases of the CNS. The matter of carcinogenicity of metronidazole has created some fear in the medical profession and in the patients, but so far no clinical evidence of cancer production in humans has been reported, in spite of the ample use of this drug throughout the world for 20 years. It is prudent to consider metronidazole as a potential carcinogenic drug, since it was found in 1971 that the incidence of naturally occurring tumors in rats and mice was increased significantly when large doses of this drug were administered to these animals for long periods of time. The drug was also shown to induce mutagenic changes in certain bacteria, a fact that has been associated with carcinogenicity.

(c) For the treatment of symptomatic intestinal amebiasis the dosage used is 30 mg/kg/day, divided in three doses after meals, during 8–10 days. For giardiasis, 15 mg/kg/day in divided doses for 5 days. The liquid preparations are recommended for children. For balantidiasis a similar treatment as for amebiasis can be used.

(d) Mass treatment or mass chemoprophylaxis with this drug are not recommended for amebiasis. For giardiasis, group treatment can be used in children institutions showing high prevalence rates.

Tinidazole [9]

(a) Chemically it is ethyl(2-(2-methyl-1,5-nitro-1-imidazolyl)-ethyl)-sulfone. This drug has similar absorption and pharmacokinetic properties as metronidazole, but the blood concentration after 24 h of administering the two drugs are twice higher for tinidazole than for metronidazole. The medium life span of tinidazole is 10–14 h, longer than for metronidazole. As opposed to metronidazole that is eliminated as a metabolite, tinidazole is eliminated as the drug itself and in less proportion through the urine.

(b) Experimental acute toxicity in rodents showed that the oral and intraperitoneal LD_{50} was higher than 2,000 mg/kg. Studies on subacute toxicity revealed that dosages of 150 mg/kg twice daily for 30 days did not produce clinical or necropsy changes in rats and monkeys. Human toxic effects have not been observed in patients receiving therapeutical dosages. Side effects are not frequently observed; when present they are mainly of the gastrointestinal tract, such as nausea and vomiting, usually transient. Although no teratogenicity has been demonstrated, the drug crosses the placenta and is excreted in the milk; for these reasons it is a good precaution not to give this drug during the first trimester of pregnancy or to nursing mothers. Disulfiram-like reactions with alcohol are observed.

(c) The most common regimens used for intestinal amebiasis are 2 g daily, as a single dose after a meal, during 2 days for adults, and 60 mg/kg in a similar way for children, during 2–3 consecutive days. These short treatments have shown comparably better results than the longer treatments with metronidazole. For both drugs the efficacy in eliminating the parasites in amebic carriers is low, since the effect on the luminal trophozoites is very little or abscent. This is the reason why a luminal amebicide should be associated when treating intestinal symptomatic cases.

For giardiasis a single dose of 2 g for adults or 60 mg/kg for children is effective.

(d) As with other nitroimidazole derivatives no mass therapy is recommended.

Ornidazole

Ornidazole [α-(chloromethyl)-2-methyl-5-nitroimidazole-1-ethanol] is similar to the two compounds already mentioned in most parmacological aspects. Some special characteristics of ornidazole presented by the producers are: high plasma concentration of the drug during 1 or 2 h after oral administration; 85 % excretion of the ingested amount during the first 5 days; 63 % elimination through the urine and 22 % through the feces; no incompatibility with alcohol; little neurotoxicity, no teratogenicity and no carcinogenicity.

Ornidazole is clinically recommended in intestinal amebiasis and giardiasis at the dosage of 500 mg twice a day during 5–10 days for adults, and at proportionally lower dosages for children. The results in cases of symptomatic intestinal amebiasis were similar for ornidazole and metronidazole; the clinical and parasitological cure rates were over 90 %. Tolerance was also similar for both drugs: 15 % had side effects usually of low intensity, consisting of dizziness, muscle and joint pains, nausea and vomiting.

Nimorazole

This drug is also called nitrimidazine [1-(N,β-ethyl-morpholine)-5-nitroimidazole]. The in vitro activity against *E. histolytica* is similar to that of metronidazole, but the blood and urine levels are higher. The recommended dosage for amebiasis and giardiasis is 40 mg/kg/day for 5–10 days. In cases of balantidiasis, similar dosages have been effective. Results and side effects seem to be similar to the other imidazoles mentioned, although less information on nimorazol was found.

Parenteral Tissue Amebicides: Emetine and Dehydroemetine

This drug has been in use for more than 50 years. Its action on *E. histolytica* in the tissues has been known for a long time. It is the methyl ester of cephaline, derived from the plant ipecac, which also can be synthesized. Emetine is freely soluble in water and is given by injection. The oral presentations are poorly tolerated and not very effective. It is stored in the tissues and eliminated slowly. For this reason the toxic action is cumulative. At therapeutic dose, side effects are not severe. They comprise pain in the area of injection, diarrhea, and nausea. The more important toxic effects are cardiovascular and neuromuscular, when the drug is used for long periods or when there are predisposing factors. The symptoms are hypotension, tachycardia, changes in cardiac rhythm and in ECG. Occasional deaths due to cardiac enlargement, congestive heart failure, or other complications have been reported. The neurological symptoms are mainly muscular weakness. Bed rest and medical supervision are recommended during treatment. In very old and debilitated patients the dose should be diminished, and it is advisable not to use emetine in patients who are pregnant or who have cardiac, renal or neuromuscular diseases.

Dehydroemetine is a synthetic substance, racemic 2-dehydroemetine-dihydrochloride, of recent appearance and considered equally effective and less toxic. This drug is excreted more rapidly. The side effects and toxicity may be similar to those of emetine, but probably occur with less frequency and severity. Both drugs are used at a dose of 1 mg/kg/day for 4–6 days.

Furazolidone

This is a synthetic nitrofuran derivative, presented as a yellow powder. It is partially soluble in water and partially absorbed from the intestine. The elimination through the kidneys may produce a brown tint to the urine. Besides the action on giardiasis it is effective on several intestinal microorganisms. Side effects are nausea, vomiting, anorexia, abdominal pain and diarrhea. Other less frequent toxic effects are cutaneous rash, agranulocytosis, hemolysis, hypertension and disulfiram-type reaction after ingestion of alcohol. Dosage for adults is 100 mg four times daily for 6 days. For children emulsion and drops are used at the dosage of 5–8 mg/kg/day divided in four doses, during 3–5 days.

Anthelmintic Drugs

Mebendazole

(a) This synthetic compound (methyl-5-benzoyl-benzimidazole-2-carbamate) pertains to the benzimidazole group. It is presented as a white to yellowish powder, very slightly soluble in water, with no special taste. Absorption from the intestine is minimal and 90% of the drug is excreted unchanged in the feces, within 24 h after oral administration. The mode of action is by inhibition of the glucose uptake by the helminths, which result in a depletion of glycogen and adenosin triphosphate contents, necessary for parasite survival, which leads to the slow death of the worms.

(b) It is generally accepted that this drug does not show toxic effects at therapeutical dosages. The LD_{50} values in mice and rats is 1,280 mg/kg and in dogs and guinea pigs 640 mg/kg. It has been observed in children heavily parasitized by *Ascaris,* that some of these worms are expelled through the mouth and nose during the treatment with mebendazole. This side effect may have to do with starvation of the parasites as a consequence of the inhibition to use exogenous glucose and the subsequent slow death. In regard to teratogenicity it was found that when the drug is administered during the organogenesis period in rodents, abnormalities of the fetuses were observed, consisting of skeletal deformities in the ribs and tail. Neither teratogenic nor embryotoxic effects were observed in dogs, sheep or horses. As a precaution, mebendazole should not be used during the first months of pregnancy.

(c) Individual treatment with mebendazole is effective for trichuriasis, ascariasis, enterobiasis and hookworms. The usual dosage is 100 mg twice daily for 3 days irrespective of the patients age. For ascariasis and enterobiasis even shorter treatments are effective. Other indications of this drug are in the treatment of *Capillaria philippinensis* infections, in which it is considered the drug of choice, at the dosage of 400 mg daily for 10–30 days. For *T. solium* and *T. saginata* the recommended dose is 300 mg twice daily for 3 days, although the results are not always good.

(d) Mass treatment with mebendazole aiminig to reduce the prevalence rates of the four common nematodes for which it is effective, has been successful. Repeated mass treatment with 1–3 months interval have shown good effects and drastic reductions of prevalence rates. It is necessary to have in mind that the ideal for mass therapy is the single dose, which is effective only for *Enterobius* and *Ascaris.* For enterobiasis a single dose of 100 mg cures 87–100%. The possible teratogenic effects and the occasional *Ascaris* migrations, are drawbacks for mass treatment with this anthelmintic.

Flubendazole [10]

This is a parafluor analogue of mebendazole showing activity against animal and human nematodes. The LD_{50} for flubendazole in acute toxicity tests is 2,560 mg/kg for several animal species. No teratological effects were observed in rats and rabbits, which seems to be an advantage over mebendazole. Flubendazole is effective for enterobiasis in single dose of 200 mg, and for ascariasis, trichuriasis and necatoriasis at the dose of 200 mg daily for 3 days or 300 mg twice a day. The results are similar, but not superior, to those found with mebendazole. Tolerance is equally good for both drugs.

Tetramisole-Levamisole

Tetramisole and its isomer levamisole have been used against a broad range of nematodal infections in animals. These two benzimidazoles are soluble in water and readily absorbed from the intestine. They act on the neuromuscular system of the worms producing paralysis. Due to the good tolerance and low single dosage, levamisole has successfully been used for mass treatment is ascariasis. At the present it is under clinical investigation for immunodeficiency diseases and some malignancies. Several cases of agronulocytosis are known after prolonged use of this drug.

Thiabendazole

This is one of the oldest benzimidazoles, absorbed from the intestine, with good activity against adult and larval forms of some tissue nematodes. It is still the drug of choice for strongyloidiasis and cutaneous larva migrans. Side effects are present in 50% or more of the treated patients, dizziness being the most common symptom. Other symptoms are nausea, vomiting, abdominal pain, anorexia and diarrhea. Headache, drowsiness, lethargy, erythema multiforme and Stevens-Johnson syndrome, with two fatalities, have been reported. The recommended dosage is 25 mg/kg/day, divided in three doses, administered with meals, during 3 or more days.

Pyrantel Pamoate

(a) This compound of the amidine group is a tetrahydropyrimidine with the chemical formula *trans*-1,4,5,6-tetrahydro-1-methyl-2(2-(2-thienyl)-vinyl)pyrimidine hydrogen pamoate. It is a crystalline powder insoluble in water and very slightly absorbed form the intestine. It has no special taste and is stable to moisture, light, and temperature. Its mode of action is inhibiting neuromuscular transmission, thus producing spastic paralysis of the worms.

(b) The oral LD_{50} for mice, rats and dogs, ranges between 2–5 g/kg. No toxic effects at therapeutic dosages have been reported and the side effects are light and transient; some reports have shown that from 4 to 20% of the patient treated present gastrointestinal symptoms such as abdominal cramps, diarrhea, nausea and vomiting. Less frequent are headache, dizziness and drowsiness. No teratogenicity has been found. There are no specific contraindications.

(c) Pyrantel is effective for ascariasis and enterobiasis at the single dose of 10 mg/kg. For hookworms the same daily dosage should be repeated for 3 consecutive days.

(d) Mass treatment with pyrantel has been effective in reducing *Ascaris* infection to very low prevalence rates. Repeated treatments every 3 months have maintained large groups of populations under control for ascariasis, since prevalences have been reduced from 80% to less than 1%.

These experiences are applicable also to groups of children infected with *Enterobius*. This drug has the advantage of being effective for these two parasites in single dose. The good tolerance and the lack of teratogenicity are in favor of the use of this drug for mass therapy, even in large scale. For hookworms it is necessary to give the treatment for 3 days to achieve appropriate worm reductions.

Oxantel Pamoate [11]

Oxantel pamoate [*trans*-1,4,5,6-tetrahydro-2-(3-hydroxystyryl)-1-methylpyrimidine hydrochloride] is used for the treatment of *T. trichiura* infections. Unlike its analogue, pyrantel, oxantel is not effective in cases of ascariasis. The combination of the two drugs widens the spectrum of activity. The possible effect on other helminths has not yet been defined. Oxantel is a crystalline salt of yellow color, practically insoluble in water; this drug is well tolerated and does not cause toxic effects.

For trichuriasis the dosage of 10–15 mg/kg/day for 2–3 days is recommended. Single doses are effective only for light infections. The combination of pyrantel and oxantel has been successfully used as a wide spectrum anthelmintic being effective for *Ascaris, Enterobius, Trichuris* and hookworms. This combination is promising for mass therapy [12, 13].

Praziquantel [14–22]

(a) Chemically this drug is 2-cyclohexylcarbonyl-1,3,4,6,7,11β-hexahydro-2H-pyrazino(2,1α-isoquinolin-4-one, a new type of acylated heterocyclic compound, an isochinolin-pyrazin-derivative. It is a colorless crystaline powder with bitter taste and insoluble in water. After oral administration the drug is rapidly absorbed from the gastrointestinal tract; maximum serum concentrations appear after 2 hours; it is metabolized in the liver and excretion is completed after 24 h, partially via the mucosal epithelia of the gastrointestinal tract, but mainly through the urine in the form of several metabolites. The intimate way of action of this drug is still under investigation, but the first studies have shown that the compound acts on the carbohydrate metabolism of the parasites.

(b) Acute toxicity tests in rats and mice showed that LD_{50} was over 2,000 mg/kg by mouth. Tolerance is good in experimental animals and in humans. Very few and transient side effects of the gastrointestinal tract, dizziness, headache and drowsiness, have been mentioned by some authors, while others report complete absence of side effects. No embryotoxic, teratogenic or mutagenic effects were found experimentally.

(c) Therapeutical efficacy has been demonstrated against *T. solium* and *T. saginata,* at the single dose of 10 mg/kg. Cure rates have been very near 100%. For *H. nana* the single dose used is 25 mg/kg with around 80% cures; probably the repetition of the treatment once or twice will produce higher cure rates. In diphyllobothriasis the single dose of 25 mg/kg is effective. The drug is also effective against cestode larval forms from different animals in experimental conditions. The efficacy on human cysticercosis seems to be promising, although clinical trials are still few. Praziquantel has been widely used in the treatment of animal cestode infections with good results. This drug is effective against the three human schistosomes. Some trials hate shown effectivity in human trematodiasis.

(d) Mass chemotherapy with praziquantel has been proved effective in animals affected by several cestode species. Due to the efficacy in single doses, the good tolerability and the lack of toxic effects, this drug promises to be adequate for mass treatment in humans.

Niclosamide

Since praziquantel is not commercially available everywhere, niclosamide is still the anticestodal drug most widely used. This drug acts against the parasites by direct contact in the intestinal lumen and produces inhibition of the oxidative phosphorylation process in the mitochondria, which release the parasites from the intestinal mucosa. This drug is well tolerated and due to the fact that it is nonabsorbable, no toxic effects are produced. The usual dosage for *T. solium* and *T. saginata* is 2 g as a single dose in an empty stomach, thoroughly chewed and passed with a little water. For *H. nana* the dosage should be repeated for 5 days and a second treatment after 3 weeks is necessary.

Piperazine

Chemically it is diethylendiamine; several salts are used, all soluble in water and absorbable from the intestine. The mechanism of action is by blocking the mioneural junctions of the helminths, producing a flaccid paralysis that permits the elimination of the living parasites by the intestinal peristalsis. Tolerance is usually good, but reported side effects are nausea, vomiting, diarrhea and allergic reactions. When inadverted large doses are ingested or in cases of renal insufficiency, dramatic symptoms may be observed that fortunately are transient and do not leave sequelae. These symptoms are muscular incoordination, ataxia, vertigo, speech difficulties, confused mental state, muscular weakness and myoclonic contractions. It may cause or exacerbate epileptic seizures in predisposed patients. Contraindications are renal or hepatic insufficiency and epilepsy. The usual dosage is 50 mg/kg/day, maximum 3.5 g daily, during 3–5 days in ascariasis and 7 days in enterobiasis.

References

1 Botero, D.: Epidemiology and public health importance of intestinal nematode infections in Latin America. Progr. Drug Res., vol. 19, pp. 28–43 (Birkhäuser, Basel 1975).

2 Bossche, H. van den: Chemotherapy of parasitic infections. Nature *273:* 626–630 (1978).

3 Botero, D.: Why the intestinal parasitic infections still persist in Latin America. Bull. Pan Am. Hlth Org. (in press 1980).

4 Botero, D.: Posibilidades de control de las geohelmintiasis mediante tratamientos en masa. Boln chil. Parasit. *34:* 39–43 (1979).

5 Botero, D.: Clinical trial methodohogy in intestinal parasitic diseases. Clin. Pharmacol. Ther. *19:* 630–637 (1976).

6 Botero, D.: Chemotherapy of human intestinal parasitic diseases. Annu. Rev. Pharmacol. Toxicol. *18:* 1–15 (1978).

7 Davis, A.: Drug treatment of intestiial helminthiasis, p. 125 (WHO, Geneva 1973).

8 A. M. A.: Drug evaluations; 4th ed., pp. 1379–1426 (American Medical Association, Chicago 1980).

9 Sawyer, P. R.; Brogden, R. N.; Pinder, R. M.; Speight, T. M.; Avery, G. S.: Tinidazole: a review of its antiprotozoal activity and therapeutic efficacy. Drugs *11:* 423–440 (1976).

10 Schenone, H.; Galdames, M.; Inzunza, E.; Jimenez, M.; Romero, E.; Bloomfield, R.: Flubendazole en el tratamiento de infecciones por nemátodes intestinales en niños. Bol chil. Parasit. *32:* 85–86 (1977).

11 Garcia, E. G.: Treatment of trichuriasis with oxantel. Am. J. trop. Med. Hyg. *25:* 914–915 (1976).

12 Amato-Neto, V.; Levi, G. C.; Stefani, H. N. V.; Konishi, S. R.; Tsukumo, M. K. K.; Avila, C. A. de; Moraes, V. M. C. de; Correa, L. de L.: Observacoes iniciaes sobre a eficacia do oxipirantel no tratamiento de tricocefaliase. Revta Inst. Med. trop. S. Paulo *18:* 261–263 (1976).

13 Rim, H. J.; Lee, S. H.; Lee, S. I.; Chang, D. S.; Lim, J. K.; Korean, J.: Effect

of oxantel/pyrantel pamoate tablets against intestinal nematodes in Korea. Korean J. Parasit. *16:* 14–20 (1978).
14 Thomas, H.; Andrews, P.: Praziquantel. A new cestocide. Pestic. Sci. *8:* 556–560 (1977).
15 Rim, H. J.: Therapeutic effects of praziquantel (Embay 8440) against *Taenia solium* infection. Korean J. Parasit. *17:* 67–72 (1979).
16 Bylund, G.; Bag, B.; Wirgren, K.: Tests with a new compound (praziquantel) against *Diphyllobothrium latum*. J. Helminth. *51:* 115–119 (1977).
17 Groll, E.: General scope of treatment with praziquantel (Embay 8440) in humans cestode infections. Bol chil. Parasit. *32:* 27–31 (1977).
18 Spina-Franca, A.; Nóbrega, J. P. S.: Neurocisticercose e praziquantel. Revta paul. Med. *95:* 34–36 (1980).
19 Robles, C.; Chavarria, M.: Un caso de cisticercosis cerebral curado médicamente. Gac. méd. Méx. *116:* 65–71 (1980).
20 Santos, A. T.; Blas, B. L.; Nosenas, J. S.; Portillo, G. P.; Ortega, O. M.; Hayashi, M.; Boehme, K.: Preliminary clinical trials with praziquantel in *Schistosoma japonicum* infections in the Philippines. Bull. Wld Hlth Org. *57:* 793–799 (1979).
21 Katz, N.; Rocha, R. S.; Chaves, A.: Preliminary trials with praziquantel in human infections due to *Schistosoma mansoni*. Bull. Wld Hlth Grg. *57:* 781–785 (1979).
22 Davis, A.; Biles, J. E.; Ulrich, A. M.: Initial experiences with praziquantel in the treatment of human infections due to *Schistosoma haematobium*. Bull Wld Hlth Org. *57:* 773–779 (1979).

Prof. D. Botero, MD, Professor of Parasitology, Universidad de Antioquia,
Apartado Aereo 1226, Medellín (Colombia)

Antibiotics Chemother., vol. 30, pp. 20–27 (Karger, Basel 1981)

Amebiasis

Francisco Biagi

Introduction

Amebiasis is the infection of man with *Entamoeba histolytica*. This infection may be asymptomatic or produce disease of variable severity, following the production of necrotic lesions in the bowel, the liver or the skin. On rare occasions secondary lesions are produced by hematogenous dissemination of the parasite or spread by contiguity of the lesions in other organs like brain, lungs, pericardium, kidney or others. Fatalities are often documented by autopsy in areas where the disease (not only the infection) is common.

Under the term amebiasis we do not include primary meningoencephalitis or brain abscess that are occasionally produced in man by free-living amebae of the genus Naegleria or Achantamoeba. The proper understanding of antiamebic treatment requires a basic knowledge about the migration of *E. histolytica* within the human body and the anatomoclinical classification dividing the infection in nine types of conditions.

Migration of the Parasite

Figure 1 shows the pattern of migration of *E. histolytica* in man. The infection is very rarely acquired by direct invasion of the teguments by trophozoites. Mostly it is due to the ingestion of cysts. The first step of the infection is the establishment of a colony of trophozoites within the lumen of the bowel. After a variable period of time and due to several associated pathogenic mechanisms [1] the trophozoite may invade the in-

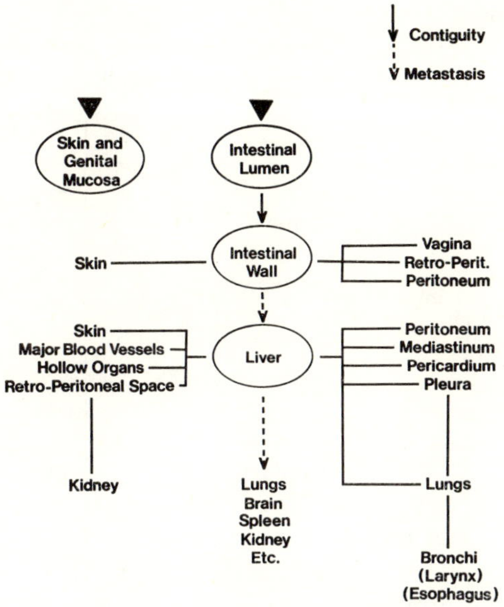

Fig. 1. Migratory pattern of *E. histolytica* in man.

testinal submucous layer. The lytic action of the parasite producing necrosis of the tissue originates in ulcers. The size of these ulcers determines the severity of the clinical picture. In about 1 out of 1,000 infected persons the parasite, spreading through the blood vessels, not only reaches but also establishes itself in the hepatic parenchyma where the necrotic lesions at the beginning are very small, multiple and disseminated, producing pain and enlargement of the liver. Later on the confluence produces clinically detectable necrotic areas called 'abscess' because the material is pus-like. Spread by contiguity of the intestinal or liver lesions produces a variety of complications; they are not primarily produced by the parasite but are rather due to the size and topography of the originating necrotic area. From the liver the parasite may spread through the bloodstream to other organs, although this event is quite uncommon even in endemic areas. Therapy of amebiasis is conditioned by the place where the parasite is established and the concentration a given drug may reach in that particular place. Decisions of the physician will also be influenced by the severity of the case.

Table I. Clinical types of amebiasis

<table>
<tr><th rowspan="2">Location of parasite[1]</th><th rowspan="2">Clinical type of amebiasis</th><th rowspan="2" colspan="2">Forms of amebiasis</th><th colspan="2">Diagnosis</th></tr>
<tr><th>PE</th><th>serology</th></tr>
<tr><td>Colonization of intestinal lumen</td><td>1 carrier[2]</td><td rowspan="2">intes-
tinal</td><td>luminal</td><td rowspan="2">+</td><td>–</td></tr>
<tr><td>Invasion of intestinal wall</td><td>2 asymptomatic
3 chronic intestinal
4 acute intestinal
5 ameboma</td><td rowspan="3">tissular[3]</td><td rowspan="3">+</td></tr>
<tr><td>Invasion of liver</td><td>6 hepatitis
7 liver abscess</td><td rowspan="2">extra-
intes-
tinal</td><td rowspan="2">–</td></tr>
<tr><td>Invasion of other organs and tissues</td><td>8 cutaneous
9 other locations</td></tr>
</table>

PE = Parasitologic examination (feces).

[1] A patient may present several locations at the same time.

[2] A patient of this type may suffer later an invasion by the parasite. It can also be the result of a clinically satisfactory treatment, but case serology might be positive for a period of time.

[3] It is also called invasive amebiasis, even though, in fact, the ameba is invasive.

Anatomoclinical Classification

A large number of terms have been used to refer to the different clinical pictures we may observe in amebiasis, although for therapeutic purposes the most rational system of language we may use is based on anatomoclinical and clinical facts. This classification is shown in table I.

Carriers of amebiasis are people having luminal infection, that is, a colony of trophozoites in the lumen of the bowel that will produce no symptoms and negative serology, but will show the parasite in the stools that is usually eliminated in cystic form as the patient does not keep the cysts when they are formed. Tissular intestinal amebiasis may appear in four main different forms. Asymptomatic amebiasis is differentiated from the carrier stage because it already shows positive serology; the invasion has already produced an immune response but a few ulcers do not produce symptoms; this has been confirmed in autopsy cases. Chronic intestinal amebiasis includes several clinical terms. These patients may have diarrhea, constipation, bloody stools, changes in evacuation schedule, headache, abdominal pain, meteorism; the disease is not severe; the patient may continue his activities; usually it lasts several weeks or even months and generally it is seen in outpatient consultations.

Acute intestinal amebiasis is a severe picture that generally demands medical care in a few days; often the patient gets hospitalized; it includes amebic dysentery, severe cases of bloody diarrhea, 'fulminant' amebiasis and acute abdomen due to complications. Ameboma is a pseudotumoral inflammatory reaction that may mimetise carcinoma.

Hepatitis produces fever, pain on the upper quadrant and enlargement of the liver, but an abscess cannot be demonstrated by clinical procedures and the biopsy might be normal as chances of hitting a necrotic site are very limited. Autopsy has sometimes documented these cases [2]. Cutaneous amebiasis appears as an ulcer of the skin or mucous membranes that grows rapidly, bleeds easily and is painful; its border is infiltrated, dark reddish and well defined. Invasive amebiasis is an unfortunate term as the parasite and not the disease is invasive.

On clinical grounds, after a good clinical history and physical examination, rectosigmoidoscopy, X-ray examination, gammagraphy or ultrasonography, and sometimes axial computerized tomography, supported by properly made fecal examinations for parasites and quantitative serology for amebiasis, all patients will fall within this classification. One must not forget the possibility that a patient may show more than one anatomo-clinical type of amebiasis. It should also be remembered that the infection is a dynamic phenomenon, so a carrier later on may have a liver abscess although the chances might be small. The selection of particular diagnostic techniques depends on the facts we obtained through the clinical history.

Choice of Drugs

According to the concentration of drugs in different sites, table II shows a pattern of selection. Emetines and imidazoles do not reach the lumen of the bowel but act through the bloodstream. They are useless in the carrier stage, have limited action on asymptomatic amebiasis and will not guarantee the parasitological cure. Chloroquines reach antiamebic concentrations only in the liver. Dichloroacetamides, oxiquinolines and

Table II. Drugs of choice in amebiasis

Location of parasite[1]	Clinical types of amebiasis	Drugs and amebicidal concentration, μg/ml					
		oxiquinolines	arsenicals	emetines	chloroquines	imidazoles	dichloroacetamides
		8	8	3	300	3	0.04 0.6
Intestinal lumen	1 carrier	×	×				×
Intestinal wall	2 asymptomatic	×	×				×
	3 chronic intestinal	×	×			×	×
	4 acute intestinal			×		×	×
	5 ameboma			×		×	×
Liver	6 amebic hepatitis			×	×	×	
	7 amebic liver abscess			×	×	×	
Others	8 cutaneous			×		×	
	9 other locations			×		×	

[1] A patient may have several locations.

arsenicals act in intestinal (invasive and noninvasive) amebiasis. The selection of drugs depends on our objectives. Carriers, asymptomatic or chronic intestinal amebiasis will be best treated by dichloroacetamides or oxiquinolines; intestinal chronic amebiasis may receive one of these drugs and imidazoles; in liver abscess we may choose among imidazoles, emetines and chloroquines; in certain cases the combination or sequence may be necessary. If the patient with a liver abscess also has an intestinal infection other types of drugs are indicated according to table II.

Imidazoles

Introduced as amebicides around 1966 [3], imidazoles are the most commonly used today. The chemical group includes metronidazole, nimorazole, tinidazole, seconidazole, carnidazole, ornidazole and others. Metronidazole is the most largely used. Its half-life is very short so dosages have to be administered every 8 h; this becomes a shortcoming for its parenteral administration. Tinidazole has a significantly larger half-life and seconidazole the largest.

Common side effects of imidazoles are related to gastritis (abdominal pain or burning, nausea, vomiting). The patients may also complain of an unpleasant metallic taste, headache, insomnia, depression, cutaneous rash, darkening of urine and diarrhea; these effects are most common for metronidazole. Ingestion of alcohol is contraindicated as imidazoles interfere with the metabolism of alcohol and produce nausea, vomiting, flushing and severe headache.

Imidazoles are contraindicated during the first trimester of pregnancy. They pass the placental barrier and are present in mother's milk. An in vitro mutagenic effect is demonstrated in anaerobic bacteria although this has not been confirmed in mammals. The dosage is from 20 to 50 mg/kg body weight/day orally during 1–3 weeks according to the severity of the case. In adults the dosage is calculated not over 60 kg body weight. The daily dosage is usually divided into three administrations for metronidazole, and nimorazole, tinidazole, ornidazole and seconidazole may be taken once a day; all administrations are given after meals. Up until today, millions of people have received these drugs and it looks evident that they are reasonably safe and effective. Proper administration produces a clinical cure in around 95 % of the patients with one single course of treatment.

Dichloracetamides

The dichloracetamide group includes etofamide, teclozan, diloxamide and clefamide. Its antiamebic action is shown at the lowest concentrations. They are almost not absorbed so they are active only in the different types of intestinal amebiasis; oral administration is at the dosage of 10–20 mg/kg body weight/day during 3–10 days and show the highest rates of cure in intestinal amebiasis. A common side effect is meteorism; sometimes the patients show loose stools. Toxic effects have not been reported in clinical experience. Side effects are not important and transient. Clinical and parasitological cure is achieved in intestinal amebiasis in more than 95 % of the patients. Taking into consideration the previous facts, and as transmission is kept by the carriers and also the infection has to start by the establishment of the parasite into the lumen of the bowel these drugs are the best for chemoprophylactic purposes. Field studies have confirmed that a dosage taken once or twice a week may stop transmission and protect people against the infection in spite of the fact that they continue living in nonsanitated towns [4].

Chloroquine

Chloroquine is one of the 4-aminoquinolines frequently used as an antimalarial. Its amebecide action was demonstrated in 1948 in vitro and its value in hepatic amebiasis is well known. It is almost completely absorbed in the small bowel and only minimal quantities are eliminated through the feces. Its deposition in tissues is remarkable, especially in the liver where it reaches larger concentrations than in plasma. Excretion of chloroquine is very slow and it occurs via the kidneys. This drug is not effective against intestinal amebiasis and its use is limited to the liver amebiasis. As there is a concomitant possibility of intestinal infection it is essential to administer systematically an effective drug against intestinal amebiasis to lower the incidence of relapses. Secondary effects include headache, nausea, vomiting, pruritus and blurring vision, all of which are transient. When the dosage is high and the administration period is long a retinopathy may develop, which is not progressive if the administration is stopped, but it is irreversible. Association of phenylbutazone, auric derivatives and chloroquine must be avoided as they produce dermatitis when used together. Chloroquines are contraindicated in porphyria and during pregnancy. The dosage for chloroquine is 10 mg/kg body weight/day orally during 5 days, continuing with half this dosage during 5–25 days. In case of persistent vomiting or when oral administration cannot be used, the intramuscular route may be employed changing to oral administration as soon as possible.

Emetine

Emetine and dehydroemetine have a direct and rapid lethal action against trophozoites of *E. histolytica.* Emetines are absorbed from parenteral sites of administration and eliminated very slowly. Its effectiveness is greater in hepatic amebiasis, acute intestinal amebiasis and cutaneous amebiasis. Side effects are diarrhea, nausea and vomiting, weakness, spontaneous pain and rigidity of skeletal muscles (especially in the neck); in some patients light-sensitive disorders and tremor may be observed. On overdosage, patients may show hypotension, precordial pain and bradycardia. Electrocardiographic findings occasionally reveal changes in the T wave, deviations in segment ST and partial blockade and prolongation of QT space, which disappear in an average period of a week after discontinuing treatment. Supervision of dosage administration and careful interrogation of the patient about having received the drug in the last 2 months are important as drug administration should not be repeated within that period of time. Emetines are administered in a dosage of 1 mg/kg body weight/day, up to 60 mg, during 10 days by deep intramuscular injection.

Oxyquinolines

A number of halogenated 8-hydroxyquinolines have been used clinically for their amebicidal action. From such compounds the two most frequently used are diiodohydroxyquinoline and iodochlorhydroxyquinoline. These agents are directly amebicidal and act only on the parasites in the intestinal tract. They are much less effective in the treatment of acute intestinal dysentery and they are recommended for asymptomatic carriers and chronic intestinal amebiasis. After oral administration a very small portion of the ingested dose is absorbed; the bulk of these drugs is passed in the feces. The most important toxic reaction, ascribed particularly to iodochlorhydroxyquinoline is a subacute myelo-optic neuropathy, the incidence of which is related to prolonged periods of administration and has had a peculiar geographic distribution. Other side effects include severe generalized furunculosis, chills, fever, wild to severe dermatitis, anal irritation and itching, transitory abdominal discomfort and headache. They are contraindicated in iodine intolerance. These drugs are administrated orally with the following dosis: diiodohydroxyquinoline 30 mg/kg body weight/day during 20 days; iodochlorhydroxyquinoline 25 mg/kg body weight/day, also for 20 days.

References

1 Biagi, F.; Beltrán-H. F.: The challenge of amebiasis; understanding pathogenic mechanisms. Int. Rev. trop. Med. *3:* 219–239 (1969).

2 Biagi, F.; Villa, S.; Navarrete, E.; García, P.: Amibiasis hepática incipiente. (Presentación de un caso de autopsia.) Rev. Latinoam. Anat. Patol. *1:* 153–167 (1957).

3 Navarrete, F.; Biagi, F.: L'utilité du métronidazole dans l'amibiase intestinale. Bull. Soc. Path. exot. *60:* 503–506 (1967).

4 Biagi, F.; López, M. R.; González C., C.; Gutiérrez, M.: Quimioprofilaxis de la amibiasis con clefamida en una comunidad abierta. Rev. Inst. Med. Trop. Sao Paulo *8:* 253–240 (1966).

Prof. Dr. F. Biagi, Cerro del Chinaco, 122-Mexico 21, D. F. (Mexico)

Antibiotics Chemother., vol. 30, pp. 28–53 (Karger, Basel 1981)

Amebic Meningoencephalitis

With 1 color plate

Clyde G. Culbertson

Lilly Laboratory for Clinical Research, Indianapolis, Ind., USA

Introduction

The purpose of this report is to record some new information, to review some of the work of others, and to present a point of view which I believe will be useful in dealing with the complicated, and as yet incompletely worked out, problem of the human ailments that are caused by free-living amebas. My point of view will be a general one, as a clinical pathologist, with the objective of persuading clinicians, clinical pathologists and microbiologists to include these organisms in their thinking when they confront disease processes, as they now do, with regard to viruses, bacteria, parasitic protozoa and pathogenic yeasts and fungi.

Comprehensive reviews of the literature concerning the pathogenic and related nonpathogenic small free-living amebas have been recently published by *Griffin* [29] and by *Schuster* [45]. As can be seen from these excellent works, the subject amebas have been extensively studied before and after some species were found to be pathogenic. In spite of all the available information, its application to clinical medicine is still undeveloped and no effective measures are generally available to the actual or potential victims of this group of diseases.

At present the total number of reported fatal cases of free-living amebic infection in man worldwide is estimated to be just over 100, which is a very small incidence compared to that of many other serious illnesses. Most of these cases were due to Naegleria. Even so, as I shall later demonstrate, this group of diseases deserves much attention since experimental evidence indicates that these amebas may well represent a greater problem than yet discovered. The dramatic meningoencephalitis has overshadowed the antecedent pathologic processes, just as happened with other well-known entities – for example, poliomyelitis and histoplasmosis.

I believe that only by serious efforts to demonstrate trophic amebas in the respiratory tract, using methods adequate to differentiate them from sojourning inhaled cysts which are generally of little significance, will the true incidence be measured. This means making careful studies of patients as well as of all the details of amebic morphology, biochemistry, and immunology. Such clinical research could lead not only to comprehension of the complete disease process but to efficient diagnostic measures, and thus to timely institution of available therapeutic measures.

Terminology

For the benefit of those who are unfamiliar with the relatively voluminous and complex literature, comments concerning terminology should be made.

(1) Some of the early reports of fatal human cases now known to have been due to Naegleria were presented as being due to Hartmannella, Acanthamoeba or Iodamoeba [22, 26, 43].

(2) Nonspecific anatomic terms such as 'primary amebic meningitis' or 'amebic granulomatous meningoencephalitis' do not indicate the causative ameba, and are in fact somewhat misleading to clinicians, since the amebic disease according to experimental evidence first attacks the respiratory system and is followed by invasion of the central nervous system.

(3) *Entamoeba histolytica,* which occasionally causes suppurative brain disease, should also be included in any scheme of classification in order to make clear the identities of various forms of 'amebic meningitis'.

(4) There are then three distinct diseases to be considered. In the following discussion we will refer to the specific entity by using the generic name of the causative ameba, compounded with the word 'amebiasis'. The following definitions briefly describe each of the three categories.

Entamebiasis [10]. *E. histolytica,* the parasitic ameba, causes infection beginning with ulceration of the colon, sometimes progressing to cause suppurative hepatitis but rarely also suppurative amebic meningoencephalitis. This disease is well known and will only be considered in this paper in comparison with the other two.

Naegleramebiasis [3, 4]. *Naegleria fowleri* infection beginning with infection of the nasopharyngeal mucosa progressing to cause amebic meningoencephalitis.

Acanthamoebiasis [32]. Infection by one of several species of Acanthamoeba beginning as nasopharyngeal mucosal infection with extension to the central nervous system. Also, possibly beginning as bronchopulmonary infection from which, via the hematogenous route, the amebas are disseminated to viscera including the central nervous system. This is not a completely proven clinical entity as yet, but is partially based upon the experimental infection.

I believe the separation of these three categories is important, since each, as will be seen, has different clinical characteristics and requires special diagnostic consideration and laboratory procedures, as well as need for specific chemotherapy.

Epidemiology

Naegleramebiasis

The worldwide distribution of the reported naegleramebiasis indicates that it occurs most often in the temperate and torrid zones. The tolerance of these amebas to warm temperatures and their rapid growth therein is well documented [30], as are the opposite effects of freezing. Most of the cases have resulted from swimming in lakes or streams or pools using natural waters in which there was sewage or organic pollution. In some instances a local increase in temperature, such as by thermal springs [20] or by discharge of hot water by a power generating plant into a polluted river was associated with fatal Naegleria infection [31].

Another known source was untreated water, piped above ground into home plumbing systems [1]. The single, well-studied swimming pool epidemic [7] was eventually traced to faulty construction that provided an unusual circumstance promoting infection. While free-living amebas of several varieties (mostly Acanthamoeba) have been found in well-cared-for swimming pools and even in drinking water, the histories of fatal cases do not indicate that standard swimming pools or water supplies are sources of the diseases. Certainly, the design and operation of swimming pools should be viewed in the light of the above-mentioned disaster. In another isolated instance, referred to below [35], the inhalation of dust containing cysts of *N. fowleri* appeared to be the cause. In this case, though the presence of trophic Naegleria in the dust is unlikely, perhaps this possibility should not be completely ruled out, since, as *Singh* [46] has shown, both cysts and trophozoites may exist together in ordinary soil. The surveys of nasal cultures in normal persons have usually not yielded Naegleria but Acanthamoeba, so that infection by Naegleria from ordinary dust would seem only a minor problem. The possible infection by gross contamination of wounds with soil containing Naegleria is suggested by the experimental production of fatal cellulocutaneous infections in guinea pigs [11].

Acanthamoebiasis

As mentioned above, in contrast to naegleramebiasis, acanthamoebiasis probably arises from the inhalation of dust [19, 47, 51]. However, since the reported number of fatal cases is very small and some Acanthamoebas are quite virulent in animals, the possibility of Acanthamoeba infection from nasal or pulmonary aspiration of water cannot be completely dismissed, although no such occurrence is now known.

Taxonomy of Pathogenic Isolates (fig. 5)

The amebas identified as the cause of fatal meningoencephalitis in man are *E. histolytica, N. fowleri* and a group comprising several species of Acanthamoeba, classified by experts according to morphologic criteria as *Entamoeba culbertsoni, Acanthamoeba polyphagia, and Acanthamoeba castellani*. From histologic studies of the brain lesions, the specific diseases caused by each genus represented can be identified with considerable accuracy. The Acanthamoeba group as now known seems to be associated with a spectrum of pathologic characteristics varying from acute amebic brain abscess to chronic granulomatous lesions associated with severe vascular injury.

Immunologic investigations of the amebas are more readily and more accurately carried out by the study of living trophozoites in cultures from the brain tissue or cerebrospinal fluid. Such studies have permitted the identification of *N. fowleri. N. fowleri* seems to be a rather homogeneous species, since the isolates from a number of fatal cases in widely scattered parts of the world are quite similar in all respects.

In the estimated 15 reported fatal cases of acanthamoebiasis discovered at autopsy [37], the study of trophic amebas has not been possible because no cultures have been isolated as yet from a human in whom the histological features suggested the cause was some species of Acanthamoeba.

In order to determine which species from which genus was responsible for many of the reported cases, immunofluorescence and immunoperoxidase have been applied as indirect tests, using rabbit antiserum against a small group of Acanthamoeba species classified morphologically. The amebas present in fixed sections of tissue from several of the reported cases have reacted to one or more of the antisera against different species of stock culture Acanthamoebas. I have used both immunofluorescence and immunoperoxidase [12, 13] and I have found the immunoperoxidase preferable because the preparations are permanent and the histologic elements are stained by the hemotoxylin and eosin (HE) counterstain. In the course of this work, it has become obvious that the fixation of the sections was extremely important, and in experiments to be published elsewhere, the inhibitory effect of heavy metals – particularly mercury and copper – either by design or accident was found to be important. By appropriate treatment of the sections to remove metals, more constant and reliable results were achieved.

The recently developed direct staphylococcus protein A coagglutination (D-SPAC) procedure [14], performed upon unfixed living amebas, has been used to test the individual amebic reactivity to a group of 14 Acanthamoebas maintained in axenic culture. With the exception of *Acanthamoeba astronyxis,* all of these reacted via the D-SPAC to either the antisera or *A. culbertsoni* or to *A. polyphagia.* This would suggest that this collection of Acanthamoebas could be separated rather sharply into two groups. Table I indicates a proposed designation as group A and group B, depending upon the reactivity as determined by the D-SPAC upon the trophozoites. Limited studies indicate that the indirect SPAC (I-SPAC) reaction reacts similarly.

Like studies with other available Acanthamoebas should be done, possibly to define other groups. These findings suggest that the present species definitions, being based only upon small morphologic differences, may not be related to pathogenicity, but rather could be related for epidemiologic purposes to serologic groupings. The D-SPAC reaction performs as well upon amebas grown on agar with bacteria, as upon bacterium-free medium, and could therefore be used upon amebas not adapted to bacterium-free medium.

My recent experience, together with published information, causes me to seriously question the ability of immunologic staining of Acanthamoebas in fixed tissue sections to determine the species of the amebas. *Willaert* et

Table I. Illustration of direct staphylococcus protein A surface coagglutination tests for serological grouping

Antiserum used in suspension		Results	
ameba	isolate	group I *A. culbertsoni*	group II *A. polyphagia*
A. culbertsoni	A-1	4+	–
A. sp.	HN-3	–	4+
A. sp.	A-5	–	4+
A. neff		–	4+
A. castellani		–	4+
A. sp.	H-1	–	4+
A. sp.	Rus 22	4+	–
A. sp.	Rus 19		4+
A. sp.	CS 21	–	4+
A. sp.	CS 22	–	4+
A. sp.	Hov 6-2	4+	–
A. sp.	Ru 32	–	4+
A. astronyxis		–	–
A. polyphagia	Tex 1	–	4+

al. [52] believe that by using antisera to a given Acanthamoeba species raised against a highly purified preparation of surface membrane, the cross reactions which occur with ordinary immune serum to the same amebas can be avoided. Although they studied but 1 case, that reported by *Jager and Stamm* [32], this may of course be a valid conclusion. The observation of *Stevens* et al. [48] that the antimembrane serum gave highly specific agglutination of live amebas may indicate that this antiserum may be active upon the same antigen as in the D-SPAC, as well as upon the antigen in the fixed amebas in the sections.

I have repeatedly tested the amebas on the fixed sections of the *Jager and Stamm* [32] case and found that they react by immunoperoxidase to antiserum against both the *A. culbertsoni* and *A. polyphagia* group. However, mouse brain sections containing only known *A. culbertsoni* react only to antiserum against *A. culbertsoni* and not to *A. polyphagia* antiserum. This may indicate the amebas in the *Jager and Stamm* [32] case are in some way atypical.

From the information available, I believe that retrospective immunologic tests on fixed amebas in sections from autopsy should not be regarded as specific except for the genus of the ameba until there is more evidence gained from concomitant morphologic and immunologic studies of fixed and trophic amebas from the same cases. This emphasizes again the importance of making cultures from patients who may possibly be suffering from acanthamoebiasis.

Morphology [4, 7, 15, 27, 42, 44, 46]

N. fowleri (fig. 2)

N. fowleri ist the smallest ameba of the pathogenic group when seen rounded up in fixed tissues, but the remarkable patterns of trophic forms under different conditions make its size widely variable. In tissue culture or on agar surfaces with bacteria, the trophozoites are 8–15 μm in greatest diameter and show a contractile vacuole. The very active motion consists of rapid appearance of lobular pseudopods, which often project in two directions producing a 'Y' form. The point-to-point migration is less noticeable than the explosive motion would suggest. In some instances Naegleria in cerebrospinal fluid has a very elongated form resembling motile larvae. The endoplasmic portion is indistinct and the nucleus cannot be seen. The cause of this unusual morphologic variation is not clear. In tissue sections *N. fowleri* is rounded and in this state the amebas measure from 8 to 12 μm in average diameter. The nuclear characteristics are described in the following paragraph, in comparison to the nuclei of Acanthamoeba.

Acanthamoeba (fig. 1)

The pathogenic *A. culbertsoni, A. polyphagia,* and *A. castellani* differ significantly only in cyst structure. The trophic forms, when attached to glass or agar surface and moving, are about twice as long as broad (18 × 8 μm) and show a fan-like, clear ectoplasmic lobopodium from which protrude sluggishly waving or moving filiform acanthopodia, which disappear posteriorly as the ameba moves. The thorn-like acanthopodia contain pinocytotic channels and become less and less numerous toward the caudal area. There is often a 'food cup' on the posterior lateral surface to which bacteria adhere and from which they are phagocytosed. In cultures grown on nonnutrient agar with bacteria, the amebas contain a multivesiculated contractile vacuole which is seen near the caudal extremity of the ameba. In bacteria-free cultures the vacuole is present but rarely con-

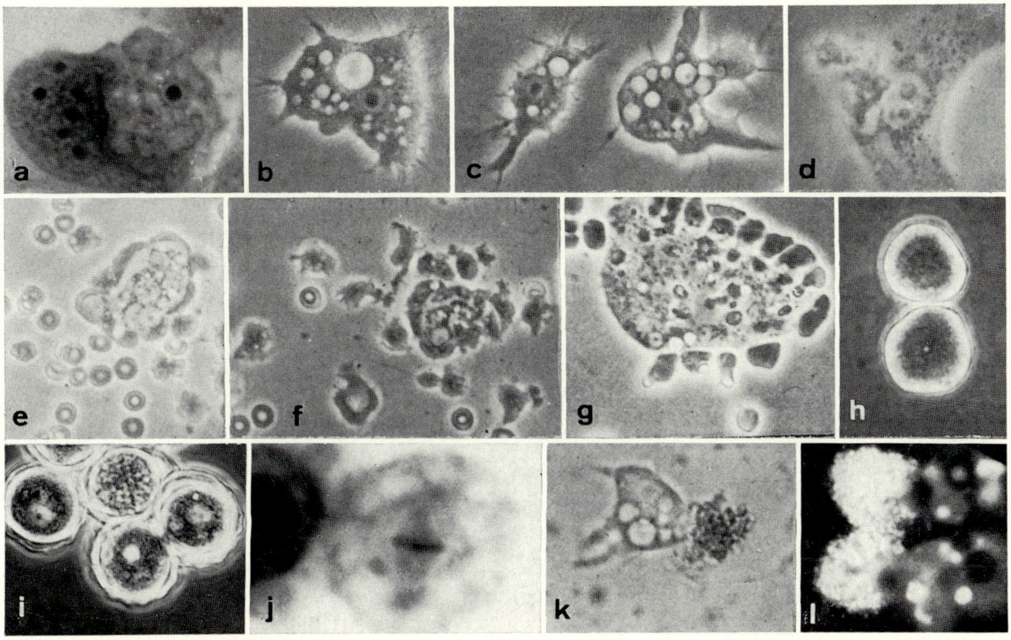

Fig. 1. Acanthamoeba morphology. *a A. culbertsoni* (A-1) tissue culture. Ameba attached to cell nucleus. HE. ×890. *b, c* Living trophozoites (A-1). Phase ×890. *d* A-1 inside partially destroyed tissue culture cell. Time lapse, phase ×355. *e* A-1 Acanthamoeba completely surrounded by neutrophils which have partially phagocytized the ameba. Time lapse. Phase ×355. *f* Same field 30 min later. Ameba nearly destroyed. Increase in attracted neutrophils. *g* A-1 Acanthamoeba showing 'piecemeal' surface phagocytosis of red blood cells. Phase ×710. *h* Two cysts of A-1 *A. culbertsoni.* Note smooth double walls. Phase ×890. *i* Cysts of (Tex) *A. polyphagia* with wrinkled cyst walls. Phase ×890. *j* A-1 *A. culbertsoni.* Typical mitotic figure. HE. ×1,070. *k* A-1 *A. culbertsoni* showing positive direct surface protein A staphylococcus coagglutination of methylene-blue-stained staphylococci. ×800. *l* Same reaction upon surface of *A. culbertsoni* when staphylococci were stained with acridine orange and viewed under fluorescence microscopy. Figures *k* and *l* are examples of the positive reaction with this method and the ameba is of the species against which the antiserum used was raised.

tracts. The nucleus is located near the center of the endoplasm, moving as the endoplasm moves into the ectoplasm in the direction of the motion. The nucleus is spherical and shows a very large nucleolus. There is a clear perinucleolar area which contains a few granules, and outside of this zone is a sharp thin nuclear membrane. This nuclear structure has about the

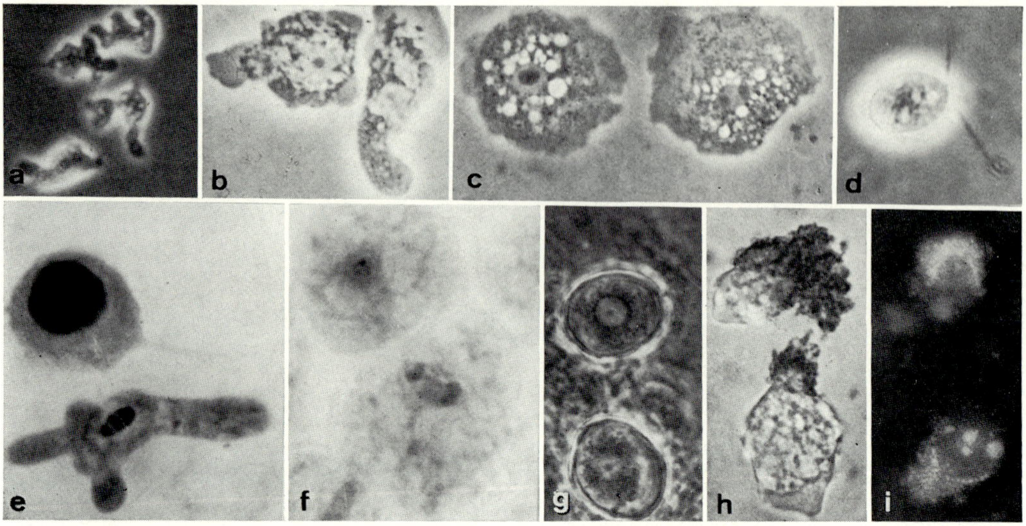

Fig. 2. N. fowleri morphology. *a–c N. fowleri* trophozoites from broth culture. *a* Phase ×710. *b* Phase ×1,070. *c* From agar culture with *E. coli.* ×1,070. *d* Flagellate form. Phase ×1,070. *e* Tissue culture. Trophozoite showing promitosis. HE. ×710. *f* Two trophozoites from agar bacterial culture. One (arrow) shows 'polar masses' and 'polar cap' of mitotic nucleus. Trichrome. ×1,070. *g N. fowleri* cysts. Phase ×1,070. *h N. fowleri* showing positive coagglutination with *N. fowleri* anti- ×1,070. *i* Same as *h* except staphylococci stained with acridine orange and viewed by fluorescence microscopy. ×890.

same appearance in the living as in the fixed stained preparations. In fixed tissue sections, the relatively large distinctive nuclei constitute the single most important feature in differentiating both Naegleria and Acanthamoeba cells from mammalian cells. In such sections they appear as 'target' or 'bull's eye' structures, whereas the mammalian nuclei are larger, usually ovoid, and have very much smaller nucleoli. In fixed tissue sections, the nuclei of Naegleria are very similar to those of Acanthamoeba. The nucleus of *E. histolytica* is easily distinguished from that of soil amebas, since *E. histolytica* has a minute nucleolus which is often difficult to identify in fixed preparations, and there may be only a uniform, slightly eosinophilic staining in contrast to the large 'bold' nucleoli of the free-living species.

Acanthamoebas divide by classical mitosis, which distinguishes them from Naegleria, which divide by a different morphologic sequence known as promitosis.

Biology [27, 45, 46]

Amebas of the genera Naegleria and Acanthamoeba are inhabitants of the soil and water and appear to be worldwide in distribution. They feed upon other microbial forms, generally more luxuriantly upon gram-negative bacilli such as *Aerobacter aerogenes* or *Escherichia coli* – thus their predilection for growth in water containing sewage or decomposing organic matter. The pathogenic amebas thrive at a warmer temperature than do the nonpathogenic ones. After feeding, and perhaps because of many other physical and chemical factors, the amebas encyst and thereby increase their resistance to cold temperature and various chemical substances. Acanthamoebas are single-form amebas, while Naegleria are biphasic with amebic trophozoites and a flagellate stage. The flagellate form develops under conditions of rapid change in the environment, such as sudden decrease in osmotic pressure. The trophic amebas transform into a small, rigid, pear-shaped organism usually with two, but sometimes more, flagellae which give it the capability of rapid movement. The flagellates do not multiply as such; they lose their flagellae and return to the amebic state. The cysts which exist in the soil, together with the trophozoites, excyst when moisture and temperature requirements are met, but the effect of associated microbiological flora, such as gram-negative bacilli, is also believed to be necessary. The amebic form of Naegleria is the pathogenic one, although some have suggested that flagellates are more pathogenic [46]. However, since they revert to the amebic state very rapidly after any kind of manipulation, and my own experiments show no difference in mouse pathogenicity between the two forms, in my opinion the relation of the flagellate to pathogenicity, if any, is uncertain. The cyst forms of either Naegleria or Acanthamoeba, while not studied sufficiently to know their part in animal infections, appear to be generally unable to excyst in vivo and cause disease when introduced alone into normal susceptible mice. However, in 1 human case of naegleramebiasis, evidence supports the probability that the inhalation of Naegleria cysts caused fatal meningoencephalitis [11]. In chronic granulomatous Acanthamoeba lesions, the formation of cysts has often been demonstrated, and in a few instances, I have seen them in the process of excystment. This is not true of Naegleria infection, but, because of the rapidity of the fatal outcome, perhaps cysts have not had a chance to develop.

An important relationship of the amebas to the human has been the repeated observation of positive Acanthamoeba cultures from the nasopharynx [47, 49]. So far as is known, live trophozoites have not been found by direct examination of nasal or other fluids of otherwise normal persons, so that the evidence generally suggests that the positive cultures may be due to cysts having been deposited upon the nasal mucosa by inhalation, with excystment when the specimen is subjected to culture. Positive nasal cultures for pathogenic Naegleria from the human have not been reported.

Pathogenesis and Pathology [16, 23, 38] (fig. 3 and 4)

In experimental Acanthamoeba and Naegleria infections in mice, the amebas are seen to multiply in the nasal mucus, to penetrate the epithelium by inserting protoplasmic processes between the epithelial cells, and to destroy the epithelium. The amebas migrate into the submucosa and into the meninges. Some may enter olfactory nerve fibers and others traverse the connective tissue into the cranial cavity via the cribriform plate. They also enter the meninges and cause small hemorrhages and a neutrophil leukocyte response. The hemorrhages enlarge until the olfactory bulb is completely hemorrhagic. The more virulent amebas multiply rapidly and spread into the cerebrum and cerebellum. In acute Naegleria infection the process is very rapid, with swarms of amebas causing massive invasive brain destruction in 2–4 days. In contrast, highly virulent Acanthamoebas produce a different lesion characterized by widespread suppuration resembling those of *E. histolytica,* and less virulent ones cause a combination of abscess and granuloma. Acanthamoebas also seriously injure the vascular structures by invasion of the arterial and vein walls, causing thrombosis and severe vascular injury. *Martinez* et al. [38] have observed even greater changes, including mycotic aneurysms in human infants. In the pulmonary vasculature of experimental mice and monkeys, the intraluminal penetration and growth of amebas cause thrombosis and give rise to systemic emboli and blood-borne spread of the amebas in the brain, heart, spleen, kidney, and perhaps other areas. In the brain, the amebas lodge in the capillaries and escape through the endothelium to proliferate and colonize in the brain tissue.

While guinea pigs may be fatally infected by subcutaneous or intramuscular injections of several thousand *N. fowleri* [11], no such lesions are known in nature. These animals show massive liver infection. The only experimental intestinal involvement yet reported has been that of blood-borne lesions in the intestinal wall of guinea pigs infected as described

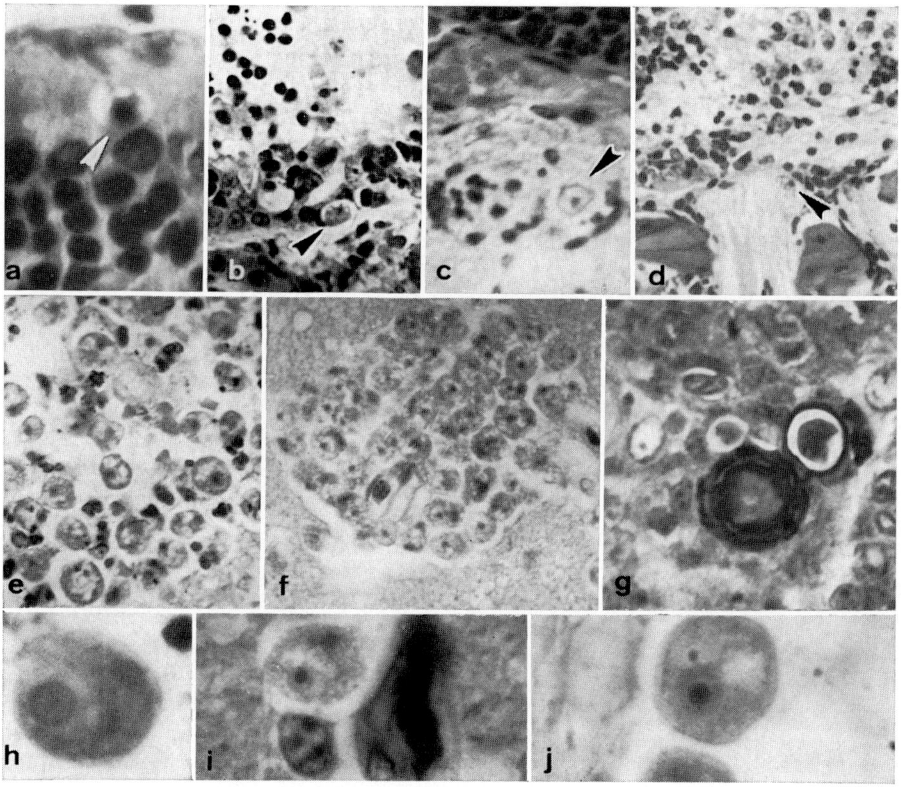

Fig. 3. Pathogenesis of experimental cerebral naegleramebiasis and acanthamoebiasis via nasal mucosa. HE. *a* Single Acanthamoeba at outset of nasal invasion. Arrow at nucleus. ×1,070. *b* Advanced nasal infection by Naegleria. Arrow at ameba in destroyed nasal epithelial layer. ×535. *c* Acanthamoeba in olfactory nerve fiber in submucosa. Arrow at ameba. ×450. *d* Small area of cribriform plate showing olfactory nerve fiber containing ameba (arrow) and olfactory bulb with many amebas. ×180. *e A. culbertsoni* in human brain in perivascular space near an abscess. ×450. *f N. fowleri* in human brain from a fatal case of naegleramebiasis. ×450. *g* Several cysts of A. sp. (HN-3) in chronic granulomatous acanthamoebiasis. ×890. *h E. histolytica* in wall of liver abscess. Note the very faint, small nucleolus. ×890. *i N. fowleri* in tissue. ×890. *j A. polyphagia.* Tissue section. ×890.

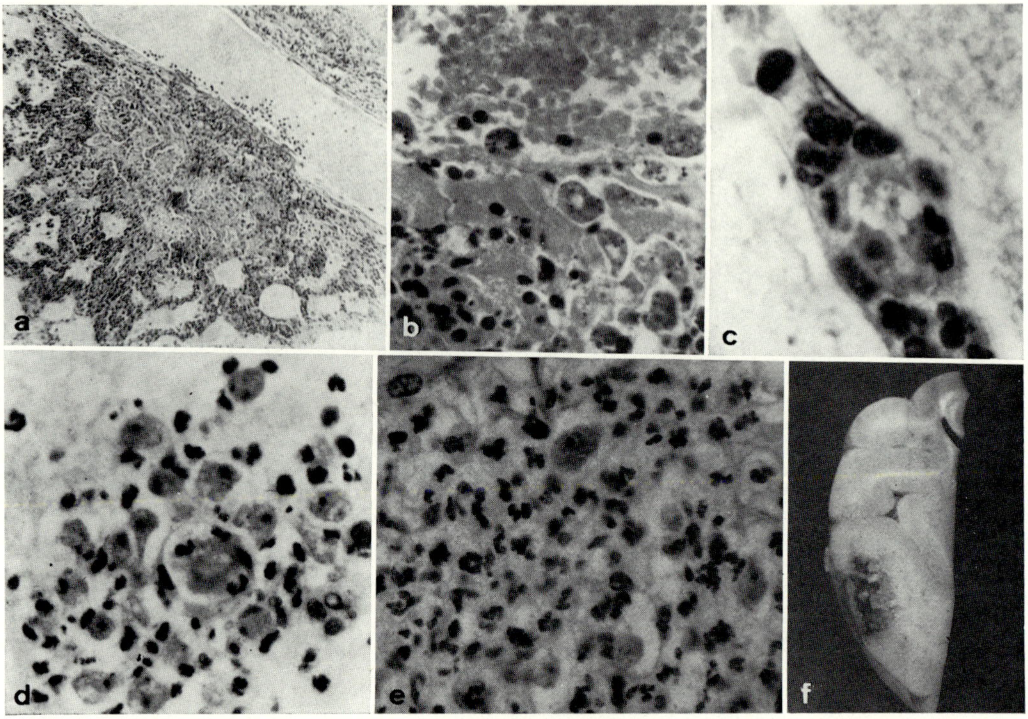

Fig. 4. Composite mouse and monkey experimental lesions to illustrate the pathogenesis of experimental acanthamoebic abscess via pulmonary hematogenous route. HE. *a* Amebic pneumonia (mouse) extending into wall of vein with leukocyte accumulation upon endothelium (arrow). ×89. *b* Acanthamoebas traversing vein wall into lumen of pulmonary vein. ×445. *c* Acanthamoeba in brain capillary, surrounded by neutrophils. ×710. *d* Acanthamoeba perivascular collection about thrombosed venule. ×535. *e* Acanthamoebic brain abscess in cortisonized monkey that developed amebic pneumonia, but without demonstrable nasal infection. ×535. *f* Gross photograph of submeningeal brain abscess of monkey, secondary to amebic pneumonia as described in *e*.

above. There was similar intestinal involvement in the first human Naegleria case reported by *Derrick* [22] as due to *Iodamoeba bütschlii,* but later shown to be Naegleria, in a patient who was dying of starvation.

Acanthamoeba and cysts thereof have been demonstrated in human corneas, in and around corneal ulcers [33], which may proceed to destruction of the globe. Whether the amebas initiate the ulcer or invade it secondarily is a question, I believe. In experimental attempts to cause

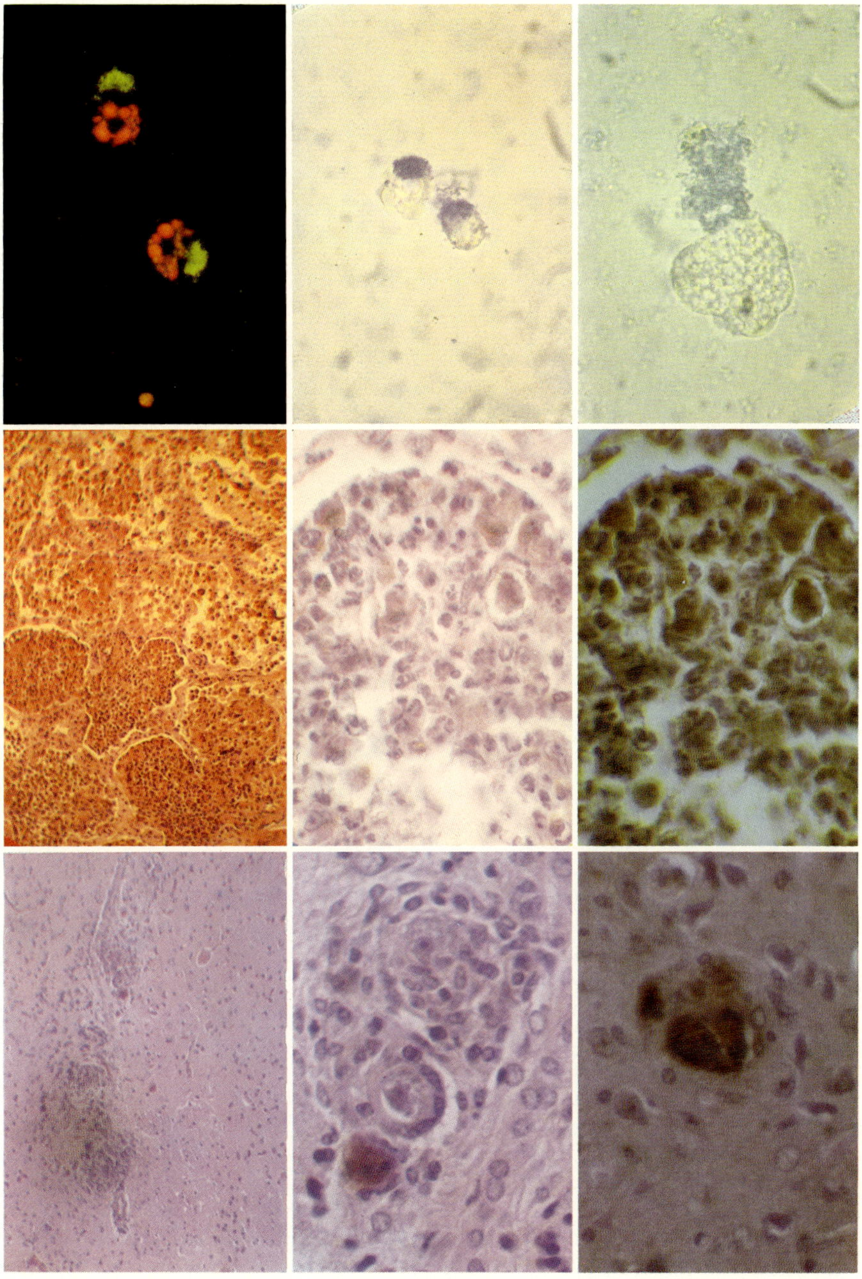

a *b, c*

d *e, f*

g *h, i*

Fig. 5. For legends see reverse side.

Fig. 5. a–c Amebas showing positive D-SPAC. ×780. *a A. culbertsoni* using acridine O and fluorescence microscopy. *b N. fowleri* using methylene-blue-stained staphylococci. *c E. histolytica* using methylene-blue-stained staphylococci. *d–f* Lung tissue from cortisonized cynomolgus monkey, anesthetized and given large dose of *A. culbertsoni* intranasally. *d* Pulmonary alveoli filled with exudate. HE. ×155. *e* Section through same alveolus, subjected to indirect immunoperoxidase procedure, plus HE counterstain results using *N. fowleri* antiserum. Note lack of any yellowish brown staining. *f* Using antiserum against *A. culbertsoni.* Note yellowish brown staining of ameba and also cytoplasm of some of tissue leukocytes. The phagocytes appear to take up amebic antigen. ×780. *g–i* Sections of mouse brain 7 months after intranasal inoculation of 2,500 HN-3 amebas *(A. polyphagia)* and sacrificed after having shown no symptoms. *g* Brain stem showing cellular infiltrate. HE. ×78. *h* Lesion in brain stem (as in *g*) showing granuloma containing two amebas. HE. ×780. *i* Lesion from same area as in *h,* subjected to indirect immunoperoxidase reaction with *A. culbertsoni* antiserum plus HE counterstain. Note intense positive reaction in two amebas and tissue in immediate vicinity. In *h* the eosinophilic mass appearing in the lower left area is an artefact and does not represent specific staining as in *i.*

amebic corneal ulcers in rabbits, I was unable [unpublished experiments] to produce them using *A. culbertsoni* following corneal epithelial scarification. However, by introduction of *A. culbertsoni* into the conjunctival sacs of rabbits with vaccinia lesions in the cornea, a general opacity developed in the cornea, an unusual result with vaccinia virus alone. Imbedded precystic trophozoites and some cysts were found in the sections.

The initial cellular response to both Naegleria and Acanthamoeba is composed of neutrophils, and in the acute infections by either, this remains the preponderant reaction. However, in the subacute and chronic lesions of acanthamoebiasis there is first a neutrophilic response, followed by the appearance of lymphocytes, plasma cells, and large mononuclear cells. Granulomata containing amebas develop with large nodules of epitheloid cells and variable numbers of multinucleated giant cells. In brains affected by destructive vascular lesions there is widespread necrosis due to infarction, and in these areas there is a lack of viable cells and even of viable amebas. In long-term mouse experiments, as well as in some of the human Acanthamoeba cases, mature, viable cysts may be seen alone in the brain tissue with no cellular reaction about them.

The demonstration of amebas in the tissue may be difficult in cases where there is a long agonal period and especially so if fixation is delayed.

The above pathological features were first seen in experimental animal infections in the early stages of this work [17]. Not surprisingly, most of the lesions have now been observed in natural disease in man and domestic animals. There are some exceptions to this, however. The expected acanthamoebic pulmonary disease has not been described in man, although it is highly probable that such exists and has not been found. The importance of the vascular disease in acanthamoebiasis has recently been noted in humans as it was in experimental mouse infections [38]. The involvement of the liver by Naegleria in the mice infected intranasally is very frequent [15], but liver involvement in human naegleramebiasis up to this time has not been observed.

Serologic Reactions (fig. 5a–c)

The determination of human antiamebic antibodies against the free-living amebas by any of the suggested methods has not been measured extensively enough to indicate their feasibility in practical diagnostic tests. One study by *Kenney* [34] resulted in the discovery of two positive results, one verified at death after testing about 1,000 random sera by complement fixation using an extract of *A. culbertsoni* as antigen. Since chronic disease is more commonly caused by the *A. polyphagia* group, the inclusion of these antigens might have doubled the number of positive results. A larger survey, preferably a more selective survey, upon subacute or chronic central nervous system disease, including cerebrovascular accidents and general vascular and pulmonary afflictions, seems to be indicated. Complement fixation, while a very satisfactory test, has been replaced generally by less complex procedures. Agglutination and immobilization reactions using fixed amebas are probably not sensitive enough for detection of low-titer antibodies. Indirect hemagglutination, as employed for anti-*E. histolytica* antibody and recently studied by *Cerva* [8] for anti-Acanthamoeba and Naegleria antibody, appears to be applicable to mass screening. Indirect and direct immunofluorescence, using formalin-fixed amebas, as devised by *Goldman* [28], is now also in general use. The recently described quantitative I-SPAC test appears also to be a simple and accurate method that compares favorably with immunofluorescence results.

In our experience with chronically infected monkeys, the complement-fixing antibody in nonfatal, long-standing or subsiding brain lesions persists for a considerable period, but diminishes to zero several months after healing of the lesion. Antibody was also detectable in the cerebrospinal fluid of one of these animals [17], and, since this fluid is less anticomplementary, larger samples of fluid could be used to obtain a more sensitive test. This monkey with the healed or subsiding nonfatal lesion which caused the positive serologic results that became negative, at autopsy showed a healed lesion with no signs of the amebas.

Host Resistance

In spite of their ubiquitous presence in the environment, the uncommon occurrence of infections caused by free-living amebas is not attributed to any single factor. The reason for the total lack of intestinal lesions caused by these amebas is still unsolved, but may be due to the unfavorable conditions in the gastrointestinal tract for the trophic free-living amebas. The presence of cystic forms in feces is well documented, but until *Schaudinn* [cited by *Culbertson,* 17] and others demonstrated rather conclusively that only *E. histolytica* was the intestinal pathogen, some workers believed that positive stool cultures for free-living forms indicated they were in fact the cause of amebic diarrhea. The factors against the growth and multiplication of Acanthamoeba and Naegleria in the intestine are the lytic effects of the gastric fluid and bile and the unfavorable anaerobic conditions prevalent, probably due to the massive bacterial flora of the large intestine. The free-living amebas are aerobic, while *E. histolytica* is reported to be anaerobic [46]. Intestinal antibodies, such as IgA, might be inhibitory to the amebas. The anti-amebic effects of complement are well known.

I have studied the interactions of living neutrophil leukocytes by cinemicrophotography in vitro with *A. culbertsoni* and *N. fowleri*. Normal human leukocytes attack, surround and destroy the Acanthamoeba. Leukocytes from the same person showed no attraction or activity against *N. fowleri* unter the same conditions. In tissue sections, however, neutrophils are easily seen surrounding individual Naegleria. Normal leukocyte function, accompanied by the known lytic and immobilizing effect of blood serum at the nasal mucosal level could probably be an effective deterrent to amebic infection. This mechanism could be most important in persons lacking normal resistance in preventing Acanthamoeba infection, but perhaps not so with Naegleria infections.

Experimental vaccination of mice with killed *A. culbertsoni* is highly successful in protecting mice from very large intranasal challenges of that ameba [17]. Some experiments have indicated that similar vaccination with *N. fowleri* was partially protective against intranasal challenge [49]. Our own tests, wherein intranasal challenge was used, were completely negative.

Another important consideration is the role of natural immunization in the possible acquired resistance which normal persons and normal monkeys appear to possess against both Naegleria and Acanthamoeba. The information relative to this question is sketchy. *Cursons* et al. [21] have suggested that natural immunity with formation of antibodies does develop and has a protective effect. Our own investigations [unpublished] would suggest that normal persons in our area have little if any specific antibody demonstrable by classical methods. Perhaps there is a difference of exposure in various regions. The incidence of positive Acanthamoeba cultures from the nasopharynx was greater in children when persons of various ages were cultured and some have attributed this finding to the development of immunity. An alternate explanation would be that children are probably more exposed to dust than adults, who are less apt to be near the floor. Furthermore, the evidence of *Skočil* et al. [47] indicates that the positive nasopharyngeal culture for Acanthamoebas in normal adults arises from the presence of inhaled cysts in the secretions from these areas. If this be true, the antibody present would not seem important in determining whether the cyst excysted under the conditions of the culture.

Finally, the types of persons susceptible to the two diseases are of both theoretical and practical interest. As reported above, naegleramebiasis is more common in children, but not exclusively so. This might indicate that children are more apt to swim in polluted water. However, adults probably being more cautious and able to control aspiration of water into the nares could conceivably escape infection when a child would not. Only a few persons who died of naegleramebiasis have had systemic disease that might have compromised their immunologic processes. Fatal acanthamoebiasis appears always to occur in patients who have somehow lost their ability to resist the infection. The presence of Acanthamoeba cysts in the nasopharynx of some persons of all ages is well documented, and excystment of these into active trophozoites is known to be stimulated by the presence of certain bacteria – usually gram-negative bacilli. One must consider therefore that the lack of resistance to these bacteria and their abnormal colonization in the nasopharynx may be crucial. If in the abnormal state the bacteria and the amebic cysts are brought together in the nasopharynx of a patient with compromised resistance, then the possibility of acanthamoebiasis becomes greater through the formation of trophozoites.

Diagnosis

Naegleramebiasis

The history of exposure to water of questionable quality by swimming should alert the physician to the possibility of amebic nasopharyngitis and meningitis. The accumulated information would indicate that only by early diagnosis and treatment is there the opportunity to prevent fatal meningoencephalitis. Thus it is advisable to evaluate the nature of upper respiratory symptoms in persons with a suggestive history of exposure, especially in areas where the disease has been known to occur.

The description of the disease as first outlined by *Carter* [4] is a guide for clinical evaluation. The patient is usually a young person, in previous good health, who in many instances after a sore throat and rhinitis suffers an abrupt onset of headache and mild fever. There is rapid development of increasing headache, vomiting and nuchal rigidity over a period of 2–3 days. The symptoms change to the point of disorientation and coma. The cerebrospinal fluid becomes more purulent and the entire picture may be mistaken for acute meningococcic meningitis.

Laboratory Findings

The cloudy cerebrospinal fluid, depending upon the stage of the disease, will contain from 1,000 to 10,000 neutrophils and often many red blood cells. Bacteria will not be found, but the highly motile Naegleria can usually be observed in the counting chamber or on a coverslip and slide preparation of the fluid or sediment. Phase microscopy is helpful but not essential. Care must be taken not to dilute or suspend the fluid in any toxic diluent, such as 2% acetic acid, which will cause the amebas to round up and appear like neutrophils. With specimens such as cerebrospinal fluid, cultures are made upon broth such as trypsinized soy peptone broth which has been prepared without the addition of NaCl but containing all the other usual ingredients. Before inoculation, sterile fetal calf serum is added to make a 10% concentration. Sustained tissue cell cultures may also be used, since the Naegleria will multiply therein and eventually destroy the mammalian cells.

Staining is occasionally desirable. Ordinary bacterial or blood stains are usually not satisfactory. The best preparations are produced by immediate fixation of the undried smear by Nissenbaum's method [41], or alcohol ether, as proposed by Papanicolaou and staining by Giemsa, HE, hematoxylin-Papanicolaou combination, or trichrome stain. These methods provide for clear distinction of the amebas from tissue cells and of course can be used for other amebas as well. I prefer Giemsa staining.

For specimens containing bacteria, such as nasal secretions or tissue samples, the amebas may be cultured with cultures of *A. aerogenes* or *E. coli*. Petri plates are prepared with 8–10 ml of sterilized 1.5% agar in distilled water. The bacterial growth from a nutrient agar culture is transferred by loop to cover a 1-cm circle in the center of the plate. The inoculum is placed upon this area and the plate sealed and incubated at 37 °C. Using subdued light, the inverted plate is examined daily for 10 days for emerging amebic growth and migration at × 100 magnification. If amebas are seen, further examination can be made by transfer to slide and coverslip preparation. This procedure has the disadvantage of obtaining amebic growth mixed with the bacteria. However, the amebas in such a culture can be identified by any of the above described immunologic methods as well as by morphology. A control culture, consisting of a plate with bacterial spot with no inoculum, should be included.

Needless to say, all specimens of this type should be cultured promptly, not frozen, but preferably kept at room temperature. If by accident the material is placed at 4 °C, it should be removed and cultured at once as the amebas will survive the refrigerator temperature for only a few hours.

If there is but a small specimen of fluid sediment available that is believed to be bacteria-free, intracerebral inoculation of one or more mice may be utilized. If the mouse succumbs, brain tissue removed aseptically may be cultured as described above.

From what has been noted concerning the rapidity of the process toward a fatal termination, diagnostic tests must be made as expeditiously as possible. The ideal procedure, it would seem, in a patient who presents with a suggestive history in the sore throat-rhinitis phase, would be to make direct examination of any obtainable nasal secretion or nasal washings. There is at present no report of having discovered the trophic amebas in nasal secretions at this stage. Since most patients are first seen with symptoms of meningeal involvement, the examination of cerebrospinal fluid is then the more appropriate procedure. The eventual ideal objective would be through public dissemination of information to recommend investigation of all rhinitis cases that occur following swimming in other than well-constructed and operated, supervised pools.

Acanthamoebiasis

Acanthamoeba infection should be suspected in serious, subacute, or chronic central nervous system disease as an alternate possibility to mycotic or viral disease. Acanthamoeba infection appears to be opportunistic in character [37], since most of the known cases have occurred in patients whose resistance has been compromised by other diseases or by immunosuppressive drugs. Since there is no report of this disease being diagnosed before autopsy, there is little to guide the investigation of living patients. The amebas, due to their entrapment in a more localized area, such as abscess or granuloma, probably will not appear in cerebrospinal fluid nearly as often as the amebas in Naegleria infection.

Studies of the patients' serum for the various types of Acanthamoeba antibodies would probably give a clue to the diagnosis, provided the patient is capable of producing antibody. Only tests showing significant increases in antibody would be of value, since some patients with disease such as Hodgkin's disease or those who have been treated with immunosuppressive drugs may not produce antibodies well.

The lack of antemortem diagnostic criteria leaves autopsy or biopsy as the only alternative. The gross cerebral lesions may suggest brain tumor. The descriptions in the few reports of human disease and of the pathology in experimental monkey infections, as described above, suggest that brains showing a combination of granuloma and hemorrhagic suppuration in the submeningeal areas of the temporal and basal regions should be suspect. Some of the brain destruction is probably due to vascular thrombosis and infarction. Definitive studies by culture and by histologic means serve to differentiate the infection from other infections or from neoplastic disease, and these should be excluded by appropriate studies. The suppurative brain abscesses due to Acanthamoeba are quite similar to those described that are due to *E. histolytica.* Therefore, to make a correct diagnosis, the type of ameba present must be determined. Cultures of fresh, aseptically obtained exudate from the lesions or cerebrospinal fluid sediment are the means of choice, and are made in the same manner as described above for Naegleria. Acanthamoebas grow well upon medium containing NaCl, but will also grow on medium without it.

Prevention

For the control of amebic infection due to exposure to water containing amebas no specific sanitary procedures are known except for ordinary purification of the water by filtration devised to remove bacteria, followed by chlorination. If the bacterial count is held to a low level the number of amebas should be expected to remain low. The highest tolerated level of chlorine in drinking water and swimming pools is not sufficient to kill the amebas.

Cerva [9] has suggested that avoiding the tracking of soil into pools and the avoidance of the presence of porous material, such as wooden steps, is important. Such procedures are customary in properly ordered pools, but perhaps not in all private or home installations. The lack of a significant number of recognized infections from modern swimming pools would at least indicate that serious infections from that source are extremely rare. There is but one additional but effective alternative – that is to prevent swimming in natural water that is polluted.

Treatment

Acanthamoebiasis

The experimental mouse infection by *A. culbertsoni* is easily prevented or cured by the administration of sulfadiazine in the diet in concentrations of 0.5–0.75 % [15, 18]. Similar experiments with *A. polyphagia* (HN-3) show activity by the drug, but with less dramatic results. Sulfapyridine and sulfamerazine were also active, but probably less so than sulfadiazine.

There is no instance in which a patient with acanthamoebiasis has been treated with sulfadiazine, since the diagnosis has never been made nor the amebas identified by culture before death.

Since acanthamoebic encephalomyelitis appears usually to be a terminal illness due to an underlying neoplastic or other debilitating process, the probability of therapeutic success is not assured even with a very active drug. In my opinion, however, sulfadiazine or other sulfa-drugs should be used if there is evidence of the presence of such an infection.

The destructive acanthamoebic keratitis reported has not yielded to any treatment. Sulfadiazine and other sulfa-drugs were slightly effective in one trial, but not curative. *Jones* et al. [33] report the use of a number of antibacterial agents, but they regard all of them as less than satisfactory.

Nagington and Richards [40] studied 24 compounds and selected 9 that showed relatively weak activity in 48-hour in vitro contact tests at 37 °C. The most active of the group that was tested against one isolate of *A. polyphagia* and two of *A. castellani,* was acriflavine. This compound was found to inhibit the trophozoite multiplication (MIC) in the range of 0.1–1.0 μg/ml and to inactivate the cysts in the range of 10–100 μg. None of the compounds were promising for systemic treatment, but several of them were believed possible candidates for local application to the cornea.

Naegleramebiasis

Several drugs have been tested, in vitro and in vivo, against *N. fowleri.* In our description of the Naegleria isolate HB-1, in 1966, we included the results of a very limited investigation by in vivo tests in mice using 0.5 % sulfadiazine in the diet plus subcutaneous injection of amphotericin B (AMP-B), which treatment proved effective [15]. Later we, and others, showed that sulfadiazine was ineffective and AMP-B was effective. *Carter* [5] reported an extensive in vitro and in vivo study and defined MIC levels.

AMP-B has now been used in a number of persons, usually unsuccessfully, for advanced cases of cerebral disease, but in a few instances patients are reported to have been cured by the use of the drug alone or in combination with some other drug [24]. The early experience is difficult to evaluate since, in some instances from reading the published reports, it appears that the diagnosis is subject to question as is the species, and in fact the origin of the cultured offending ameba. Combining the experimental evidence supporting the definite effectiveness of AMP-B with the somewhat sketchy clinical evidence results in the definite impression that the drug is clinically useful for the treatment of the disease. *Carter* [6] has called attention to the advisability of using the intravenous route and reported administration of very small doses intraventricularly. He called attention to the case reported by *Apley* et al. [2] wherein the intravenous use of AMP-B resulted in a concentration of nearly 0.2 μg in the cerebrospinal fluid, which is probably a minimal effective level against the ameba. *Carter* [6] cited 1 patient apparently cured by AMP-B. Thus, careful administration of 1 mg/kg of AMP-B daily by intravenous drip would seem to be a therapeutic procedure of value. This should prove important if one were to discover a patient with active Naegleria in nasal secretions in the initial stage of the infection – before the extension of the disease to the central nervous system. Nasal irrigation with an active drug might even be considered in addition to intravenous administration.

Recently, 1 patient has been reported to have recovered from naegleramebiasis when treated with intravenous and intrathecal AMP-B, miconazole and oral rifampin [39]. Miconazole was reported by *Duma and Finley* [25] to have in vitro anti-Naegleria activity, but to have somewhat less effect on a weight basis than AMP-B. There are as yet no published in vivo tests that would serve to evaluate the relative value of miconazole and AMP-B or a combination thereof.

The intraventricular administration of AMP-B as practiced in myotic infections has been used in one or two instances with questionable results. The toxicity of the preparation prevents intraventricular administration beyond very small doses; it is not an approved procedure in the United States. We found that intracerebral doses in both normal and infected mice caused choroid plexus injury and ventricular enlargement [19]. We do not know whether this was due to the added bile acid or the drug. There is no information as to the occurrence of similar effects in man. However, in later [unpublished] experiments, a single dose of 7.50 μg in 0.03 ml volume given 1 day after intranasal inoculation of 100 and 200 Naegleria saved most of the mice, whereas all the untreated mice injected intracerebrally with saline became infected and died.

The above information suggests that aggressive clinical and laboratory diagnostic studies, combined with prompt use of AMP-B in recommended fashion, are probably capable of preventing death or serious injury from naegleramebiasis. The observation by *Thong* [50] that AMP-B acted synergistically with tetracycline and also rifamycin against *N. fowleri* in mice infected intranasally was also reported by *Lee* et al. [36] who tested the two drugs in vitro. They also stated that minocycline and tetracycline were synergistic with AMP-B but that miconazole was not. These findings may be of clinical importance.

Summary

As the result of research by many workers, information as to the accurate diagnosis and possibly effective treatment has accumulated. While much more definitive academic investigation will aid in improving the results of medical management, the next objective should be the serious study of patients with suggestive histories and with acute and chronic respiratory ailments for the possible role of free-living amebas therein.

The state of the art has reached the point where the two free-living amebic infections can probably be diagnosed by direct examination of exudates from the respiratory tract before the diseases become serious and beyond treatment. At present, the lack of effort to do this is as if one were trying to diagnose amebic dysentery without examination of fecal or sigmoidoscopic specimens for the presence of *E. histolytica* in the diagnosis of entamebiasis. There is need for increased effort by local health officials, parents, clinicians and laboratory scientists to attempt to prevent the tragic consequences of naegleramebiasis by all possible means, at facilities near the patient's home. While the prospects of effectively handling the problem of acanthamoebiasis are less promising, earlier recognition of it in patients now known likely to develop such an infection might lead to better understanding the approaches to its treatment.

References

1 Anderson, K.; Jamieson, A.: Primary amoebic meningoencephalitis. Lancet *i:* 902–903 (1972).

2 Apley, J.; Clarke, S. K. R.; Rome, A. P. C. H.; Sandry, S. A.; Daygi, G.; Silk, B.; Warhorst, D. C.: Primary amoebic meningoencephalitis in Britain. Br. med. J. *i:* 596–599 (1970).

3 Butt, C. G.: Primary amebic meningoencephalitis. New Engl. J. Med. *274:* 1473–1476 (1966).

4 Carter, R. F.: Primary amoebic meningo-encephalitis: clinical, pathological, and epidemiological features of six fatal cases. J. Path. Bact. *96:* 1–25 (1968).

5 Carter, R. F.: Sensitivity to amphotericin B of a Naegleria sp. isolated from a case of primary amoebic meningoencephalitis. J. clin. Path. *22:* 470–474 (1969).

6 Carter, R. R.: Primary amoebic meningo-encephalitis. An appraisal of present knowledge. Trans. R. Soc. trop. Med. Hyg. *66:* 193–213 (1972).

7 Cerva, L.; Novák, K.; Culbertson, C. G.: An outbreak of acute, fatal amebic meningoencephalitis. Am. J. Epidem. *88:* 436–444 (1968).

8 Cerva, L.: Detection of antibody against *Limax amoebae* by means of the indirect haemagglutination test. Folia parasit., Praha *24:* 293–299 (1977).

9 Cerva, L.: Studies of limax amoebae in a swimming pool. Hydrobiologia *38:* 141–161 (1971).

10 Connor, A. H.; Neafie, R. C.; Meyers, W. M.: Amebiasis; in Binford, Connor, Pathology of tropical and extraordinary diseases, pp. 308–316 (AFIP, Washington 1976).

11 Culbertson, C. G.; Ensminger, P. W.; Overton, W. M.: Amebic cellulocutaneous invasion by *Naegleria aerobia* with generalized visceral lesions after subcutaneous inoculation. An experimental study in guinea pigs. Am. J. clin. Path. *57:* 375–386 (1972).

12 Culbertson, C. G.: Soil ameba infection. Specific indirect immunoenzymatic (peroxidase) staining of formalin-fixed paraffin sections. Am. J. clin. Path. *63:* 475–482 (1975).

13 Culbertson, C. G.; Harper, K.: Immunoperoxidase staining of *E. histolytica* and soil amebas in formalin-fixed tissue. Am. J. clin. Path. *68:* 529 (1977).

14 Culbertson, C. G.; Harper, K.: Surface coagglutination with formalinized, stained protein A staphylococci in the immunologic study of three pathogenic amebae. Am. J. trop. Med. Hyg. *29:* 785–794 (1980).

15 Culbertson, C. G.; Ensminger, P. W.; Overton, W. M.: Pathogenic Naegleria sp. Study of a strain isolated from human cerebrospinal fluid. J. Protozool. *15:* 353–363 (1968).

16 Culbertson, C. G.: Amebic meningoencephalitides; in Binford, Connor, Pathology of tropical and extraordinary diseases, pp. 317–324 (AFIP, Washington 1976).

17 Culbertson, C. G.: The pathogenicity of soil amebas. A. Rev. Microbiol. *25:* 231–254 (1971).

18 Culbertson, C. G.; Holmes, D. H.; Overton, W. M.: *Hartmannella castellani* (Acanthamoeba Sp.). Am. J. clin. Path. *43:* 361–364 (1965).

19 Culbertson, C. G.; Overton, W. M.; Ensminger, P. W.: Pathogenic Hartmannella (Acanthamoeba) and Naegleria; studies on experimental chemotherapy and pathology; in Hejzlar, Semonsky, Masák, Advances in antimicrobial and antineoplastic chemotherapy. Proc. VIIth Int. Congr. Chemother., Prague 1971, pp. 433–434 (Urban & Schwarzenberg, München 1972).

20 Cursons, R. T. M.; Brown, T. J.; Bruns, B. J.; Taylor, D. E. M.: Primary amoebic meningoencephalitis contracted in a thermal tributary of the Waikato river – Taupo: a case report. N. Z. med. J. *84:* 479–481 (1976).

21 Cursons, R. T. M.; Brown, T. J.; Keys, E. A.: Immunity to pathogenic free-living amoebae. Lancet *ii:* 875 (1977).

22 Derrick, E. H.: A fatal case of generalized amoebiasis due to a protozoan closely resembling, if not identical with, *Iodamoeba bütschlii.* Trans. R. Soc. trop. Med. Hyg. *42:* 191–198 (1948).

23 Duma, R. J.; Helwig, W. B.; Martinez, A. J.: Meningoencephalitis and brain abscess due to a free-living amoeba. Ann. intern. Med. *88:* 468–473 (1978).

24 Duma, R. J.; Rosenblum, W. I.; McGehee, R. F.; Jones, M. M.; Nelson, E. C.: Primary amoebic meningoencephalitis caused by Naegleria – Two new cases, response to amphotericin B, and a review. Ann. intern. Med. *74:* 923–931 (1971).

25 Duma, R. J.; Finley, R.: In vitro susceptibility of pathogenic Naegleria and Acanthamoeba species to a variety of therapeutic agents. Antimicrob. Agents Chemother. *10:* 370–376 (1976).

26 Fowler, M.; Carter, R. F.: Acute pyogenic meningitis probably due to Acanthamoeba sp.: a preliminary report. Br. med. J. *ii:* 740–742 (1965).

27 Fulton, C.: Amebo-flagellates as research partners: the laboratory biology of Naegleria and Tetramitus; in Prescott, Methods in cell physiology, vol. 4, pp. 341–476 (Academic Press, New York 1970).

28 Goldman, M.: Evaluation of a fluorescent antibody test for amebiasis using two widely differing ameba strains as antigen. Am. J. trop. Med. Hyg. *15:* 694–700 (1966).

29 Griffin, J. L.: Pathogenic free-living amoebae; in Krier, Parasitic protozoa, vol. 2 (Academic Press, New York 1978).

30 Griffin, J. L.: Temperature tolerance of pathogenic and nonpathogenic free-living amoebas. Science *178:* 869–870 (1972).

31 Jadin, J. B.; Hermanne, J.; Robyn, G.; Willaert, E.; Van Maercke, Y.; Stevens, W.: Trois cas de méningo-encéphalite amibienne primitive observés à Anvers (Belgique). Annls Soc. belge Méd. trop. *51:* 255–266 (1971).

32 Jager, B. V.; Stamm, W. P.: Brain abscesses caused by free-living amoeba probably of the genus Hartmannella in a patient with Hodgkin's disease. Lancet *ii:* 1343–1345 (1972).

33 Jones, D. B.; Visvesvara, G. S.; Robinson, N. M.: *Acanthamoeba polyphaga* keratitis and Acanthamoeba uveitis associated with fatal meningoencephalitis. Trans. ophthal. Soc. UK *95:* 221–232 (1975).

34 Kenney, M.: The micro-Kolmer complement fixation test in routine screening for soil ameba infection. Hlth Lab. Sci. *8:* 5–10 (1971).

35 Lawande, R. V.; Abraham, S. N.; John, I.; Egler, L. J.: Recovery of soil amebas from the nasal passages of children during the dusty Harmattan period in Zaire. Am. J. clin. Path. *71:* 201–203 (1979).

36 Lee, K. K.; Karr, S. L., Jr.; Wong, M. M.; Hoeprich, P. D.: In vitro susceptibilities of *Naegleria fowleri* strain HB-1 to selected antimicrobial agents, singly and in combination. Antimicrob. Agents Chemother. *16:* 217–220 (1979).

37 Martinez, A. J.: Is Acanthamoeba encephalitis an opportunistic infection? Neurology, Minneap. *30:* 567–574 (1980).

38 Martinez, A. J.; Sotelo-Avila, C.; Alcalá, H.; Willaert, E.: Granulomatous encephalitis, intracranial arteritis, and mycotic aneurysm due to a free-living ameba. Acta neuropath. *49:* 7–12 (1980).

39 Primary amebic meningoencephalitis. Morb. Mort. Week. Rep. *27:* 343 (1978).

40 Nagington, J.; Richards, J. E.: Chemotherapeutic compounds and Acanthamoebae from eye infections. J. clin. Path. *29:* 648–651 (1976).

41 Nissenbaum, G.: A combined method for the rapid fixation and adhesion of ciliates and flagellates. Science *118:* 31–32 (1953).

42 Page, F. C.: Taxonomic criteria for limax amoebae, with descriptions of three new species of Hartmannella and three of Vahlkampfia. J. Protozool. *14:* 499–521 (1967).

43 Patras, D.; Andujar, J. J.: Meningoencephalitis due to Hartmannella (Acanthamoeba). Am. J. clin. Path. *46:* 226–233 (1966).

44 Rafalko, J. S.: Cytological observations on the amoeboflagellate, *Naegleria gruberi* (protozoa). J. Morph. *81:* 1–44 (1947).

45 Schuster, F. L.: Small amebas and ameboflagellates; in Biochemistry and physiology of protozoa, vol. 1; 2nd ed., pp. 215–285 (Academic Press, New York 1979).

46 Singh, B. N.: Aerobic small free-living amoebae; in Pathogenic and non-pathogenic amoebae, pp. 3–4 (Wiley, New York 1975).

47 Skočil, V.; Serbus, C.; Cerva, L.: Epidemiological study of the incidence of amoebae of the limax group in military communities. VI. Relation between the finding of amoebas of the limax group in nasal swabs and some epidemiological indices. J. Hyg. Epidem. Microbiol. Immun. *16:* 226–230 (1972).

48 Stevens, A. R.; Kilpatrick, T.; Willaert, E.; Capton, A.: Serologic analysis of cell surface antigens of Acanthamoeba spp. with plasma membrane antisera. J. Protozool. *24:* 316–324 (1977).

49 Thong, Y. H.; Shepherd, C.; Ferrante, A.; Rowan-Kelly, B.: Protective immunity to *Naegleria fowleri* in experimental amebic meningoencephalitis. Am. J. trop. Med. Hyg. *27:* 238–240 (1978).

50 Thong, Y. H.: Primary amoebic meningoencephalitis: fifteen years later. Med. J. Aust. *i:* 352–354 (1980).

51 Wang, S. S.; Feldman, H. A.: Isolation of Hartmannella species from human throats. New Engl. J. Med. *277:* 1174–1179 (1967).

52 Willaert, E.; Stevens, Z. R.; Healy, G. R.: Retrospective identification of *Acanthamoeba culbertsoni* in a case of amoebic meningoencephalitis. J. clin. Path. *31:* 717–720 (1978).

C. G. Culbertson, MD, Lilly Laboratory for Clinical Research,
1001 West Tenth Street, Indianapolis, IN 46202 (USA)

Antibiotics Chemother., vol. 30, pp. 54–114 (Karger, Basel 1981)

Cestodes

M. A. Gemmell, P. D. Johnstone

Hydatid Research Unit, Research Division, Ministry of Agriculture and Fisheries, University of Otago Medical School, Dunedin, New Zealand;
Research Division, Ministry of Agriculture and Fisheries, Invermay Agricultural Research Centre, Mosgiel, New Zealand

1. Introduction and Historical Comment

About 30 species of tapeworm involve man to a greater or less extent in their life cycles. Recent estimates suggest that more than 100 million people are parasitized with tapeworms [120]. The majority of important cyclophyllidean human tapeworm infections occur with the family Taeniidae. These include the ubiquitous *Taenia saginata* and the less common *Taenia solium* for which man is the obligatory definitive host, with cattle and pigs acting respectively as the intermediate hosts for the larval (metacestode) phase. Infection occurs by the ingestion of undercooked meat. Man can also act as the intermediate host for *T. solium* following the ingestion of its eggs and this can have serious, even fatal, consequences.

Among the Hymenolepididae, *Hymenolepis nana,* a common parasite of rodents, also frequently parasitizes man. This life cycle may be direct or indirect and involve the ingestion of beetle-derived cysticercoids or the ingestion of eggs. *Hymenolepis diminuta,* also a common parasite of rodents, occasionally parasitizes man following the ingestion of beetles harbouring cysticercoids. A similar invasion of the human gut may occur with the common dog-tapeworm *Dipylidium caninum* following the ingestion of parasitized fleas.

Apart from larval tapeworm infections with *T. solium* and *H. nana,* man frequently becomes infected with metacestodes following the ingestion of eggs of the ubiquitous dog tapeworm *Echinococcus granulosus.* Similarly, man can act as an accidental host for *Echinococcus multilocularis,* a common tapeworm of foxes and cricetid rodents in the northern hemisphere. Both species may be lethal to man.

Among the pseudophyllidean tapeworms, *Diphyllobothrium latum* and to a lesser extent *Diphyllobothrium pacificum* are important human parasites. Their life cycle involves copepods (procercoid), then fish (plerocercoid) and this can be followed either by: (i) survival, but not reorganization in paratenic hosts (e. g. larger predatory fish) or (ii) growth to the adult phase in the gut of fish-eating mammals including man. Plerocercoids of *Spirometra* develop in reptiles, amphibeans, birds and mammals including man.

Historically, the treatment of tapeworm infections in man must have been regarded as a most disquietening experience (fig. 1). Prior to 1956, when the introduction of dichlorophen marked the beginning of drug treatment without the need for special preparation and hospitalization, drugs such as carbon tetrachloride, pelletierine, extract of male fern *(Dryopteris filix-mas),* kamala, pomegranate bark, pumpkin seeds and hexylresorcinol were commonly used. During the 1950s, a derivative of acridine mepacrine hydrochloride (Quinacrin, Atabrin), extract of male fern and tin compounds provided the main groups of drugs for treating human tapeworm infections. These drugs had severe disadvantages as was pointed out in 1960: 'Traditional methods of expelling tapeworms made it something of an ordeal even to a patient in good health and a procedure only undertaken reluctantly in elderly or frail persons or in children' [413]. Similarly in veterinary medicine, the principal drugs available for the treatment of tapeworm infections including *Echinococcus* spp in dogs, were the arecoline salts. While these are useful in the diagnosis of echinococcosis, there are also contraindications to their use [172].

Several studies have been undertaken using in vitro techniques, but they have not revealed important new compounds. The commonest method by which potentially useful compounds have been found is through a rational exploitation of an empirical screening programme usually involving tapeworm such as *H. nana* and *H. diminuta* in rodents [70, 115, 120, 416, 428]. This may be followed by evaluations using target organisms such as *Taenia hydatigena, Taenia ovis* and *Taenia pisiformis* and *D. caninum* in dogs and *Taenia taeniaeformis* in cats. Subsequent studies may involve *Echinococcus* spp, but these require special facilities, if patent infections are to be used. Following appropriate toxicity and pharmacokinetic studies in animals, the candidate compound may be evaluated for efficacy against human tapeworm infections.

Data collected in trials to establish the efficacy of a drug may be highly variable and worm counts in both the untreated and treated groups

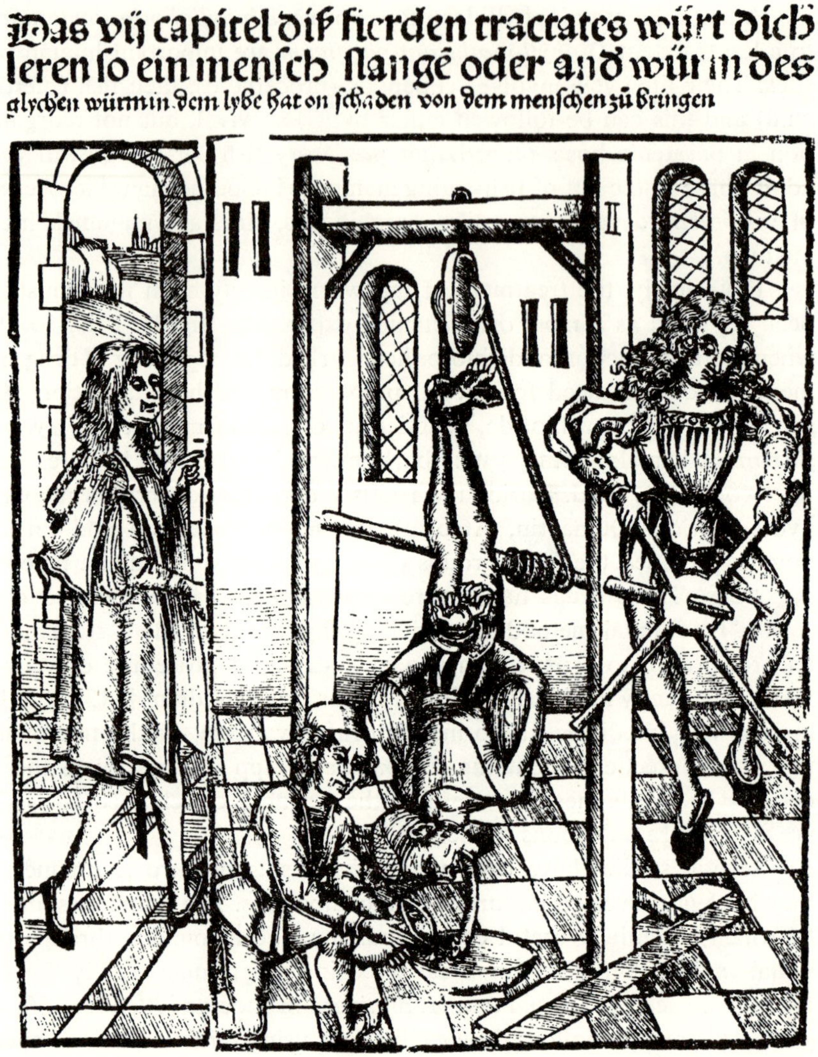
Das vij capitel diß fierden tractates würt dich
leren so ein mensch slangē oder and' würm in des
glychen würmin dem lybe hat on schaden von dem menschen zū bringen

Fig. 1. Hieronymus Brunschwig (1450–1533): Das Buch der Cirurgia des Hieronymus Brunschwig; Strassburg, publisher Johann Grüninger (1497); in Carl Kuhn (ed.): Alte Meister der Medizin und Naturkunde, vol. 3, p. 257 (München, 1911). Reproduced from copy in University of Otago Medical School Library, New Zealand and first cited in ref. 419.

may vary from nil to several thousand. Because of this, researchers have found biometry most helpful in designing and enterpreting drug trials. For example, the estimation of a dose-response curve for those animals freed from infection following drug therapy has been used to identify dose rates and treatment schedules likely to achieve predictable levels of parasite control. Despite the availability of these methods for analysis and evaluation [156, 157] throughout the period under review (1956–1980) there is for various reasons, a substantial literature that does not go beyond case history studies.

With regard to drugs that kill the larval phase (metacestode), this is a relatively new field. Here again, several small and large animal models are available, for example, laboratory rodents for studies on echinococcosis, pigs for studies on *T. solium,* sheep for studies on *T. hydatigena* and *T. ovis* and cattle for studies on *T. saginata.* The results from these models may be useful in designing trials of drugs to combat human echinococcosis and cysticercosis. Again, design and analyses are similar to those required for the evaluation of drugs for adult tapeworm infections.

During the past three decades, several comprehensive reviews have dealt specifically with cestocidal drugs [104, 120, 170, 264, 361, 386, 476] including larvacides [41], of medical and veterinary significance; others have been concerned with cestocidal drugs amongst parasiticides [89, 118, 145, 197, 210, 428, 470]. In this review, covering the period from 1956, an era of remarkable progress in chemotherapy of the cestode zoonoses, emphasis has been placed on identifying the merits and shortcomings of the drugs studied. Where possible, the criterion upon which a drug has been assessed for efficacy is an estimate of the single dose required to free 90 % of the hosts from infection together with a 95 % confidence interval. Alternatively, the number of treatments required to achieve the ED_{90} and falling within the non-toxic dose range has been found. Where the original papers have not provided these estimates, but the data allow them to be made, the present authors have undertaken the necessary calculations.

In the preparation of this review, more than 2,000 publications dealing with cestocides were consulted. Limitations of space have restricted the number cited to some of those that have contributed to knowledge on dose rates, toxicity or drug-orientated control programmes. The chemical formulae have been adopted from either the Merck Index, 9th Edition, 1976 or Chemical Abstracts. The principal adult tapeworm infections covered include rodent hymenolepiasis, canine/feline taeniasis and dipylidiasis, canine echinococcosis, human hymenolepiasis, taeniasis and diphyllobothriasis. The larval infections studied include murine, ovine, porcine, bovine and human echinococcosis and cysticercosis. Following this introductory section, the drugs are described in the approximate order in which they were first reported as having cestocidal activity. In the third and fourth sections, progress in research on larvacides and ovicides is discussed. In the fifth section, brief consideration is given to the role of drugs in control programmes and in the final section, some future research goals are outlined.

2. Drugs for the Treatment of Adult Tapeworm Infections

2.1 Dichlorophen and Trichlorophen

Dichlorophen (Anthiphen, Dicestal, Didroxane, Diphenthane-70, Hyosan, Parabis, Plath-Lyse, Preventol G-D, Teniathane, Teniatol), 2,2′-dihydroxy-5,5′-dichlorophenylmethane
Trichlorophen (G-610), 2,6-bis(2′-oxy-5-chlorobenzyl-4-chlorophenol)

Dichlorophen was first introduced into veterinary medicine in 1946 [84, 114]. At that time it was regarded as an important advance in the treatment of taeniasis and dipylidiasis. The drug was introduced into human medicine 10 years later [327, 412]. This marked the beginning of a new era in the treatment of human tapeworm infections. In the words of one author [414]: 'The patient is told to swallow a dozen 0.5-gramme tablets with tea or water before breakfast, which is then taken in the usual way.'

2.1.1 Cestodes in Laboratory Rodents

Hymenolepiasis. Dichlorophen appears to be more active against older *H. nana* of about 14 days than younger organisms in mice [42], but a single dose at 2,000 mg/kg was reported to have low activity against *H. nana* in naturally infected rats [32]. A dose rate of 500 mg/kg was reported to be effective in light, but not heavy infections in mice [207]. At a dose rate of 400 mg/kg, only 1 of 7 mice was cleared of infection and the drug showed variable activity from 45 to 90% in worm removal in different experiments [70]. The LD_{50} for mice was estimated at 1,670 mg/kg [46]. Trichlorophen was reported to be slightly more active against *H. nana* and less toxic to mice than dichlorophen [57]. Insufficient data are available to determine the ED_{90} or the number of treatments required to achieve strong lethal effects of either compound.

2.1.2 Cestodes in Domestic Carnivores

Taeniasis and Dipylidiasis. During the decade following the introduction of dichlorophen 9 case history reports provided conflicting evidence on its efficacy [142, 169, 352]. A mixture of dichlorophen with toluene was studied for broad-spectrum activity [69], but no evidence could be found to indicate a synergistic effect against canine cestodiasis. The recommended dose rate for dichlorophen was of the order of 150–300 mg/kg. The drug appeared to be tolerated within this dose range. The lethal dose was of the order of 2,000–3,000 mg/kg. Symptoms at these dose levels included tremors, dullness, vomiting and diarrhoea.

An estimate of the single dose ED_{50} for dichlorophen against *T. hydatigena* in dogs was 101 (16–653) mg/kg [author's unpublished data]. Within this dose range strong destrobilating effects were observed. The ED_{90} was outside the dose rates tested.

Echinococcosis. No evidence could be found indicating that dichlorophen was active in eliminating *E. granulosus* or *E. multilocularis* [169, 310, 326, 357, 358, 381, 398]. Indeed, following two treatments at 280 mg/kg, *E. granulosus* was still present in all the treated dogs [169].

2.1.3 Cestodes in Man

Hymenolepiasis. Low efficacy was usually recorded for dichlorophen in the treatment of *H. nana* even after several treatments were administered [65, 247, 418]. For example, two 0.5-gramme tablets were given three times daily for 5 days to 20 students with *H. nana* infections and this regime was repeated on two further occasions within 35 days [247]. With 90 tablets per patient over 35 days, a cure rate of only 90% was achieved.

Taeniasis. More than 20 clinical trials were reported on the use of dichlorophen in the treatment of *T. saginata* and *T. solium* infections [11, 12, 64, 135, 221, 299, 327, 335, 408, 412–414, 418]. Assessing them as a group, the results were extremely variable with cure rates ranging from 30 to 90%. For example, in one study, all 8 cases of *T. saginata* treated at 75 mg/kg were still found to be parasitized 3 months after treatment [64]. It is possible with some of the more positive claims that destrobilating effects were interpreted as cures.

Although several authors [299, 418] regarded dichlorophen as the drug of choice for the treatment of *T. saginata* taeniasis, others considered that the older remedies such as extract of male fern, mepacrine [249, 335] and tin compounds [360] were more effective. Dichlorophen was extensively used in mass drug treatment programmes in the USSR, but it seems that an intolerance developed to the dose rate used (600–900 mg) and the drug was relegated to a secondary role or combined with other compounds [282]. Nausea, intestinal colic, vomiting and diarrhoea were fairly common sequelae.

Diphyllobothriasis. Too few studies were undertaken with dichlorophen in the treatment of diphyllobothriasis to determine efficacy [218, 355, 469], but it seems that the cure rate was no greater than against taeniasis.

2.2 Bithionol and Bithionol Sulphoxide

Bithionol (Actamer, Bithin, Bitin, Lorothidol), 2,2′-thiobis(4,6-dichlorophenol)
Bithionol sulphoxide (Bitin-S, Disto-5), 2,2′-sulphinyl-bis(4,6-dichlorophenol)

Bithionol was first synthesized in Japan in 1955. This compound and bithionol sulphoxide have been studied more for their activity against trematodes than cestodes. Nevertheless, bithionol has been used successfully in the treatment of human tapeworm infections.

2.2.1 Cestodes in Laboratory Rodents

Hymenolepiasis. Bithionol and/or bithionol sulphoxide have been reported as being active against *H. nana* infections in mice [9, 264, 281, 349, 428]. The LD_{50} for mice was estimated to be 1,080–1,920 mg/kg, and the single dose ED_{50} was estimated to be 78–90 mg/kg for 20-day-old infections [281]. Single doses of 500 mg/kg and 200 mg/kg, but not 100 mg/kg, cleared *H. nana* from mice. Data for an estimate of the ED_{90} for both single and multiple doses are not available for any parasite age-group.

2.2.2 Cestodes in Domestic Carnivores

Taeniasis and Dipylidiasis. Assessments against *T. pisiformis, T. hydatigena* and *D. caninum* in dogs indicate that these drugs have a strong and consistent activity [143, 181, 223]. An estimate of the ED_{90} for a single treatment against *T. hydatigena* infections was 36 (24–55) mg/kg [181].

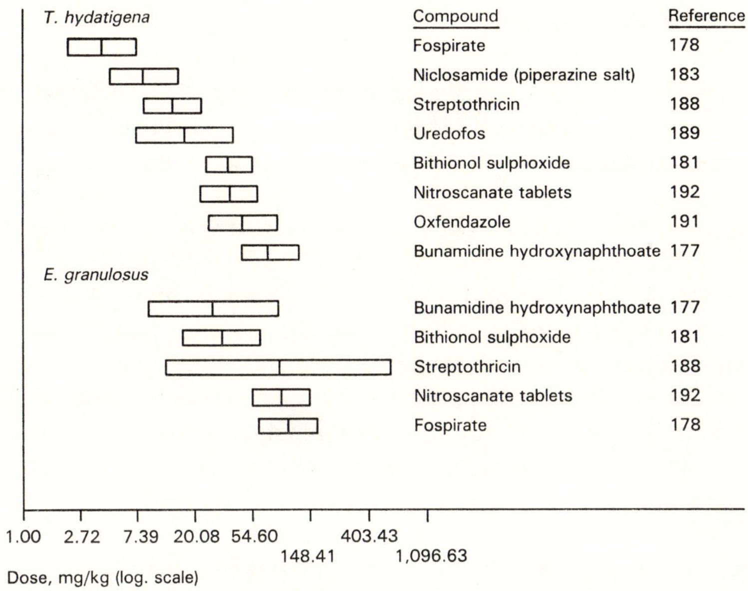

Fig. 2. The single oral dose ED_{90} and ED_{50}, with their 95% confidence intervals, for the treatment by specified compounds of *T. hydatigena* and *E. granulosus* infections, respectively, in dogs.

Vomiting and/or diarrhoea were relatively common sequelae, but deaths were not recorded within this dose range.

Canine Echinococcosis. Several studies have been recorded on the lethal effects of bithionol and/or bithionol sulphoxide against *Echinococcus* spp infections in dogs [181, 310, 381, 398, 487]. The results were relatively consistent. For example, a single dose of 300 mg/kg reduced *E. granulosus* infections by 99% [487].

Although three doses of bithionol at 200 mg/kg were not completely successful against *E. multilocularis,* three doses of bithionol sulphoxide were effective [398]. An estimate of the single dose ED_{90} against *E. granulosus* was 152 (71–325) mg/kg [181]. At this dose level deaths were reported [181, 398]. Estimates of the number of treatments required to reach the ED_{90} at safe dose levels cannot be made from the literature cited. The comparative efficacy, based on the single dose ED_{90} and ED_{50} for *T. hydatigena* and *E. granulosus,* respectively, of bithionol sulphoxide with other cestocidal compounds is illustrated in figure 2.

2.2.3 Cestodes in Man

Hymenolepiasis. Too few studies have been reported on the efficacy of bithionol against *H. nana* [134] for estimates to be made of the number of treatments required to reach the ED_{90} at safe dose levels.

Taeniasis. Bithionol has been used successfully in the treatment of *T. saginata* taeniasis [9, 22, 94, 95, 134, 135, 163, 341, 456]. The usual dose rate was of the order of 40–60 mg/kg with a maximum of 4,000 mg. Taking these case history studies as a group, the cure rate for a single treatment was consistent and of the order of 80–90 %. Fasting prior to treatment was regarded as important, but the need was not proven. Mild side effects such as nausea, anorexia, abdominal discomfort and diarrhoea were fairly common sequelae. The safety of the drug has been queried [361].

Diphyllobothriasis. The limited trials undertaken with bithionol against *D. latum* infections [298, 341, 390], suggest that it may be as efficacious as it is against *T. saginata.* For example, all 8 cases of *D. latum* and all 8 cases of *T. saginata* were cured with a single treatment at 50–66 mg/kg [341]. Again no estimates of the single dose ED_{90} can be made from the literature cited.

2.3 Niclosamide

Niclosamide (Bayer 2353, Cestocid, Devermin, Lintex, Mansonil, Nasemo, Phenasal, Radeverm, Sagimid, Sulqui, Tredermine, Vermitin, Yomesan, Zemun)
2′,5-dichloro-4′-nitrosalicylanilide
N-(2′-chlor-4′-nitrophenyl)-amine-5-chlorosalicylic acid (Phenasal USSR)

Niclosamide was introduced into human and veterinary medicine for the treatment of tapeworm infections in 1960 following studies on this compound against *H. diminuta* [203, 232, 431]. Further studies on its mode of action on tapeworms and absorption by the host were made during the next 10 years [105, 200, 204, 432].

2.3.1 Cestodes in Laboratory Rodents

Hymenolepiasis. Niclosamide was found to be least effective against cysticercoids and most effective against mature *H. nana* [42, 47]. The minimum effective single dose against 10-day-old and 16-day-old infections was estimated to be 2,000 and 1,000 mg/kg, respectively. However, restrobilation frequently occurred at 1,000 mg/kg [244]. Several factors were reported to influence efficacy [70, 207, 286, 485]. For example, possibly associated with a circadian rhythm, niclosamide was reported to be more effective when given in the evening than in the morning [286]. It was found that continuous therapy for 1 week followed by a further 7-day treatment schedule was sufficient to eliminate *H. nana* from rats [242] and a 7-day course removed *H. nana* from hamsters [389]. The single dose ED_{50} for niclosamide against 10-day-old and 16-day-old infections in mice was estimated to be 360–540 mg/kg and 150–290 mg/kg, respectively [284]. Estimates of the single or multiple treatments required to reach the ED_{90} cannot be determined from the literature reviewed.

Daily therapy for 1 week followed by a further 7-day treatment schedule eliminated *H. diminuta* from rats [242]. An estimate or a single dose ED_{90} of niclosamide against this species was 83 (53–130) mg/kg [203].

2.3.2 Cestodes in Domestic Carnivores

Taeniasis, Dipylidiasis. More than 30 studies have been reported on the efficacy of niclosamide in the treatment of *T. hydatigena, T. pisiformis, Taenia multiceps* and *D. caninum* in dogs and *T. taeniaeformis* in cats [31, 103, 112, 122, 158, 183, 208, 222, 343, 354, 371, 385, 424, 437, 474]. Most writers agreed that the drug is safe and without serious side effects. Transient vomiting and/or diarrhoea were recorded as relatively common sequelae at and above 32 mg/kg. Death was reported in 4 dogs shortly after treatment [246], but the association with the drug was not clearly established. The dose rates tested in these studies varied from 2–500 mg/kg. In only one of them sufficient data were reported to estimate the single dose ED_{90}. This was 8 (5–15) mg/kg against *T. hydatigena* in dogs [183]. The efficacy of niclosamide compared to other drugs in the treatment of *T. hydatigena* infections is illustrated in figure 2.

The efficacy of niclosamide against *D. caninum* infections is variable. In several trials the drug was found to be almost ineffictive [371, 385, 424]. It is possible that the drug is less effective against this species than against *Taenia* spp. However, in the absence of controlled trials, this remains unproven. Variable effects against *Mesocestoides* spp were also reported [453].

Echinococcosis. The erratic effect of niclosamide against canine echinococcosis has been well documented. Some of the 30 reports examined suggested that the compound was effective and recommended it for control purposes. Others, however, concluded that the drug was ineffective. The possibility exists that the age of the organisms at the time of treatment may modify efficacy and this may account for the conflicting results. This, however, has not been proven experimentally. Most reports examined included too few dogs and dose rates for the single dose ED_{50} to be estimated [31, 96, 110, 122, 123, 126, 158, 183, 222, 261, 277, 296, 310, 326, 357, 358, 380, 381, 398] For 28-day-old *E. granulosus,* the single dose ED_{50} does not lie within the dose range 75–1,200 mg/kg [198]. Certainly, the erratic nature of the drug does not warrant any positive recommendation for use in control programmes.

2.3.3 Cestodes in Man

Hymenolepiasis. More than 70 case history studies were reported on the efficacy of niclosamide against *H. nana* infections [7, 26, 28, 39, 43, 45, 48–50, 61–63, 66, 67, 166, 244, 245, 259, 260, 267, 282, 306, 308, 309, 336, 342, 366, 402, 421]. Most writers agree that one or more 5- to 7-day courses of treatment are required to achieve high cure rates. Most observed few side effects and no known contraindications to its use have been determined. A death was recorded on the 16th day of niclosamide (Phenasal) treatment, but this was attributed to anaphylaxis from the tapeworm infection [27].

Only four reports were cited where specific dose rates were recorded. Here it was found that a single treatment of 40–60 mg/kg failed to cure most patients of hymenolepiasis [342]. However, a single dose rate at 100–130 mg/kg for children and 70 mg/kg for adults cured all of 25 patients [7]. This result was considered to be due to the high dose rate used. In contrast, only 2 of 10 children were successfully treated with a dose rate of 100 mg/kg [336]. In the same study, it was found that 40–50 mg/kg for 5 days cured only 8 of 10 children and that 60–80 mg/kg for 5 days cured only 47 of 52 patients. That relatively long treatment schedules are required is also indicated in a study where a dose of 60 mg/kg was administered initially and followed by 15 mg/kg each day for one week. Only 60 of 68 patients were cured [267]. While a cure rate of 70–80% with one or more treatment schedules was demonstrated in a number of studies, the ED_{90} for single or multiple doses could not be determined from the literature examined.

Studies on the treatment of *H. diminuta* infections with niclosamide are equivocal, but they do suggest that a series of treatments may be required against this organism in man [195, 248]. In one study it was found that only 17 of 19 patients were cured with a 5- to 7-day course of niclosamide, but a further course was effective.

Taeniasis. Following the introduction of niclosamide for the treatment of tapeworm infections in man, more than 120 case history studies on *T. saginata* and *T. solium* infections were reported [1–3, 5, 6, 11, 13, 55, 56, 67, 109, 129, 133, 148, 149, 154, 155, 166, 196, 250, 252, 258, 267, 273–275, 282, 311, 325, 339, 360, 366, 409, 414, 415, 419–423, 454]. This is an indication that niclosamide has been considered to be the drug of choice for the treatment of human tapeworm infections during the past 20 years. Almost all writers confirmed that there were no important side effects and no contraindications to the use of niclosamide in the treatment of human taeniasis. The generally adopted dose was of the order of 2,000 mg for adults and about half this amount for children. Only one report was cited where a specific dose rate was administered [267]. This was 60 mg/kg in a divided dose treatment schedule over 1 h and only 11 of the 13 patients were cured. Although it was considered that well-checked clinical investigations indicated a cure rate of 90%, the single treatment cure rate usually varied between 50 and 100%, but in one study only a 7% cure rate was achieved [258]. Evidence was reported that some batches of Phenasal and Vermitin were less effective than expected [58, 258, 360], possibly due to particle size effects [282]. Some other factors were considered important in drug failures [250], but these were not confirmed by experimentation. Despite the voluminous literature, the ED_{90} for niclosamide could not be defined for the treatment of human taeniasis.

Diphyllobothriasis. Case history studies on niclosamide in the treatment of *D. latum* infections also showed variation in cure rates [4, 67, 131–133, 196, 251, 366, 390]. For example, single treatment at 2,000 mg gave a cure rate of 77% and a second treatment of 1,000 mg only increased this rate to 85% [4]. A slightly higher cure rate was achieved by chewing rather than swallowing the tablets, but fasting did not increase efficacy [251]. While the ED_{90} could not be determined from the literature cited, it seems likely that niclosamide has similar advantages and shortcomings in the treatment of diphyllobothriasis as in taeniasis.

Other Cestodiasis. Other reports included studies on the efficacy of niclosamide in the treatment of *D. caninum* infections [60, 248], *Inermicapsifer madagascariensis* [202], *Mesocestoides* [201] and *Bertiella studieri* infections [450]. Most infections with these rarely recorded parasites appear to have been removed successfully by a single treatment.

2.4 Niclosamide and Combinations

2.4.1 Cestodes in Laboratory Rodents

Hymenolepiasis. The introduction of dichlorophen, bithionol and niclosamide permitted out-patient treatment. None of them were always effective at the recommended dose rate, particularly not against *H. nana* infections. This prompted a series of studies, mainly in the USSR, on combining them; early emphasis was placed on evaluations of their efficacy against *H. nana* in mice. The question has frequently been raised as to whether a failure was due to an inadequate dose rate or to reinfection [26, 28, 43, 63, 244, 443]. Reference should be made to the biology of *H. nana* in its normal hosts with regard to modes of infections, strain differences, worm burden variations, immunity, circadian rhythm, autoinfection and sites of predilection [25–28, 234, 286, 307, 309, 443, 472]. These factors present problems in the interpretation of results in both rodent and human *H. nana* infections.

Niclosamide and Dichlorophen (Dichlosal). As previously stated, the efficacy of niclosamide and dichlorophen appears to be associated inter alia with the age of the organisms. The ED_{50} for niclosamide against 20- to 22-day-old infections was estimated to be 420 mg/kg and that of dichlorophen to be 110 mg/kg. When these were mixed in the ratio of 4:1, the ED_{50} for each was reduced to 63 and 16 mg/kg, respectively [42, 47]. It was also observed that a divided dose schedule over 4 days gave high cure rates with 9-day-old *H. nana* infections [216].

Niclosamide and Bithionol. Niclosamide was also studied in combination with bithionol [199, 281, 349]. Here, it was observed that with 20-day-old *H. nana* that the ED_{50} for niclosamide was 200–440 mg/kg and for bithionol was 78–90 mg/kg. When combined, the ED_{50} was reduced to 44 and 21 mg/kg, respectively [281].

Niclosamide and Other Combinations. The therapeutic index (LD_{50}/ED_{50}) was estimated for a number of drugs combined with niclosamide [44, 279, 280, 283, 285, 348, 349]. These included acrichin, aminoacrichin, extract of male fern, kamala and trichlorophen. Synergistic effects without an increase in toxicity were reported for some of these combinations.

2.4.2 Cestodes in Man

Niclosamide and Dichlorophen (Dichlosal) and Trichlorophen (Trichlosal). At the same time as the drug combinations were being studied for activity against *H. nana* in mice, they were also being evaluated in the treatment of human tapeworm infections. Dichlosal was usually used at dose rates of 1,000–2,000 mg niclosamide with 500–1,000 mg dichlorophen given together or separately. More than 35 studies were reported on *H. nana* [211, 214, 215, 282]; on *T. saginata* [2, 121, 130, 160–162, 211, 213, 257, 258, 275, 282, 283, 313, 334, 368, 433] and on *D. latum* infections [72, 218, 219, 268, 276, 282, 378]. Similar studies were undertaken with Trichlosal against *H. nana* [214], against *T. saginata* [283, 323, 340] and against *D. latum* [276, 283, 378, 390]. Several authors considered that the combination of niclosamide and dichlorophen was contraindicated in patients with liver and kidney disorders. At least one study reported severe side effects including nausea and dizziness [130].

Niclosamide and Bithionol. This combination was reported to be active against both *T. saginata* taeniasis [9] and *D. latum* infections [298, 390]. No toxic sequelae were reported.

Other Combinations. Other combinations with reported activity against *H. nana, T. saginata* and *D. latum* infections included niclosamide with acrichin and aminoacrichin [2, 131, 132, 162, 212, 213, 257, 258, 334, 433], with extract of male fern [212, 213], with kamala [132] and paromomycin [369]. Some of these combinations cause severe side effects such as headache, epigastric pain and vomiting. There is very little evidence that any of these mixtures show important synergistic effects or that they were more effective than niclosamide on its own. In no case was it possible to define the single dose ED_{90}.

2.5 Antibiotics

One of the more important antibiotics showing cestocidal activity is paromomycin (Humatin, Monomycin A, Pargonyl) from *Streptomyces rimosus* var *paromomycinus*. It was first suggested that this antibiotic might be used in the treatment of human taeniasis following the observation that patients treated for intestinal amoebiasis also eliminated tapeworms [167, 403]. Since that time, several antibiotics, particularly the streptothricins, have been examined for cestocidal activity and it has been suggested that they may interfere with protein synthesis in cestode metabolism [85].

2.5.1 Cestodes in Laboratory Rodents

Hymenolepiasis. Several antibiotics including paromomycin, axenomycin from *S. lisandri,* thaimycin from *S. michiganensis* var *amylolyticus* and kanamycin from *S. kanamyceticus* have been shown to have some activity against *H. nana* in mice or *H. diminuta* in rats [53, 54, 102, 106, 124, 125, 466]. Of the antibiotics studied, paromomycin was one of the least active against rodent hymenolepiasis [106, 466]. However, all three fractions of thaimycin were particularly active at 5 mg/kg daily for 5 days and removed all *H. nana* from 10 mice [102]. The ED_{50} for a single treatment of thaimycin A was estimated at 19 (11–32) mg/kg and for 3 treatments the ED_{90} was 40 (18–90) mg/kg. The LD_{50} for mice for fractions A, B, C was of the order of 100, 250 and 1,000 mg/kg, respectively.

Fraction A of axenomycin was virtually inactive against 12-day-old *H. nana* infections. However, the single dose ED_{50} for fractions B and D were estimated at 14 (12–16) mg/kg and 10 (7–13) mg/kg, respectively [124]. Axenomycin was virtually inactive when administered at the same time as the eggs. The oral LD_{50} was estimated to be 100 mg/kg, but when given by the subcutaneous route was 1 mg/kg [124]. Fractions A and B, but not C and D of the antibiotic complex SQ21,704 from *S. griseocarneus* strain S15-1, identified as having antiviral activity, also proved active against *H. nana,* but the ED_{50} could not be determined from the data presented [85].

2.5.2 Cestodes in Domestic Carnivores

Taeniasis and Dipylidiasis. Paromomycin showed some activity against *T. taeniaeformis* in cats, but a dose rate of 200 mg/kg for 5 days eliminated the worms from only 3 of 4 animals [466]. On the other hand, a single treatment of axenomycin at 5 mg/kg was strongly active against *D. caninum, T. pisiformis* and *Diphyllobothrium* spp in dogs [124]. There were insufficient data to determine the ED_{90}. The antibiotic complex SQ21,704 also showed strong activity against canine taeniasis and dipylidiasis [85, 116]. Estimates of the ED_{90} for *T. pisiformis* and *T. hydatigena* were similar at 16 (11–22) mg/kg and 14 (9–24) mg/kg, respectively [188, 434]. A higher dose rate was required for the treatment of *D. caninum* and the ED_{90} was estimated to be 52 (20–136) mg/kg [434]. Vomiting and diarrhoea were reported at low dose rates in one [188], but not the other study [434].

Echinococcosis. The streptothricin complex SQ21,704 is the only antibiotic tested for activity against *Echinococcus* spp and it is marginally active, with an estimated ED_{50} for a single treatment of 84 (12–570) mg/kg [188]. The efficacy of this streptothricin complex compared to other cestocides against *T. hydatigena* and *E. granulosus* is illlustrated in figure 2.

2.5.3 Cestodes in Man

Hymenolepiasis. In contrast to rodent hymenolepiasis, high human cure rates were reported for paromomycin with a 5-day treatment schedule [78, 369, 404, 459, 484]. For example, a 100% cure rate was reported with a single 5-day treatment schedule at 45 mg/kg [484]. Untoward sequelae with this schedule included abdominal pain, nausea, diarrhoea, vomiting and dizziness.

Taeniasis. Almost invariably high cure rates were recorded in clinical studies on the treatment of *T. saginata* and *T. solium* with paromomycin [78, 105, 167, 168, 356, 403, 404, 427, 458, 459, 484]. Neomycin and kanamycin, but not streptomycin also showed activity against *T. saginata* infections [168].

A 100% cure rate was reported for paromomycin against *T. saginata* when it was administered at a dose of 50 mg/kg on 5 consecutive days [404]. However, a single dose of 30 mg/kg or less was not always successful [404], but a 100% cure rate was achieved in a small number of cases with a single dose at 75 mg/kg [78, 484]. The drug was well tolerated even by the young children when administered for a period of 3–5 days in daily doses of 15–45 mg/kg [458]. Case history studies do not suggest that side effects such as diarrhoea and less frequently nausea and vomiting prevented patients from continuing treatment [404, 484]. Some authors considered paromomycin to be an alternative to niclosamide for the treatment of taeniasis [361].

Diphyllobothriasis. Paromomycin has also been used successfully in the treatment of *D. latum* infections [243, 256, 484]. Too few studies have been reported to estimate the effective single dose cure rate, but efficacy appears to be similar to that for taeniasis.

2.6 Bunamidine Hydrochloride (Scolaban)

N,N-dibutyl-4-(hexyloxy)-1-naphthalenecarboximidamide hydrochloride

In 1965 naphthamidines were reported to have cestocidal activity [34]. The introduction of two of the series represented an important advance in the treatment of canine tapeworm infections, because they provided the first commercial compounds other than the arecoline salts, for the treatment of *Echinococcus* spp. Both of them were unsuitable for use against human tapeworm infections.

2.6.1 Cestodes in Laboratory Rodents

Hymenolepiasis. A comprehensive research programme evaluating 45 naphthamidines against *H. nana* in mice was undertaken [226]. Structure-activity relationships were sometimes quite different between the various tapeworm species and bunamidine was selected as having the widest range of activity. The LD_{50} for bunamidine in mice was estimated to be 540 mg/kg and the drug was effective against mature *H. nana* at 200 mg/kg [89, 226, 264, 265].

2.6.2 Cestodes in Carnivores

Taeniasis and Dipylidiasis. Bunamidine hydrochloride was studied for activity against *T. hydatigena, T. pisiformis, T. taeniaeformis, D. caninum, Diphyllobothrium* spp and *Mesocestoides* spp in dogs and cats appropriately [90, 91, 173, 227, 228, 241, 265, 271, 302, 385, 453]. The drug almost invariably demonstrated strong activity at 25–50 mg/kg against all the above, but could not always be relied upon to eliminate all worms in all animals. Indeed, in one study, two treatments at 25 mg/kg failed to remove all *T. hydatigena* from dogs [173]. Some strains of *Taenia* were regarded as being less sensitive to bunamidine than others [91]. Despite these extensive studies, the single dose ED_{90} could only be estimated for *T. pisiformis* and this was 21 (14–32) mg/kg [228]. Vomiting and diarrhoea were fairly common sequelae following doses of 25 mg/kg.

Echinococcosis. Bunamidine hydrochloride was studied for activity against *E. granulosus* [16, 30, 35, 71, 76, 126, 170, 176, 261, 277, 379, 455, 479, 490] and *E. multilocularis* in dogs [398]. The drug is regarded as having an ovicidal effect against free eggs of *E. granulosus* [480], but not those contained in proglottids [440]. It was also not ovicidal against the eggs of *E. multilocularis* [398].

Most studies involved very few animals and/or dose rates. Taking them as a group, the evidence suggests that at 25–50 mg/kg the drug can usually be expected to reduce worm burdens by about 90%. The drug, however, is somewhat erratic in its action. This may be associated with a number of factors including the age of the worms at the time of treatment [16, 35, 176]. The ED_{50} for two treatments against 28-day-old *E. granulosus* was estimated to be 55 (27–113) mg/kg [176].

As with bithionol, bunamidine hydrochloride is toxic to dogs. Deaths were recorded in laboratory studies at 200 mg/kg [176]. However, field studies showed that deaths (about 1/3,000 treatments) occurred at and above 25 mg/kg under circumstances where substantial amounts of catecholamines are liberated into the blood – as in excitement [68, 150–153, 330, 465]. Deaths were also reported in veterinary practice [481].

2.7 Bunamidine Hydroxynaphthoate (Buban)

N,N-dibutyl-4-(hexyloxy)-1-Naphthalenecarboximidamide 3-hydroxy-2-naphthoate

2.7.1 Cestodes in Domestic Carnivores

Taeniasis and Dipylidiasis. Bunamidine hydroxynaphthoate was relatively extensively studied for activity against *T. pisiformis, T. hydatigena, T. multiceps* and *D. caninum* in dogs [177, 180, 225, 228, 344, 488, 489]. Reviewing these studies as a group, it seems that, as with the hydrochloride, the hydroxynaphthoate at 50 mg/kg is strongly active against *Taenia* spp, but not sufficiently active to remove all worms with a single treatment.

An estimate for the single dose ED_{90} against *T. hydatigena* was 53 (41–67) mg/kg. For two and three treatment schedules the estimates for the ED_{90} were 45 (34–61) mg/kg and 31 (21–44) mg/kg, respectively [177, 180]. The numbers of treatments required to reach the upper limit of the 95% confidence interval of the ED_{90} at 32, 48 and 64 mg/kg were 5, 2 and 2, respectively. Insufficient data are available to define efficacy against *D. caninum.*

Echinococcosis. Following a report in 1967 that bunamidine hydroxynaphthoate was more active when given in food than when dogs were starved [228], several studies were undertaken to develop a medicated food for the treatment of canine echinococcosis and taeniasis [177, 180, 225, 261, 262, 344, 379, 380, 488, 489]. An estimate of the single dose ED_{50} against *E. granulosus* infections was 27 (9–83) mg/kg. The number of treatments required to reach the upper limit of the 95% confidence interval of the ED_{90} at 32, 48 and 64 mg/kg were 4, 3 and 3 respectively [177, 425]. Vomiting and/or diarrhoea were common sequelae at and above 32 mg/kg. Deaths, however, were not recorded even at 100 mg/kg. Bunamidine hydroxynaphthoate has a bitter taste and it seems that the concentration in food and the type of food influences the rate of refusal and some dogs, even when hungry, soon learn to recognise the taste. An effective long-term treatment schedule was not determined [177, 180]. The efficacy of bunamidine hydroxynaphthoate in the treatment of *T. hydatigena* and *E. granulosus* is compared with other drugs in figure 2.

2.8 Bunamidine *p*-Toluene Sulphonate

N,N-dibutyl-4-(hexyloxy)-1-naphthalenecarboximidamide p-toluene sulphonate

This compound was studied for activity against *T. pisiformis* [228]. It was regarded as being as effective as bunamidine hydrochloride, but was strongly emetic in action.

2.9 Nitroscanate (Lopatol, Echinon)

1-isothiocyanato-4-(4-nitrophenoxy)benzene

Various formulations of nitroscanate were first shown in 1973 to have a wide spectrum of activity against nematode and cestode infections of dogs [75]. The use of this compound was limited to carnivores.

2.9.1 Cestodes in Domestic Carnivores

Taeniasis and Dipylidiasis. Since 1973, the drug has been extensively evaluated for activity against *T. hydatigena, T. ovis, T. pisiformis* and *D. caninum* infections [74–76, 179, 184, 192]. When administered as a powder (particle size 2–3 μm), the drug is strongly active against *T. hydatigena.* An estimate of the ED_{90} was 8 (6–12) mg/kg [184]. However, when the drug (particle size 2–3 μm) was incorporated into a tablet, the ED_{90} approximated that for the powder of particle size 10–20 μm, with an ED_{90} for the tablet of 37 (23–60) mg/kg. A dose rate of 50 mg/kg given with food has been recommended for the treatment of common dog tapeworm such as *Taenia* spp and *D. caninum* [74, 76].

Diarrhoea and/or vomiting and temporary tranquilizing effects were observed in a few dogs at and above 62 mg/kg [179, 184, 192]. However, a group of dogs was treated with nitroscanate at 1,000 mg/kg every 2 weeks for 1 year without clinical signs of toxicity [74, 76].

It was also pointed out that the additional value of regular treatments with nitroscanate included the control of *Ancylostoma caninum, Uncinaria stenocephala, Toxocara canis* and congenital toxacarosis [74, 76].

Echinococcosis. Nitroscanate was also extensively studied for activity against *E. granulosus* in dogs [35, 74–76, 179, 184, 192, 261, 262, 377, 379, 406]. Differences in efficacy were observed between micronized and non-micronized powder. While the former was strongly active at 65 mg/kg, the latter and the commercial tablet had single dose ED_{50} estimates of 115 (66–200) mg/kg and 89 (56–142) mg/kg, respectively. The number of treatments required to reach the upper limit of the 95 % confidence interval of the ED_{90} for the micronized powder at 32 mg/kg was 5 doses [184]; whereas for the non-micronized powder given at four or eight times that dose rate these estimates were 4 and 3, respectively [179]. Agglomeration of particles during the manufacture of the tablets was regarded as a possible explanation for the reduced efficacy [192]. The efficacy of the tablets in the treatment of *T. hydatigena* and *E. granulosus* infections is compared with other drugs in figure 2.

2.10 Mebendazole (Telmin, Vermox) and Other Benzimidazoles

Methyl 5-benzoyl-2-benzimidazole carbamate

The benzimidazoles have a broad spectrum of activity, and within this group, the greatest interest has been shown in the cestocidal activity of mebendazole.

2.10.1 Cestodes in Laboratory Rodents

Hymenolepiasis. Some of the benzimidazoles have shown activity against *H. nana* in mice. These include thiabendazole [435, 436], oxfendazole [29], parbendazole [295] and mebendazole [107, 290]. Several treatments are required to achieve strong activity, but the number reported to reach the ED_{90} could not be estimated from the literature cited.

2.10.2 Cestodes in Domestic Carnivores

Taeniasis and Dipylidiasis. A study of the activity of fenbendazole, parbendazole, oxibendazole, cambendazole and thiabendazole against *T. hydatigena* indicated that the first three-named were more active than the last two-named compounds, but several treatments are required to achieve strong activity [185]. Oxfendazole appeared to be more effective and the single dose ED_{90} for this compound against *T. hydatigena* was estimated to be 47 (25–84) mg/kg [191]. Oxfendazole also showed weak activity against *E. granulosus* infections [191].

Activity for mebendazole against *T. pisiformis, T. hydatigena* and *D. caninum* was first recorded in 1973 [462]. In that study, using micronized mebendazole in tablet formulation at 100 mg/kg twice daily for 5 days, 8 of 10, 7 of 9 and 3 of 8 dogs were cleared of infection, respectively. Subsequent studies confirmed that several treatments were required to eliminate these tapeworms [198, 220].

In a series of studies with *T. hydatigena* [182, 185, 197], it was determined that the single dose ED_{90} for micronized mebendazole powder (particle size 86% $<20\ \mu m$ and 55% $<10\ \mu m$) was 8 (3–18) mg/kg. It was also strongly active when given in a prepared medicated food. However, with the non-micronized powder (particle size 40% $<21\ \mu m$ and 18% $<10\ \mu m$) only the single dose ED_{50} could be determined within the dose range tested and this estimate was 40 (13–126) mg/kg. As with nitroscanate, it was suggested that cestocidal efficacy may be a function of particle size.

Echinococcosis. When mebendazole tablets were administered to dogs at 40 mg/kg for 5 consecutive days, only half the population of *E. granu-*

losus was removed [209]. In a series of studies it was found that the single dose ED_{90} for micronized powder was 56 (14–218) mg/kg. When, however, the tablet with micronized mebendazole was used, there was a loss of activity and the ED_{50} could not be determined within the dose range tested [182, 185, 187]. Again it was suggested that the loss of activity might be associated with the agglomeration of particles during the manufacture of the tablets.

2.10.3 Cestodes in Man

Mebendazole has been shown to have a wide margin of safety in animals [324]. The oral LD_{50} exceeds 1,280 mg/kg in mice and 640 mg/kg in dogs and cats. It has been widely used in the treatment of nematode infections in man [86]. Studies with ^{14}C-labelled mebendazole in human volunteers have shown that the drug is poorly absorbed and is excreted in the urine within 24–48 h [86]. Its possible modes of action and effects on ultrastructure have been described [461, 463]. The drug is well tolerated and there are virtually no side effects.

Hymenolepiasis. Mebendazole administered twice daily at 100 mg/kg for 3 days was not particularly effective in the treatment of *H. nana* infections [331]. Too few studies have been cited to determine treatment schedules against *H. nana* in man.

Taeniasis. Successful treatment of *T. saginata* and *T. solium* taeniasis with mebendazole at 200 mg twice daily for 4 days has been reported [263]. Another study reported that 300 mg twice daily for 3 days was effective in most cases [365]. A 95% cure rate was achieved with 41 patients with *T. saginata* when they were dosed with 300 mg twice daily for 3 days [23]. However, in another trial, a treatment schedule of 300 mg twice daily for 4 days completely failed to cure *T. saginata* or *T. solium* taeniasis [460]. The drug was given in tablet form and information on the nominal particle size was not recorded.

2.11 Fospirate (Dowco 217)

0,0-demthyl-0-3,5,6-trichloro-2-pyridyl phosphate

Fospirate was originally investigated as an insecticide for flea control. The compound was shown to be active against nematodes. Activity against cestodes was demonstrated in 1975. The LD_{50} for rats and mice was estimated at 869 and 668 mg/kg, respectively. Due to emesis, it was not possible to establish the LD_{50} for dogs.

2.11.1 Cestodes in Domestic Carnivores

Taeniasis. An estimate of the single dose ED_{90} for fospirate was 4 (2–7) mg/kg against *T. hydatigena* [178]. Vomiting and diarrhoea were fairly common sequelae at 20 and 40 mg/kg, respectively.

Echinococcosis. Two studies were undertaken to determine the efficacy of fospirate against *E. granulosus* in dogs [178, 405]. The single dose ED_{50} was estimated to be 101 (61–168) mg/kg. The number of treatments required to reach the upper limit of the 95% confidence interval of the ED_{90} at 40 mg/kg was estimated to be 4. The efficacy of fospirate against *T. hydatigena* and *E. granulosus* is compared with other drugs in figure 2.

2.12 Uredofos (Diuredosan, RH 565, Sansalid

Diethyl-[thio-0-[3-(*p*-tolylsulphonyl)ureido]-phenyl]-carbamoyl phosphoramidate

Between 1975 and 1978, several reports indicated that uredofos showed a wide range of activity against nematodes and cestodes [385–387, 426, 453]. The oral LD_{50} for rats and dogs was estimated to be 102 and 1,000–1,500 mg/kg, respectively. Clinical signs of toxicity at high dose levels included diarrhoea, vomiting, muscular tremors and impaired motor reflexes.

2.12.1 Cestodes in Laboratory Rodents

Hymenolepiasis. The drug was reported to be highly active against *H. nana* in mice a 12 mg/kg [426, 438]. No evidence has been cited in the literature indicating that it was effective against cysticercoids or immature organisms.

2.12.2 Cestodes in Domestic Carnivores

Taeniasis and Dipylidiasis. Uredofos was considered to be strongly active in the treatment of *Taenia* spp and *D. caninum* and *Mesocestoides*

corti infections when it was given at 50 mg/kg [385–387, 426, 453]. An estimate of the single dose ED_{90} against *T. hydatigena* was 17 (7–40) mg/kg [189]. In that study it was estimated that about 6 and 2% of dogs may still harbour tapeworms following a single treatment at 25 and 50 mg/kg, respectively. The efficacy of uredofos in the treatment of *T. hydatigena* infections is compared with other drugs in figure 2. Vomiting and diarrhoea were common sequelae at 50 and 25 mg/kg, respectively [189]. Toxic side effects have been reported at therapeutic dose rates [76].

Echinococcosis. In 1975, it was considered that three treatments of uredofos at 25 mg/kg were sufficient for the treatment of *E. granulosus* infections [426]. In a subsequent study, however, the single dose ED_{50} could not be determined within the dose range 12.5–100 mg/kg [189]. Estimates of the number of treatments required to reach the upper limit of the 95% confidence interval of the ED_{90} at 50 and 100 mg/kg were 5 and 4, respectively [189].

2.13 Praziquantel (EMD 29810, Embay 8440, Droncit)

2-(cyclohexylcarbonyl)-4-oxo-1,2,3,6,7,11b-hexahydro-4H-pyrazino[2,1-a]-isoquinoline

The strong cestocidal activity of praziquantel was first reported in 1975 [444]. Extensive studies have been made on the pharmacokinetic and other properties of the compound in vitro and in vivo [20, 128, 303, 417, 429, 430]. Investigations of acute, subacute and subchronic toxicity, including teratogenicity, embryotoxicity, peri- and post-natal toxicity and mutogenicity have shown that the drug has no known serious side effects [40, 320, 337, 350]. Clinical pharmacological trials with volunteers suggest that there may be no contraindications to the use of praziquantel in healthy persons [304]. Side effects are usually gastro-intestinal in nature and are not infrequent at high dose rates (50 mg/kg) in the treatment of schistosomiasis [119]. These types of side effects were observed in 17 of 392 patients over a period of 24 h following treatment for cestodiasis [217]. Patient tolerance was regarded as good.

2.13.1 Cestodes in Laboratory Rodents

Hymenolepiasis. Extensive studies have been reported on the activity of praziquantel against *H. diminuta, H. nana* and *H. microstoma* in rats and mice appropriately [446, 447, 452]. Estimates of the oral single dose ED_{90} for adult and juvenile (2- to 10-day-old) *H. diminuta* were 2.7 (2.2–3.4) mg/kg and 6.3 (2.9–13.7) mg/kg, respectively. In contrast, the ED_{90} for a single oral treatment against 7- to 10-day-old *H. nana* infections was 19.8 (15.1–26.1) mg/kg. When the drug was administered by the subcutaneous route, the ED_{90} against *H. diminuta* and *H. nana* infections were 3.9 (2.3–6.7) mg/kg and 6.5 (4.0–10.7) mg/kg, respectively [446, 447].

The drug is rapidly absorbed, metabolized and excreted from the body [20]. Sex and strain of host and intensity of infection did not modify the efficacy of the drug. Its effect on the worms is rapid and they are immobilized, contracted and excreted in the faeces within a few hours of treatment [446, 447].

Diphyllobothriasis. The drug was active against *D. latum* in hamsters, but the estimate of the ED_{90} was 35.9 (26.9–48.0) mg/kg [92, 93].

2.13.2 Cestodes in Domestic Carnivores

Taeniasis, Dipylidiasis and Diphyllobothriasis. Many reports are now available confirming the strong cestocidal activity of praziquantel against *T. pisiformis, T. hydatigena, T. ovis, T. taeniaeformis, D. caninum, D. latun* and *M. corti* in dogs and cats pappropriately [33, 35, 41, 108, 127, 186, 224, 225, 388, 394, 401, 446, 448]. Estimates of the ED_{90} against 2- to 28-day-old and 28-day-old *T. hydatigena* infections were 1.8 (1.0–3.1) mg/kg [33] and 0.5 (0.3–1.1) mg/kg [186], respectively. Estimates for *T. taeniaeformis* and *M. corti* in cats and dogs were 0.7 (0.4–1.4) mg/kg and 1.9 (0.8–4.1) mg/kg, respectively [394]. A preliminary estimate suggests that the ED_{90} for dipylidiasis is about the same as that for taeniasis [127]. The drug can be given with equal efficacy by the oral, intramuscular or subcutaneous routes [41]. It is well tolerated by each route and no side effects have been reported.

Echinococcosis. Special attention has been given to the evaluation of praziquantel against *E. granulosus* [17, 18, 24, 35, 41, 111, 127, 186, 193, 224, 225, 269, 270, 439, 441, 477, 491] and *E. multilocularis* [388, 394, 401, 446, 448]. Estimates of the ED_{90} for a single treatment against naturally acquired and 28-day-old *E. granulosus* were similar at 2.3 (1.5–3.7) mg/kg [127], 2.7 (2.1–3.5) mg/kg [186] and 3.2 (1.8–5.6) mg/kg [439], respectively. The single dose ED_{90} for *E. multilocularis* was estimated at 4.6 (2.1–10.1) mg/kg [394], suggesting that a slightly higher dose rate may be required against this species.

Praziquantel was of similar efficacy against *E. granulosus* when administered by the intramuscular and oral routes [17, 18, 41, 193]. Efficacy was reduced, however, following injection by the subcutaneous route and the ED_{90} was estimated at 7.6 (3.1–18.6) mg/kg [193]. The drug is equally effective when administered with or without food [439]. It can also be successfully incorporated into a medicated food retaining high palatability and acceptability for dogs [author's unpublished data]. The drug does not have a practical ovicidal effect [440].

2.13.3 Cestodes in Man

Hymenolepiasis. The drug is highly effective against *H. nana* [38, 101, 144, 217, 383, 384, 407]. Estimates of the single dose ED_{90} were 12.6 (10.1–15.7) mg/kg [407]; 16.1 (13.3–19.5) mg/kg [101] and 19.7 (14.6–26.3) mg/kg [217]. These estimates are fairly close to those for oral treatment of *H. nana* in mice [447].

Taeniasis. Praziquantel is highly active when given as a single dose at 10 mg/kg in the treatment of *T. saginata* and *T. solium* [38, 101, 144, 217, 364, 383]. The lowest dose rate tested was 5 mg/kg and this was successful in 9 patients with *T. saginata,* but unsuccessful in 1 patient with *T. solium.* The highest dose rate tested was 10 mg/kg and this was successful in all 158 patients with either *T. saginata* or *T. solium.*

Diphyllobothriasis. Several reports have shown that praziquantel is active against diphyllobothriasis in man [21, 93, 144, 217]. The drug eliminated *D. latum* from all 33 patients at 25 mg/kg and *D. pacificum* from all 25 patients at 10 mg/kg [144, 217].

2.13.4 Species and Dose-Response Effects

Figure 3 summarizes the observed single dose ED_{90}'s for praziquantel against various species of cestode. It is interesting to note that all but *H. nana* and *D. latum* have a single dose ED_{90} of less than 10 mg/kg and that the ED_{90}'s for both *T. hydatigena* and *E. granulosus* are less than 5 mg/kg. This situation does not arise with any other drug for which data are available (see fig. 2).

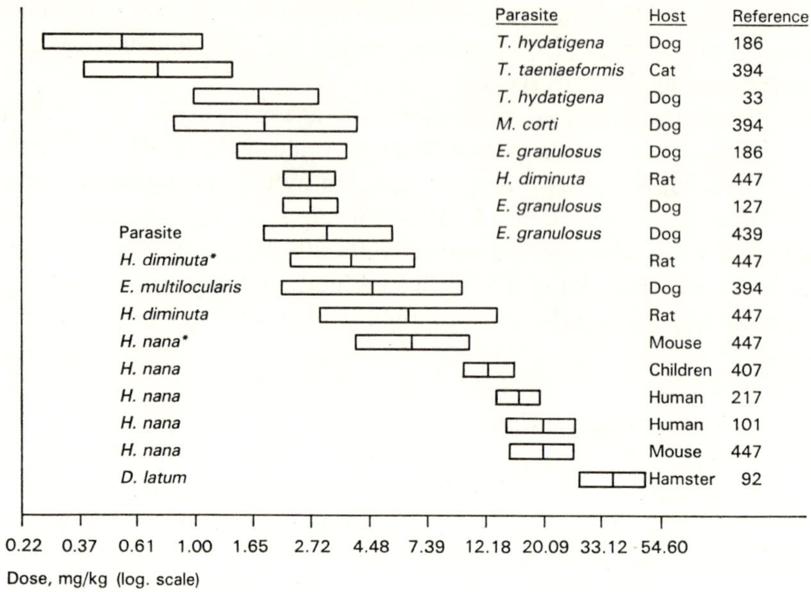

Fig. 3. The single dose ED_{90} and the 95% confidence interval of praziquantel against specified tapeworm infections in various hosts. * Subcutaneous, remainder oral treatment.

3. Drugs for the Treatment of Larval Tapeworm Infections

Over the past two decades, there have been attempts to find effective scolicides for use in the surgical treatment of echinococcosis or killing larval *H. nana* [287]. Both in vitro and in vivo screening programmes have been undertaken [159, 233, 235–237, 253, 254, 314, 315, 317, 318, 333, 391–393, 396, 397, 399, 400, 411, 486]. It was not, however, until the mid 1970s when mebendazole and praziquantel were shown to have larvacidal activity, that a major effort was initiated to identify the value and shortcomings of larvacides in the treatment of echinococcosis and cysticercosis. This work has recently been reviewed [141].

3.1 Mebendazole and Other Benzimidazoles

Several benzimidazoles including albendazole, cambendazole, fenbendazole and thiabendazole have been studied for larvacidal activity in laboratory and large animals [37, 51, 97, 98, 100, 113, 136, 238, 288, 289, 293, 312]; most research effort has been directed towards mebendazole and fluoro-mebendazole (= Flubendazole).

3.1.1 Metacestodes in Laboratory Animals

Hymenolepiasis. A novel approach to the study of larvacides includes the treatment of cysticercoids by feeding the drug to hymenolepid-infected beetles. Several studies have shown that mebendazole can motify the survival of cysticercoids in beetles [146, 147, 347].

Cysticercosis. About 20 studies on the efficacy of mebendazole administered by oral and/or parenteral routes against *T. pisiformis, Taenia crassiceps, T. taeniaeformis* and *M. corti* infections in rodents and rabbits appropriately have been reported [37, 77, 83, 100, 137, 229, 231, 239, 297, 442]. These show that the drug can cause the death of metacestodes. Progressive changes in the micromorphology suggest that the primary site of damage involves the tegument and alteration to the microtubule system [77, 463, 464]. Up to a point this effect appears to be reversible. Treatment schedules to achieve lethal effects cannot be determined from the literature cited.

Echinococcosis. The efficacy of mebendazole against secondary *E. granulosus* infections [139–141, 229, 255, 478] and *E. multilocularis* infections in rodents [37, 73, 88, 99, 100, 137–141, 272, 288, 289, 291–293, 319, 322] appear to differ. There is strong evidence with the former of limitations to growth, altered osmo-regulatory capabilities and death of some cysts. Most can be severely damaged by an 80-day treatment schedule [140, 141]. The drug permeates through the cyst wall by simple diffusion [382]. With *E. multilocularis,* however, evidence of lethal effects is less convincing. In some cases damaged parasites resumed growth after transplantation into naive recipient hosts. For example, treatment with mebendazole for 167–330 days with 500 ppm in food (about 30 mg/kg/day), resulted only in inhibition of proliferation and formation of metastases [139–141].

Intraperitoneal injections of mebendazole into laboratory animals were reported to cause complete growth inhibition and tissue destruction of even large conglomerates; deep injections of the same suspension into the conglomerates did not affect viability [291]. In albino mice daily oral doses of 25 mg/kg inhibited larval development by up to 90%, but its effect was temporary. In cotton rats and hamsters, in which the metacestode develops much faster than in albino mice, mebendazole was less effective [291].

3.1.2 Metacestodes in Domestic Food Animals

Cysticercosis. Incomplete kills have been reported for *T. hydatigena* and *T. saginata* with short-term treatment (about 5–14 days) in sheep, pigs and cattle appropriately [164, 194, 230, 239, 240, 297, 351, 363]. When, however, daily treatments of 50 mg/kg were extended to 1 month, no *T. hydatigena* survived [194].

Echinococcosis. Young experimental infections in sheep and pigs with thin-walled *E. granulosus* survived daily short-term treatment schedules [230, 362]. With naturally acquired infections of thick-walled metacestodes in aged sheep, a model that may approximate human echinococcosis more closely than infections with young larvae, daily treatments at 50 mg/kg for 5 days were without effect [194]. At 1 month considerable damage was observed, but some protoscoleces survived and were infective to a dog. None, however, survived daily treatment for 3 months [194]. It seems that to achieve high cure rates a much longer treatment schedule is required for echinococcosis than for cysticercosis in sheep.

3.1.3 Metacestodes in Man

Several case history studies on *E. granulosus* and *E. multilocularis* have reported regression of cyst size, but many have been inconclusive [8, 10, 14, 15, 52, 59, 79, 80, 87, 117, 140, 206, 266, 278, 316, 329, 338, 353, 376, 451, 457, 473, 483]. For example, in one study with *E. granulosus,* protoscolices were still viable following daily treatment for 1 month at 30 mg/kg [15] (as observed in sheep) [194]. A similar result was obtained following three 15-day treatment periods [376]. A 2-year treatment schedule has been suggested [451]. With *E. multilocularis,* daily treatments for 30 days to 3.5 years have provided evidence of stabilization in some cases only [8, 316, 483]. The real problem of evaluating the efficacy of chemotherapy from these case history studies is that very little is yet known about drug levels in serum and in cyst fluid as well as normal patterns of growth and regression of matacestodes.

3.2 Praziquantel

Larvacidal activity was first reported in 1975 [445]. Reference has already been made to the larvacidal activity against cysticercoids of *H. nana* [446]. In these studies, evidence was provided that the drug was more effective against older (70–90 h) than younger (24–48 h) organisms. A single dose at 25 mg/kg was effective against fully developed cysticercoids.

3.2.1 Metacestodes in Laboratory Animals

Cysticercosis. Studies have been reported on the efficacy of praziquantel against *T. pisiformis, T. taeniaeformis, T. crassiceps* and *M. corti* [37, 239, 240, 297, 346, 395, 445, 446, 449]. Also, evidence has been provided in some studies of an age dependent effect. For example, 4-week-old *T. taeniaeformis* were insusceptible and 4- to 7-week-old organisms were only partially susceptible, but older organisms were fully susceptible [446, 449]. Estimates of the single dose ED_{90} for oral or parenteral treatments have yet to be determined for each species. An immobilizing effect has been observed [346, 446]. In some cases when death did not ensue, the organisms failed to reorganize in the definitive host [36, and authors' unpublished data].

Echinococcosis. Praziquantel showed slight or negligeable effects with short-term treatment schedules against secondary *E. granulosus* and *E. multilocularis* infections in rodents [37, 395, 445, 449, 478].

3.2.2 Metacestodes in Domestic Food Animals

Cysticercosis and Coenurosis. Praziquantel has been shown to be active against *T. hydatigena, T. ovis, T. multiceps* and *T. saginata* in sheep, pigs and cattle appropriately [36, 82, 165, 230, 239, 240, 297, 351, 363, 445, 446, 449, 467, 468]. Again, age dependent effects were evident in some studies [165, 449]. For example, there was no obvious lethal effect of praziquantel against 4- to 10-week-old *T. saginata,* but a strong effect was observed against 12-week-old and older organisms [165]. Also with *T. hydatigena* up to 12 weeks old many larvae are killed by the drug, but this is not dose-rate-dependent within the dose range 25–200 mg/kg. In contrast, the single dose ED_{90} for *T. hydatigena* in aged sheep was estimated to be 9.4 (5.1–17.4) mg/kg [authors' unpublished data].

Echinococcosis. Praziquantel has no obvious lethal effects on thick-walled *E. granulosus* in aged sheep [authors' unpublished data].

3.2.3 Metacestodes in Man

Cysticercosis. The efficacy of praziquantel against *T. solium* cysticercosis in man is not yet known. On many occasions, comment has been made on the potential risk of *T. solium* cysticercosis following the anteriad movement of proglottids during drug treatment. Self-infection was first postulated in 1856, but subsequent studies have failed to substantiate the hypothesis [205, 471]. Cysticercosis is only likely to occur in those patients who have not previously been immunized by the ingestion of eggs from self-infection (from anus to mouth) prior to treatment. It is not yet known if the larvadical activity of praziquantel will alleviate this rate phenomenon.

4. Drugs for the Treatment of Eggs

4.1 Ovicidal Cestocides

There are two main circumstances when ovicides may be useful. The first is concerned with killing eggs during drug therapy. This is important during the early stages of echinococcosis control as there may be a mass release of viable eggs post-treatment. No cestocides have been shown to have a practical ovicidal activity [398, 440, 480]. However, in the case of echinococcosis arecoline hydrobromide can be used simultaneously with the cestocide and the purged material incinerated or deep buried. This problem has not yet been solved inter alia for *T. saginata,* because there is a massive increase in eggs expelled for up to 3 days after treatment [274].

4.2 Environmental Ovicides

The second use for an ovicide is in the destruction of eggs particularly those of *Echinococcus,* adhering to dogs or scattered around kennels, or for the treatment of eggs, particularly those of *T. saginata, T. solium* and

D. latum, in sewage. Extensive in vitro studies have revealed no compounds with reliable ovicidal activity [300, 301, 321, 332, 345, 359, 367, 482].

5. Drug-Orientated Field-Trials and Control Programmes

An understanding of the dynamics of transmission and the inter-relationships of the factors that modify it in the face of perturbation, is fundamental to the planning and assessment of drug-orientated field-trials and control programmes. The stability of a parasite population describes its ability to survive perturbation in the form of, for example, environmental change without either becoming extinct or reaching plague proportions. This involves biotic characteristics, such as egg production, which influence infection pressure and the development of acquired immunity [19, 81, 174, 190]. Drug-orientated control programmes directed against the adult and/or larval populations are man-made perturbations and the stability of the host-parasite system determines to a major extent the effort required for success. In the words of one author: 'one can only measure stability by giving the system a push and seeing what happens' [81].

5.1 Treatment Programmes Directed against Cestodes

Echinococcosis control programmes, such as those in Cyprus, New Zealand and Tasmania, have primarily used an educational approach, and as part of it, have utilised arecoline hydrobromide as a diagnostic agent to identify dogs that have obtained access to raw infective offal. This has been administered at intervals varying from 3 months to 1 year [172]. Others, such as the Falkland Islands have used a 3-monthly treatment programme with bunamidine hydrochloride. Whatever methods have been used, all of them stress education in prevention and all have shown evidence of a reduction in echinococcosis in intermediate hosts including man in a relatively short period of time [174, 175, 190, 328, 370]. It is not possible to separate the role played by drugs from that played by, inter alia, the educational programme in achieving this reduction in prevalence.

The Styx field-trial carried out in New Zealand over a period of more than 30 years, has shown that echinococcosis can be controlled by a combination of education and the use of drugs against the tapeworms in dogs [171, 173]. In contrast, the same methods employed against ovine cysticercosis *(T. hydatigena* and *T. ovis)* have been unsuccessful (see also the Manypeaks Trial in Western Australia) [475]. Similarly, in the Styx trial, these ovine cysticercoses survived a 4-weekly dog-dosing programme with bunamidine hydrochloride and nitroscanate carried out over periods of 9 years and 4 years, respectively. This was due to the occasional introduction of untreated dogs and failure of the drug to kill all tapeworms. Indeed, due to the loss of the immunizing dose of eggs, it was found that if the interval between drug failures was long enough (about 1 year), a second larval population imposed itself upon, and survived with, the original metacestodes thereby doubling the larval population. It seems, therefore, that due to high egg production, ovine cysticercoses with dogs as the definitive host are much more stable and less susceptible to perturbation with drugs than is echinococcosis.

Many reports are available on the use of drugs, such as dichlorophen and niclosamide and their mixtures, in human hymenolepiasis, taeniasis and diphyllobothriasis control programmes [294, 305, 372–375]. Some of these programmes have shown promise with regard to a reduction in human tapeworm carriers. All stress the need for educational programmes on prevention of infection as well as improved sanitation standards. As was observed with the ovine cysticercoses involving dogs as the definitive host, drug-orientated programmes are unlikely to control human tapeworm infections where health-education and sanitary disposal of faeces do not exist. It was also observed that due to the high egg production and rapid spread of eggs from dogs in ovine cysticercosis a single infected animal can contaminate a large area [173, 174, 190]. Likewise, a single human tapeworm carrier practising promiscuous defaecation can initiate a devastating bovine 'cysticercosis storm', particularly in modern feed-lots [410]. The introduction of highly effective drugs, such as praziquantel, does not reduce the need for other control measures.

5.2 Treatment Programmes Directed against Metacestodes

The introdoction of larvacides provides a major new option in any cost/benefit approach to control involving food animals [174]. In this regard, they should remove the larval population in all age cohorts with a single treatment. There are problems with residues, and where wild animals are involved. Such limitations do not apply to the therapy of human echinococcosis and cysticercosis.

Several benzimidazoles have been shown to be larvacidal, but none are completely effective when used as a single treatment. On the other hand, praziquantel given once is rapidly eliminated and kills larvae causing cysticercosis provided the population is fully susceptible. As yet no field-trials have been reported describing 'endemic' or 'epidemic'-type situations where larvacidal programmes have been applied.

6. Future Research Requirements

Regulations in many countries now insist on adequate evidence of efficacy vis-à-vis toxic sequelae before a drug can be registered. Valuable lessons can be learnt from the research programmes undertaken over the past two decades, particularly with regard to models, protocols, screening procedures and the need to identify dose rates and treatment schedules having predictable effects.

6.1 Cestode Research

While the introduction of dichlorophen and bunamidine can be regarded as milestones in out-patient chemotherapy and in echinococcosis control, respectively, the introduction of praziquantel with its predictable activity can be regarded as the highlight of cestode drug research. With regard to the last-named drug, there is a need to: (a) consolidate data on dose response curves and safety in the treatment of human tapeworm infections; (b) exploit the strong echinococcicidal effects by developing medicated foods for animals; (c) combine the drug with nematocides for broad-spectrum activity. Benefits that may accrue from such programmes include for example, an attack on wild life echinococcosis with the 'baiting' of foxes or dog populations owned by nomadic tribes in highly endemic zones. Broad-spectrum activity may achieve control over such zoonoses as visceral larval migrans in echinococcosis control programmes.

Several antibiotics have shown promise as cestocides. Detailed comparative evaluations on isolated fractions in laboratory rodents may provide compounds with a wide range of activity for the treatment of gastrointestinal conditions also involving tapeworms.

Several benzimidazoles have shown cestocidal activity. There is a need to re-examine the importance of such factors as particle size with the objective of attempting to formulate 'one-hit' compounds with a wide range of activity. Such compounds could be used with advantage in many mass-treatment situations such as, for example, the treatment of gastro-intestinal parasites in refugee camps where many parasite species may be present. Prevention of reinfection by providing slow release drug depots may also have application in the control of parasites of veterinary and medical importance.

6.2 Metacestode Research

The finding in 1974 that mebendazole showed larvacidal activity, particularly against *Echinococcus* spp can be regarded as a milestone in metacestode research. It has, however, been pointed out that mebendazole was developed for use against gastro-intestinal parasites and is poorly absorbed from the gut. Mebendazole, like dichlorophen in human tapeworm infections, may not itself assume an important role in the chemotherapy of human echinococcosis. However, the demonstration that metacestodes can be killed in situ opens up a most exciting field of research. Several authors have pointed out the need for international co-ordination.

The finding in 1975 that praziquantel showed larvacidal activity against the cysticercoses of domestic food animals, also opens up another exciting field of research. Here, extensive research is required on: (a) dose response effects against larvae of different ages; (b) cost-benefit field trials defining the role of larvacides in the control of bovine, ovine and porcine cysticercoses.

6.3 Ovicide Research

The lack of chemicals with ovicidal activity seriously hampers an attack on eggs in sewage. As the human population increases and tourism expands, sewerage systems may become overloaded and pose a threat to pasture-reared animals, in the case of *T. saginata* and to fish stocks in the case of *D. latum*. There is a need to expand research in this important field of veterinary public health.

Co-operation between international agencies, the pharmaceutical industry and individual researchers having specialized facilities and with emphasis on action-orientated programmes, could lead to a reduction in the prevalence of many of the important cestode parasitisms of man and animals to a negligeable level before the end of the twentieth century.

7. Summary

A review has been made of the advances in knowledge on the treatment of tapeworm infections of man and animals from the time of the introduction of dichlorophen in 1956. This opened up the era of out-patient treatment for human tapeworm infections. The drugs studied have been compared, where possible, on the basis of estimates of the single dose ED_{90} or the number of treatments required to reach that efficacy at safe dose levels.

During the period under review, niclosamide, introduced in 1960, has been regarded as the drug of choice for the treatment of human tapeworm infections with paromomycin as a possible alternative. The bunamidine salts, introduced in 1966, permitted the treatment of *Echinococcus* spp in dogs. Several treatments were required to achieve acceptable efficacy. In 1975 praziquantel was introduced and based on the ED_{90}, a single dose at no more than 10 mg/kg removed all tapeworms responsible for the cestode zoonoses and for which data are available with the exception of *H. nana* and *D. latum;* these require a higher dose rate. In the mid 1970s, several benzimidazoles and praziquantel were shown to have activity against metacestodes. This has opened up a new field of research promising a practical outcome. No progress has been made during the period under review in finding effective ovicides.

References

1 Abdallah, A. et al.: The efficacy of *N*-(2′chloro-4′-nitrophenyl)-5-chlorosalicylamide in the treatment of taeniasis. J. Egypt. med. Ass. *44:* 379–381 (1961).

2 Abdiev, T. A.: Experimental mass treatment of *Taenia saginata* with phenasal alone or in combination with dichlorophen and acrichin. Mater. nauch. Konf. vses. Obshch. gel'mint. Pt *1:* 3–7 (1968).

3 Abdullaev, A. M.: Studies on the efficiency of phenasal in treatment of patients with taeniarhynchosis. Medskaya Parazit. *35:* 484–485 (1966).

4 Abdullaev, A. M.: Phenasal treatment for diphyllobothriasis. Medskaya Parazit. *36:* 394–395 (1967).

5 Abrams, G. J. et al.: The treatment of human tapeworm infections with 'Yomesan'. S. Afr. med. J. *37:* 6–8 (1963).

6 Ahkami, S. et al.: The appearance of the scolex of *Taenia saginata* in the stool after the eradication of the parasite by niclosamide. Tropenmed. Parasitol. *20:* 341–345 (1969).

7 Ahkami, S. et al.: Radical treatment of *Hymenolepis nana* with niclosamide. J. trop. Med. Hyg. *73:* 258–259 (1970).

8 Akovbiantz, A. et al.: Gibt es eine Chemotherapie der Echinokokkose des Menschen? Schweiz. med. Wschr. *108:* 1101–1103 (1978).

9 Akuginova, Z. D.: A new combination of anthelmintics (Phenasal with bithionol) for the treatment of cestodiasis. II. Study on the efficiency of bithionol alone and mixed with Phenasal against *Taenia saginata* infections. Medskaya Parazit. *38:* 545–548 (1969).

10 Al-Moslih, M. I. et al.: Treatment of hydatidosis. Br. med. J. *ii:* 1435 (1978).

11 Alterio, D. L.: Tratamento das teníases pela clorossalicilamida e pelo difentano. Revta Hosp. Clín. Fac. Med. Univ. S. Paulo *23:* 259–261 (1968).

12 Amato-Neto, V. et al.: Resultados obtidos como diclorofen no tratamento das teníases. Hospital, Rio de J. *60:* 271–275 (1961).

13 Amato-Neto, V. et al.: Tratamento, por um derivado da salicilamida, de infestaçoes causadas por *Taenia saginata* e *Taenia solium*. Revta Inst. Med. trop. S. Paulo *6:* 297–299 (1964).

14 Ammann, R. et al.: Chemotherapie der Echinokokkose des Menschen mit Mebendazol (Vermox). Schweiz. med. Wschr. *109:* 148–151 (1979).

15 Anon: Medical treatment for hydatid disease. Br. med. J. *ii:* 563 (1979).

16 Andersen, F. L. et al.: Efficacy of bunamidine hydrochloride against immature and mature stages of *Echinococcus granulosus*. Am. J. vet. Res. *36:* 673–675 (1975).

17 Andersen, F. L. et al.: Efficacy of injectable and tablet formulations of praziquantel against mature *Echinococcus granulosus*. Am. J. vet. Res. *39:* 1861–1862 (1978).

18 Andersen, F. L. et al.: Efficacy of injectable and tablet formulation of praziquantel against immature *Echinococcus granulosus*. Am. J. vet. Res. *40:* 700–701 (1979).

19 Anderson, R. M.: The regulation of host population growth by parasitic species. Parasitology *76:* 119–157 (1978).

20 Andrews, P.: Pharmacokinetic studies with Droncit® in animals using a biological assay. Vet. Med. Rev. *ii:* 154–165 (1976).

21 Apajalahti, J.: Tratamiento de infecciones por *Diphyllobothrium latum* con una dosis oral única de praziquantel. Boln chil. Parasit. *32:* 43 (1977).

22 Arambulo, P. V. et al.: Studies on the zoonotic cycle of *Taenia saginata* taeniasis and cysticercosis in the Philippines. Int. J. Zoon. *3:* 77–104 (1976).

23 Arambulo, P. V. et al.: The use of mebendazole in the treatment of *Taenia saginata* taeniasis in an endemic area in the Philippines. Acta trop. *35:* 281–286 (1978).

24 Arru, E. et al.: Valutazione dell'efficacia del praziquantel (Droncit) contro *Echinococcus granulosus* del cane. Comm. Svolta 30th Cong. Soc. Ital. Sci. Vet., Taormina (CT) (1976).

25 Astaf'ev, B. A.: Main results of studies on the morphology, biology and pathogenesis of hymenolepids in the past 10 to 15 years and future tasks. Medskaya Parazit. *40:* 730–736 (1971).

26 Astaf'ev, B. A. et al.: On the problems of remote relapses after treatment of patients with *Hymenolepis* infections. Medskaya Parazit. *40:* 131–136 (1971).

27 Astaf'ev, B. A. et al.: The pathology of human hymenolepiasis; in Probl. Para-

zit. Mater. VIII nauch. Konf. Parazit. UkSSR. Izdatel'stvo 'Naukova Dumka', pp. 41–43 (1975).

28 Astaf'ev, B. A. et al.: Duration of the follow-up period in outpatients after treatment against Hymenolepis infections. Medskaya Parazit. *45:* 739–743 (1976).

29 Averkin, E. A. et al.: Methyl 5(6)-phenylsulphinyl-2-benzimidazolecarbamate, a new, potent anthelmintic. J. med. Chem. *18:* 1164–1166 (1975).

30 Azimov, S. A. et al.: The efficacy of arecoline and bunamidine hydrochloride against Echinococcus infection. Veterinariya No. 10, pp. 81–82 (1974).

31 Bábos, S. et al.: Összehasonlító vizsgálatok a Devermin A (Chinoin) és Yomesan (Bayer) ebek galandférgessége elleni hatásaról, különös tekintettel az echinococcosisra. Magy. Allatorv. Lapja *19:* 472–474 (1964).

32 Balazs, T. et al.: A comparative study of hymenolepicides in *Hymenolepis nana* infestation of rats. Can. J. comp. Med. *26:* 160–162 (1962).

33 Baldock, F. C. et al.: Efficiency of praciquantel, a new cestocide, against *Taenia hydatigena* in the dog. Res. vet. Sci. *23:* 237–238 (1977).

34 Baltzly, R. et al.: A series of compounds active against cestodes. Nature, Lond. *206:* 408–409 (1965).

35 Bankov, D. E.: Comparative assessment of anthelmintics against *Echinococcus granulosus*. Vet. Med. Rev. *ii:* 145–148 (1977).

36 Bankov, D.: Trials for therapy and chemoprophylaxis of coenurosis in sheep. Vet. Med. Rev. *i:* 79–80 (1979).

37 Barandun, G.: Untersuchungen zur Chemotherapie der alveolären Echinokokkose und der *Mesocestoides corti*-Infektion bei Labortieren; vet. Diss. Zürich (1978), p. 76.

38 Baranski, M. C.: Tratamiento de teniasis e himenolepiasis humanas con praziquantel (Embay 8440). Boln chil. Parasit. *32:* 37–39 (1977).

39 Baranski, M. C. et al.: Tratamento da himenolepíase nana com um derivado da salicilamida *(N*-(2′cloro-4′-nitrofenil)-5-clorosalicilamida). Hospital, Rio de J. *67:* 593–599 (1965).

40 Bartsch, H. et al.: Absence of mutagenicity of praziquantel, a new, effective, anti-schistosomal drug, in bacteria, yeasts, insects and mammalian cells. Mutat. Res. *58:* 133–142 (1978).

41 Bauditz, R. et al.: Droncit® injectable: new possibilities of tapeworm control. Vet. Med. Rev. *ii:* 129–133 (1979).

42 Bayandina, D. G.: The effect of a series of anthelmintics on the different stages of *Hymenolepis nana* in white mice. Medskaya Parazit. *34:* 556–562 (1965).

43 Bayandina, D. G.: The causes of relapse in hymenolepid infection. Medskaya Parazit. *40:* 137–140 (1971).

44 Bayandina, D. G. et al.: Experimental studies of a new anthelmintic yomesan and its combination with acrichine. Medskaya Parazit. *31:* 673–677 (1962).

45 Bayandina, D. G. et al.: Treatment of hymenolepiasis with Yomesan. Medskaya Parazit. *33:* 411–415 (1964).

46 Bayandina, D. G. et al.: Experimental study of the anthelmintic properties of dichlorophen. Medskaya Parazit. *33:* 591–594 (1964).

47 Bayandina, D. G. et al.: The combined effect of phenasal and dichlorophen on the imago stages of *Hymenolepis nana* in white mice. Medskaya Parazit. *34:* 107–109 (1965).

48 Bayandina, D. G. et al.: Efficiency of new methods of treatment of *Hymenolepis nana*. Medskaya Parazit. *35:* 412–413 (1966).
49 Bayandina, D. G. et al.: An improved method for diagnosing *Hymenolepis nana* infection. Medskaya Parazit. *39:* 239–240 (1970).
50 Bayandina, D. G. et al.: Phenasal treatment of hymenolepidiasis. Medskaya Parazit. *41:* 411–413 (1972).
51 Beal, C. B. et al.: Experimental alveolar hydatid disease. J. Am. med. Ass. *198:* 75 (1966).
52 Beard, T. C. et al.: Medical treatment for hydatids. Med. J. Aust. *i:* 633–635 (1978).
53 Beaudoin, R. L.: The effect of altering the intestinal flora in *Hymenolepis diminuta* populations in rats. Diss. Abstr. *22:* 2915 (1962).
54 Beaudoin, R. L.: Action of selected antibiotics on *Hymenolepis diminuta* in the rat host. J. Parasit. *51:* 34 (1965).
55 Beier, A.: Die *Taenia-saginata*-Infektion und ihre Behandlung mit Acranil und Yomesan. Münch. med. Wschr. *105:* 2075–2083 (1963).
56 Beier, A.: Therapeutische Erfahrungen mit Yomesan (Bayer) bei menschlichen Bandwurminfektionen. Tropenmed. Parasitol. *17:* 50–57 (1966).
57 Bekhli, A. F. et al.: Preparation G-610, a new anthelmintic, an analogue of dichlorophen. Medskaya Parazit. *38:* 192–193 (1969).
58 Bekhli, A. F. et al.: The anthelmintic activity of polymorphous modifications of phenasal. Medskaya Parazit. *45:* 228 (1976).
59 Bekhti, A. et al.: Treatment of hepatic hydatid disease with mebendazole: preliminary results in four cases. Br. med. J. *ii:* 1047–1051 (1977).
60 Belmar, R.: *Dipylidium caninum* en niños. Comunicación de 13 casos y tratamiento con un derivado de la Salicilamida. Boln chil. Parasit. *18:* 63–67 (1963).
61 Belmar, R. et al.: Ensayo terapéutico de la teniasis por *Hymenolepis nana* con un derivado de la salicilamida (Yomesan Bayer 2353). Boln chil. Parasit. *17:* 69–71 (1962).
62 Besedina, T. K. et al.: On the treatment of hymenolepidiasis with phenasal. Medskaya Parazit. *42:* 160–162 (1973).
63 Besedina, T. R. et al.: Duration of follow-up period in out-patients after anthelmintic treatment against Hymenolepis infection. Medskaya Parazit. *45:* 738–739 (1976).
64 Bhaduri, N. V. et al.: Dichlorophen in the treatment of *Taenia saginata* infection. Bull. Calcutta Sch. trop. Med. Hyg. *6:* 19 (1958).
65 Biagi, F. et al.: Efectividad del dichlorofen contra *Hymenolepis nana*. Boln méd. Hosp. infant., Méx. *16:* 113–116 (1959).
66 Biagi, F. et al.: Tratamiento de la himenolepiasis nana con una nueva substancia tenicida. Med. Rev. Méx. *41:* 241–243 (1961).
67 Billerau, M.: Le niclosamide nouvel antihelminthique actif sur les taenias; thèse, Faculté mixte de Médicine et de Pharmacie de Lyon (1964), p. 42.
68 Bills, G. N. B. et al.: Possible role of the liver in bunamidine toxicity. Proc. Univ. Otago med. Sch. *48:* 59–60 (1970).
69 Blair, H. E.: Vermiplex, a new anthelmintic for dogs. N. Am. Vet. *30:* 306 (1949).

70 Blakemore, R. C.: A comparison of in vitro and in vivo methods for determining anthelmintic activity using *Hymenolepis* var. *fraterna*. J. Inst. Sci. Technol. *12:* 114–126 (1966).

71 Blood, B. D. et al.: Evaluation of selected drugs for the treatment of canine echinococcosis. Bull. Wld Hlth Org. *39:* 67–72 (1968).

72 Bolt, A. S. et al.: Treatment of diphyllobothriasis patients with Dichlosal. Medskaya Parazit. *37:* 486 (1968).

73 Bolshakova, G. M. et al.: Cellular and humoral immunity responses before and after chemotherapy in white mice infected with hydatid *(Echinococcus multilocularis)*. Medskaya Parazit. *46:* 176–181 (1977).

74 Boray, J. C.: Nitroscanate (lopatol) – a new broad spectrum anthelmintic against nematodes and cestodes in dogs. Proc. 54th Conf. Aust. Vet. Ass. (1977), pp. 123–126.

75 Boray, J. C. et al.: The role of broad spectrum anthelmintics in the control of zoonoses due to helminths of dogs. 6th Symp. Wld Ass. Adv. Vet. Parasit., Vienna 1973.

76 Boray, J. C. et al.: Nitroscanate, a new broad spectrum anthelmintic against nematodes and cestodes of dogs and cats. Aust. vet. J. *55:* 45–53 (1979).

77 Borgers, M. et al.: Morphological changes in cysticerci of *Taenia taeniaeformis* after mebendazole treatment. J. Parasit. *61:* 830–843 (1975).

78 Botero, D.: Paromomycin as effective treatment of *Taenia* infections. Am. J. trop. Med. Hyg. *19:* 234–237 (1970).

79 Bouree, P. et al.: Echinococcoses multiples. Essais thérapeutiques avec le fluro-mébendazole. Bull. Soc. Path. exot. *70:* 365–371 (1977).

80 Bouree, P. et al.: Treatment of echinococcosis. Br. med. J. *i:* 301 (1978).

81 Bradley, D. J.: Regulation of parasite populations. A general theory of the epidemiology and control of parasitic infections. Trans. R. Soc. trop. Med. Hyg. *66:* 697–708 (1972).

82 Brglez, J. et al.: Pokusaj lijecenja eksperimentalne misicne cysticerkoze teladi novim anthelmintikom praziquantelom. Acta parasitol. iugosl. *7:* 103–107 (1976).

83 Brichko N. V.: Therapeutic efficacy of mebendazole against *Cysticercus pisiformis* in rabbits. Sb. nauch. Trud. Mosk. vet. Akad. *86:* 97–98 (1976).

84 Brinkner, W. O. et al.: Some observations on the efficiency of Di-phenthane-70 in canine teniasis. Mich. St. Coll. Vet. *6:* 57–86 (1946).

85 Brown, W. E. et al.: Taeniacidal activity of streptothricin antibiotic complex S15-1(SQ21,704). J. Antibiot. *30:* 886–889 (1977).

86 Brugmans, J. P. et al.: Mebendazole in enterobiasis. Radiochemical and pilot clinical study in 1,278 subjects. J. Am. med. Ass. *217:* 313–316 (1971).

87 Bryceson, A.: Mebendazole and hydatid disease. Br. med. J. *i:* 796 (1980).

88 Budanova, I. S.: Histological changes in *Echinococcus multilocularis* cysts in laboratory animals caused by mebendazole and levamisole; in Probl. parasit. Mater. VIII nauch. Konf. Parasit. UkSSR Izdated'stvo 'Naukova Dumka', pp. 80–81 (1975).

89 Burrows, R. B.: Human and veterinary anthelmintics. Prog. Drug Res. *17:* 108–209 (1973).

90 Burrows, R. B. et al.: Treatment of canine and feline tapeworm infections with bunamidine hydrochloride. Am. J. vet. Res. *27:* 1381–1384 (1966).

91 Burrows, R. B. et al.: Cestocidal activity of 4-alkoxy-1-naphthamidines against dog and cat tapeworms. J. med. Chem. *14:* 87–90 (1971).

92 Bylund, G. et al.: Evaluación experimental del efecto de praziquantel contra *Diphyllobothrium latum* in vivo e in vitro. Boln chil. Parasit. *32:* 7–10 (1977).

93 Bylund, G. et al.: Tests with a new compound (Praziquantel) against *Diphyllobothrium latum.* J. Helminth. *51:* 115–119 (1977).

94 Cabrera, B. D.: The treatment of taeniasis saginata with bithionol (Bitin) in Jaro, Leyte. Acta med. philipp. *9:* 139–143 (1973).

95 Cabrera, B. D. et al.: Studies on the epidemiology and transmission of human taeniasis in the Philippines – a paradoxical public health problem. J. Philipp. med. Ass. *53:* 105–130 (1977).

96 Cacho Lopez, W. N. et al.: Terapia comparativa del Yomesan y el bromhidrato de arecolina en la echinococcosis canina. An. Cient., Lima *1:* 275–290 (1963).

97 Campbell, W. C. et al.: Prevention and cure of hepatic cysticercosis in mice. J. Parasit. *60:* 1049–1052 (1974).

98 Campbell, W. C. et al.: Treatment of the cystic stage of *Taenia crassiceps* and *Echinococcus multilocularis* in laboratory animals. J. Parasit. *60:* 1053–1054 (1974).

99 Campbell, W. C. et al.: Therapy of hydatid disease. J. Am. med. Ass. *230:* 825 (1974).

100 Campbell, W. C. et al.: Effect of parenterally injected benzimidazole compounds on *Echinococcus multilocularis* and *Taenia crassiceps* metacestodes in laboratory animals. J. Parasit. *61:* 844–852 (1975).

101 Canzonieri, C. J. et al.: Ensayos terapéuticos con praziquantel en infecciones por *Taenia saginata,* e *Hymenolepis nana.* Boln chil. Parasit. *32:* 41–42 (1977).

102 Casinelli, G. et al.: Thaimycins, new anthelmintic and anti-protozoal antibiotics produced by *Streptomyces michiganensis* var *amylolyticus* var *nova.* Arch. Mikrobiol. *70:* 197–210 (1970).

103 Castillo, V. H. T.: Eficacia de la niclosamida sobre el *Dipylidium caninum* en perros. Gac. vet., Buenos Aires *31:* 107–114 (1969).

104 Cavier, R.: Les nouveaux médicaments utilisables dans le traitement du téniasis chez l'homme. Prod. Prob. pharm. *21:* 581–592 (1966).

105 Cavier, R. et al.: Essai pharmacologique de quelques anthelminthiques agissant sur les cestodes de l'intestin de l'homme. Annls pharm. fr. *26:* 603–606 (1968).

106 Cavier, R. et al.: Sur les propriétés anthelminthiques du sulfate de paromomycine. Annls pharm. fr. *28:* 729–732 (1970).

107 Cavier, R. et al.: Etudes pharmacologiques des propriétés ténicides de deux anthelmintiques dérivés du benzimidazole: mébendazole et flubendazole. Annls pharm. fr. *37:* 33–36 (1979).

108 Chawla, J. S. et al.: Effectiveness of Embay 8440 in experimental *Taenia hydatigena* infection in dogs. Indian J. Parasitol. *1:* 19–20 (1977).

109 Chularerk, P. et al.: Some aspects of epidemiology and mass treatment of taeniasis in Ban Tard; Udorn Thani. J. med. Ass. Thailand *50:* 666–670 (1967).

110 Cordero del Campillo, M.; et al.: Ensayo experimental de *N*-(2'chlor-4-nitrofenil)-5-chlorsalicilamida frente a *Echinococcus granulosus* (Batsch, 1786) adultos en el intestino del perro. Revta ibér. Parasit. *25:* 119–129 (1965).

111 Cordero del Campillo, M. et al.: Eficacia de droncit-Bayer (Praziquantel) contra *Echinococcus granulosus* juveniles y adultos, en perros experimentalmente infectados. An. Fac. Vet. León *22:* 39–46 (1976).

112 Cox, D. D. et al.: The anthelmintic activity of Yomesan against *Taenia* spp of dogs and cats. Vet. med. Rev. *1:* 49–55 (1966).

113 Craig, T. M. et al.: Preliminary studies on the effect of albendazole on the cysticerci of *Taenia saginata.* SWest. Vet. *31:* 121–124 (1978).

114 Craige, A. A. et al.: Teniacidal action of Di-phenthane-70. A. Am. Vet. *27:* 26–30 (1946).

115 Crowley, J.: An in vivo screening method for anthelmintic activity using *Hymenolepis nana* var *fraterna* in mice. Parasitology *51:* 339–345 (1961).

116 Cruthers, L. R. et al.: Taeniacidal efficacy of SQ21,704 in dogs by various types of oral administration and in comparison with niclosamide and bunamidine hydrochloride. Am. J. vet. Res. *40:* 676–678 (1979).

117 Danis, M. et al.: Treatment of hepatic hydatid disease. Br. med. J. *ii:* 1356 (1977).

118 Davis, A.: Drug treatment in intestinal helminthiasis. World Health Organization WHO/HELM/72.1, p. 100 (1972).

119 Davis, A.: Efficacy and acceptability of praziquantel in patients infected with schistosome species other than *S. mansoni.* 14th Congr. Braz. Soc. Trop. Med. Brazil (1978).

120 de Carneri, I. et al.: Drugs used in cestode diseases; in IEPT Sect. 64, pp. 145–213 (Pergamon Press, Oxford 1973).

121 Dedov, V. S. et al.: The effect of dichlosal in man. Medskaya Parazit. *37:* 209–212 (1968).

122 Deiana, S. et al.: Azione del Mansonil (Bayer) nelle infestioni da cestodi del cane. Parassitologia *14:* 269–273 (1972).

123 Delak, M. et al.: Istraživanje djelatnosti *N*-(2′klor-4′-nitrofenil)-5-klorsalicilamida na trakovičavost pasa uzrokovanu s *Echinococcus granulosus.* Vet. Arh. *33:* 57–62 (1963).

124 Della Bruna, C. et al.: Axenomycins, new cestocidal antibiotics. Antimicrob. Agents Chemother. *3:* 708–710 (1973).

125 Demidov, N. V. et al.: Cestocidal properties of antibiotics. Byull. nauchnotekh. inf. vses. Inst. gel'mint. K. I. Skryabina *14:* 14–15 (1974).

126 Demidov, N. V. et al.: An improved method for anthelmintic treatment of dogs with *Echinococcus.* Veterinariya Moscow *10:* 80–81 (1974).

127 Dey-Hazra, A.: The efficacy of Droncit® (praziquantel) against tapeworm infections in dog and cat. Vet. Med. Rev. *ii:* 134–141 (1976).

128 Diekmann, H. W. et al.: The fate of praziquantel in the organism. III. Metabolism in rat, beagle dog and rhesus monkey. Eur. J. Drug Metab. Pharmacokinet. *2:* 107–112 (1976).

129 Ditzel, J. et al.: Worm cure without tears. The effect of niclosamide on taeniasis saginata in man. Acta med. scand. *182:* 663–664 (1967).

130 Doroshak, O. F. et al.: Side effects of the application of phenasal and dichlorophen. Medskaya Parazit. *37:* 110 (1968).

131 Dovzhenko, V. A.: Timing of control examination in the treatment of diphyllobothriasis with phenasal alone and in combination with other drugs. Medskaya Parazit. *42:* 222–223 (1973).

132 Dovzhenko, V. A.: Therapy of diphyllobothriasis with phenasal in combination with aminoacrichin and kamala. Medskaya Parazit. *42:* 738–741 (1973).

133 Dovzhenko, V. A. et al.: The effect of phenasal on different areas of the strobilar of cestodes. Medskaya Parazit. *45:* 169–173 (1976).

134 Drouet, T. W. L.: Bithionol en el tratamiento de la infestacion humana por Teniasis saginata, solium e *Himenolepis nana.* Rev. ecuat. Hig. Med. trop. *28:* 95–97 (1971).

135 Dufek, M. et al.: Experience with modern treatment of taeniasis. Rev. Czech. Med. *15:* 29–32 (1969).

136 Duwel, D.: Activity of fenbendazole on metacestodes of different tapeworms in small and domestic animals. Curr. Chemotherapy *1978:* 142–144.

137 Eckert, J. et al.: Zur Wirkung von Mebendazol auf Metazestoden von *Mesocestoides corti* und *Echinococcus multilocularis.* Tropenmed. Parasitol. *27:* 247–262 (1976).

138 Eckert, J. et al.: Untersuchungen zur Chemotherapie der Echinokokkose. Tropenmed. Parasitol. *28:* 274–275 (1977).

139 Eckert, J. et al.: Chemotherapie der larvalen Echinokokkose bei Labortieren. Schweiz. med. Wschr. *108:* 1104–1112 (1978).

140 Eckert, J. et al.: Immunodiagnose und Therapie der Echinokokkose. Ther. Umsch. *35:* 766–776 (1978).

141 Eckert, J. et al.: New aspects of larval cestode infections. Report on Workshop CII, 7: Echinococcosis and other larval cestode infections. Proc. 4th Int. Congr. Parasit, Warsaw (in press, 1978).

142 Enzie, F. D. et al.: Taeniacides in dogs and cats. N. Am. Vet. *38:* 119–128 (1957).

143 Enzie, F. D. et al.: Preliminary trials with bithionol against tapeworm infections in cats, dogs, sheep and chickens. Am. J. vet. Res. *21:* 628–630 (1960).

144 Espejo, H.: Tratamiento de infecciones por *Hymenolepis nana, Taenia saginata, Taenia solium* y *Diphyllobothrium pacificum* con praziquantel (Embay 8440). Boln chil. Parasit. *32:* 39–40 (1977).

145 Euzeby, J.: La thérapeutique anthelminthique. Cah. Méd. vét. *47:* 165–184 (1978).

146 Evans, W. S. et al.: The effect of Mebendazole on the development of *Hymenolepis diminuta* in *Tribolium confusum.* Can. J. Zool. *54:* 1079–1083 (1976).

147 Evans, W. S. et al.: Effect of mebendazole on the larval development of three hymenolepidid cestodes. J. Parasit. *65:* 31–34 (1979).

148 Faiguenbaum, J. et al.: Tratamiento de las teniasis con un derivado de la salicilamida (*N*-(2′cloro-4′-nitrofenil)5-clorosalicilamida). Boln chil. Parasit. *18:* 30–32 (1963).

149 Farahmandian, I. et al.: A comparison of stool examination and mass treatment for indication of the prevalence of *Taenia saginata.* Trop. geogr. Med. *25:* 171–173 (1973).

150 Fastier, F. N.: Pharmacological aspects of bunamidine dosing of dogs. N. Z. vet. J. *20:* 148–150 (1972).

151 Fastier, F. N. et al.: Induction of ventricular fibrillation with adrenaline in dogs pretreated with bunamidine hydrochloride. Proc. Univ. Otago med. Sch. *46:* 64–66 (1968).

152 Fastier, F. N. et al.: Toxicity of bunamidine. 3. Trial of propranolol as antidote. N. Z. vet. J. *21:* 216–217 (1973).

153 Fastier, F. N. et al.: Toxicity of Bunamidine. I. Cardiovascular effects. N. Z. vet. J. *21:* 201–204 (1973).

154 Fazakas, B. et al.: Klinikai megfigyelesek emberi galandfergessegben. Parasitol. hung. *2:* 195–208 (1969).

155 Ferreira, F. S. Da C. et al.: Ensaios terâpeuticos com o Bayer 2353 (Yomesan) na teníase *(Taenia saginata).* Anais Inst. Med. trop., Lisb. *17:* 1009–1016 (1960).

156 Finney, D. J.: The application of the probit method to toxicity test data adjusted for mortality with controls. Ann. appl. Biol. *31:* 68–74 (1944).

157 Finney, D. J.: Probit analysis (Cambridge University Press, Cambridge 1971).

158 Forbes, L. S.: The efficiency of *N*-(2′-chlor-4′-nitrophenyl)-5-chlor-salicylamid against *Taenia hydatigena* and *Echinococcus granulosus* infections in dogs. Vet. Rec. *75:* 321–324 (1963).

159 Fraya, G. J. et al.: Systematic search for a systemic hydatid scolicide. 1. In vitro screening of chemicals against the scolices of hydatid cysts *(Echinococcus granulosus).* Chemotherapy *16:* 371–379 (1971).

160 Frolova, A. A.: The period of dispensary follow-up of patients with *Taenia saginata* infections. Medskaya Parazit. *39:* 108–109 (1970).

161 Frolova, A. A.: Epidemiological efficiency of Dichlosal treatment of patients with taeniasis. Medskaya Parazit. *40:* 453–455 (1971).

162 Frolova, A. A. et al.: Treatment of *Taenia saginata* with phenasal (Yomesan) in combination with dichlorophen or acrichin. Medskaya Parazit. *36:* 149–151 (1967).

163 Fujimori, I. et al.: Treatment of *Diphyllobothrium latum* and *Taenia saginata* with 2,2′-thiobis (4,6-dichlorophenol) (Bitin, bithionol, Actamer). Jap. J. Parasit. *14:* 573–576 (1965).

164 Gallie, C. J. et al.: The effect of mebendazole on the cysticerci of *Taenia saginata* in calves. Trop. Anim. Hlth Prod. *9:* 24 (1977).

165 Gallie, G. J. et al.: The efficacy of praziquantel against the cysticerci of *Taenia saginata* in calves. Trop. Anim. Hlth Prod. *10:* 36–38 (1978).

166 Ganozzi-Blanc, J.: Le traitement des taeniasis par la tredermine; thèse de médecine Paris (1967), p. 41.

167 Garin, J. P. et al.: Le sulfate de paromomycine antibiotique actif sur les protozoaires du tube digestif se révèle aussi un bon taenicide. Lyon méd. *215:* 979–992 (1966).

168 Garin, J. P. et al.: Action de quatre antibiotiques du groupe des oligosaccharides sur *Taenia saginata.* Lyon méd. *215:* 123–129 (1971).

169 Gemmell, M. A.: The efficiency of Dichlorophen (2,2′-dihydroxy-5,5′-dichlorodiphenyl methane) against *Echinococcus granulosus* infestations in dogs. Aust. vet. J. *34:* 249–252 (1958).

170 Gemmell, M. A.: Screening of drugs and their assessment for use against the strobilate stage of *Echinococcus.* Bull. Wld Hlth Org. *39:* 57–65 (1968).

171 Gemmell, M. A.: The Styx field-trial. A study on the application of control measures against hydatid disease caused by *Echinococcus granulosus.* Bull. Wld Hlth Org. *39:* 73–100 (1968).

172 Gemmell, M. A.: Surveillance of *Echinococcus granulosus* in dogs with arecoline hydrobromide. Bull. Wld Hlth Org. *48:* 649–652 (1973).

173 Gemmell, M. A.: The Styx field-trial. Effect of treatment of the definitive host for tapeworms on larval forms in the intermediate host. Bull. Wld Hlth Org. *56:* 433–443 (1978).
174 Gemmell, M. A.: Perspective on options for hydatidosis and cysticercosis control. Vet. Med. Rev. *i:* 3–48 (1978).
175 Gemmell, M. A.: Hydatidosis control – a global view. Aust. vet. J. *55:* 118–125 (1979).
176 Gemmell, M. A. et al.: Bunamidine hydrochloride: its efficiency against *Echinococcus granulosus.* Vet. Rec. *82:* 252–256 (1968).
177 Gemmell, M. A. et al.: Treatment of *Echinococcus granulosus* and *Taenia hydatigena* with bunamidine hydroxynaphthoate in a prepared food. Res. vet. Sci. *16:* 85–88 (1974).
178 Gemmell, M. A. et al.: The effect of fospirate on *Echinococcus granulosus* and *Taenia hydatigena* infections in dogs. Res. vet. Sci. *19:* 216–217 (1975).
179 Gemmell, M. A. et al.: The effect of nitroscanate on *Echinococcus granulosus* and *Taenia hydatigena* infections in dogs. Res. vet. Sci. *19:* 217–219 (1975).
180 Gemmell, M. A. et al.: Treatment of *Taenia hydatigena* infections in dogs with bunamidine hydroxynaphthoate incorporated in food. N. Z. vet. J. *23:* 142–144 (1975).
181 Gemmell, M. A. et al.: The effect of bithionol sulphoxide on *Echinococcus granulosus* and *Taenia hydatigena* infections in dogs. Res. vet. Sci. *18:* 109–110 (1975).
182 Gemmell, M. A. et al.: The effect of mebendazole on *Echinococcus granulosus* and *Taenia hydatigena* in dogs. Res. vet. Sci. *19:* 229–230 (1975).
183 Gemmell, M. A. et al.: The effect of niclosamide on *Echinococcus granulosus, Taenia hydatigena* and *Taenia ovis* infections in dogs. Res. vet. Sci. *22:* 389–391 (1977).
184 Gemmell, M. A. et al.: The effect of micronised nitroscanate on *Echinococcus granulosus* and *Taenia hydatigena* infections in dogs. Res. vet. Sci. *22:* 391–392 (1977).
185 Gemmell, M. A. et al.: The lethal effect of some benzimidazoles on *Taenia hydatigena* in dogs. Res. vet. Sci. *23:* 115–116 (1977).
186 Gemmell, M. A. et al.: The effect of praziquantel on *Echinococcus granulosus, Taenia hydatigena* and *Taenia ovis* infections in dogs. Res. vet. Sci. *23:* 121–123 (1977).
187 Gemmell, M. A. et al.: The effect of mebendazole in food on *Echinococcus granulosus* and *Taenia hydatigena* infections in dogs. Res. vet. Sci. *25:* 107–108 (1978).
188 Gemmell, M. A. et al.: The effect of an antibiotic of the streptothricin family against *Echinococcus granulosus* and *Taenia hydatigena* infections in dogs. Res. vet. Sci. *25:* 109–110 (1978).
189 Gemmell, M. A. et al.: The effect of diuredosan on *Echinococcus granulosus* and *Taenia hydatigena* infections in dogs. Res. vet. Sci. *25:* 111–112 (1978).
190 Gemmell, M. A. et al.: Experimental epidemiology of hydatidosis and cysticercosis. Adv. Parasitol. *15:* 311–369 (1977).
191 Gemmell, M. A. et al.: The effect of oxfendazole on *Echinococcus granulosus* and *Taenia hydatigena* infections in dogs. Res. vet. Sci. *26:* 389–390 (1979).

192 Gemmell, M. A. et al.: The effect of nitroscanate tablets on *Echinococcus granulosus* and *Taenia hydatigena* infections in dogs. Res. vet. Sci. *27:* 255–257 (1979).

193 Gemmell, M. A. et al.: The effect of route of administration on the efficacy of praziquantel against *Echinococcus granulosus* infections in dogs. Res. vet. Sci. *29:* 131–132 (1980).

194 Gemmell, M. A. et al.: Effect of mebendazole against *Echinococcus granulosus* and *Taenia hydatigena* cysts in naturally infected sheep and relevance to larval tapeworm infections in man. Z. ParasitKde (in press, 1980).

195 Ghadirian, E. et al.: Human infection with *Hymenolepis diminuta* in villages of Minab, Southern Iran. Int. J. Parasitol. *2:* 481–482 (1972).

196 Gherman, I.: Observations sur le traitement du téniasis par le *N*-2′-chloro-4′-nitrophénil-5-chloro-salicyl amide. Bull. Soc. Path. exot. *61:* 432–434 (1968).

197 Gibson, T. E.: Veterinary anthelmintic medication; 2nd ed., pp. 144–173, Commonwealth Agricultural Bureau Technical Communication, No. 33 (Commonwealth Agricultural Bureau, 1965).

198 Girardi, C. et al.: Il mebendazolo nei piccoli animale. Tossicita-assorbimento ed eliminazione-attività antielmintica. Annali Fac. Med. vet. Torino *24:* 82–113 (1977).

199 Gladkikh, V. F. et al.: Pharmacological investigation of combination of bithionol with phenasal. Medskaya Parazit *37:* 675–677 (1968).

200 Gladkikh, V. F. et al.: Investigation of absorption of phenasal administered orally to white rat. Medskaya Parazit. *39:* 88–91 (1970).

201 Gleason, N. N. et al.: Mesocestoides (Cestoda) in a child in New Jersey treated with Niclosamide (Yomesan). Am. J. trop. Med. Hyg. *22:* 757–760 (1973).

202 Goldsmid, J. M. et al.: *Inermicapsifer madagascariensis* (Davaine, 1870), Baer, 1956 (Platyhelminthes Cestoda) as a parasite of man in Rhodesia. Cent. Afr. J. Med. *18:* 205–207 (1972).

203 Gönnert, R. et al.: Experimentelle Untersuchungen mit (*N*-(2′-chlor-4′-nitrophenyl)-5-chlorsalicylamid, einem neuen Bandwurmmittel. 1. Mitteilung: Chemotherapeutische Versuche. Arzneimittel-Forsch. *10:* 881–884 (1960).

204 Gönnert, R. et al.: Konstitution und cestocide Wirkung in der Yomesan-Reiche. Medizin Chem. *7:* 540 (1963).

205 Gönnert, R. et al.: Biologische Probleme bei *Taenia solium*. Tropenmed. Parasitol. *18:* 76–81 (1967).

206 Goodman, H. T.: Mebendazole. Med. J. Aust. *2:* 662 (1976).

207 Gras, G. et al.: Chimiothérapie expérimentale des helminthiasis. Contribution à l'étude de la technique pharmacologique utilisant la souris parasitée par: *Hymenolepis nana* var. *fraterna*. Archs Inst. Pasteur Tunis *44:* 141–154 (1967).

208 Gregor, W. W.: A clinical assessment of 5-chloro N-(2-chloro-4-nitrophenyl) salicylamide as a taeniacide for dogs and cats. Vet. Rec. *75:* 1421–1422 (1963).

209 Grevel, V. et al.: Untersuchungen über Mebendazol, ein neues Breitspektrum-anthelminthikum für die Kleintierpraxis. Schweizer Arch. Tierheilk. *115:* 559–578 (1973).

210 Griffiths, R. B.: The application of some anthelmintics in veterinary practice. J. Pharm. Pharmac. *6:* 921–943 (1954).

211 Grinenko, N. V.: The effect of anthelmintics and of their combinations upon cestodes in vitro. Medskaya Parazit *33:* 87–92 (1964).

212 Grinenko, N. V.: Combined methods of taeniarhynchosis treatment. Medskaya Parazit. *33:* 221–225 (1964).

213 Grinenko, N. V.: Treatment of taeniasis with phenasal (Yomesan) alone or in combination with other anthelmintics. Medskaya Parazit. *33:* 599–602 (1964).

214 Grinenko, N. V. et al.: Data on the efficiency of and tolerance to divided doses of phenasal, dichlosal and trichlosal in hymenolepid infections in man. Medskaya Parazit. *42:* 163–167 (1973).

215 Grinenko, N. V. et al.: Treatment of hymenolepis in man with 5- or 7-day courses of Dichlosal and Trichlosal administered in split doses. Medskaya Parazit. *45:* 101–103 (1976).

216 Grinenko, N. V. et al.: The effect of divided doses of phenasal, trichlorophen, dichlosal or trichlosal on the cysticercoids and juvenile forms of *Hymenolepis nana* in white mice. Medskaya Parazit. *45:* 176–178 (1976).

217 Groll, E.: Panorama general del tratamiento de las infecciones humanas por cestodes con praziquantel (Embay 8440). Boln chil. Parasit. *30:* 27–31 (1977).

218 Gromova, V. K.: The efficiency of various schedules for the treatment of diphyllobothriasis with phenasal and dichlorophen. Medskaya Parazit. *37:* 397–399 (1968).

219 Gromova, V. K.: The effect of dichlosal and phenasal on the development of *Diphyllobothrium latum* eggs. Medskaya Parazit. *37:* 544–546 (1968).

220 Guerrero, J.: Telmintic (mebendazole) powder, a new broad spectrum anthelmintic for canine use. Practicing Vet. *49:* 15–17 (1978).

221 Guilhon, J. et al.: Essais de traitement du téniasis humain par le 5,5′-dichloro-2,2′-dihydroxydiphénylméthane. Bull. Soc. Path. exot. *53:* 697–703 (1960).

222 Güralp, N. et al.: Yomesan in köpek ve kedi cestod'larina etkisi. Vet. Fak. Derg. Ankara Üniv. *13:* 253–267 (1966).

223 Güralp, N. et al.: The efficiency of bithionol in the treatment of dog tapeworms. Arzneimittel-Forsch. *19:* 831–832 (1969).

224 Güralp, N. et al.: Preliminary studies on the effect of Droncit® against different tapeworms in dogs and cats. Vet. Med. Rev. *ii:* 129–133 (1976).

225 Gyul'gyuzli, G. S.: Tests with bunamidine oxynaphthoate and Droncit in intestinal cestode infections in dogs. Byull. nauchno-tekh. inf. vses. Inst. gel'mint. K. I. Skryabina No. 20, pp. 9–12 (1977).

226 Harfenist, M. et al.: Synthesis and anthelmintic activity of 4-alkoxy-1-naphthamidines. J. med. Chem. *14:* 97–103 (1971).

227 Hatton, C. J.: A new taeniacide, bunamidine hydrochloride: its efficiency against *Taenia pisiformis* and *Dipylidium caninum* in the dog and *Hydatigera taeniaeformis* in the cat. Vet. Rec. *77:* 408–411 (1965).

228 Hatton, C. J.: Efficiency of bunamidine salts against tapeworms. Vet. Rec. *81:* 104–106 (1967).

229 Heath, D. D. et al.: The lethal effect of mebendazole on secondary *Echinococcus granulosus,* cysticerci of *Taenia pisiformis* and tetrathyridia of *Mesocestoides corti.* Parasitology *70:* 273–285 (1975).

230 Heath, D. D. et al.: The effect of mebendazole and praziquantel on the cysts

of *Echinococcus granulosus, Taenia hydatigena* and *T. ovis* in sheep. N. Z. vet. J. *26:* 11–15 (1978).

231 Heath, D. D. et al.: A single oral treatment with mebendazole for the control of *Taenia crassiceps* larval infections in rats. Int. J. Parasitol. *9:* 73–76 (1979).

232 Hecht, G. et al.: Experimentelle Untersuchungen mit *N*-(2′-chlor-4′-nitrophenyl)-5-chlorsalicylamid, einem neuen Bandwurmmittel. Mitteilung 2: Toxicologische Untersuchungen. Arzneimittel-Forsch. *10:* 884–885 (1960).

233 Heslop, J. H.: An assessment of the efficacy of hydatid scolicidal agents used locally in surgery. Aust. N. Z. J. Surg. *37:* 205–208 (1967).

234 Heyneman, D.: Host-parasite resistance patterns – some implications from experimental studies with helminths. Ann. N. Y. Acad. Sci. *113:* 114–129 (1963).

235 Hinz, E.: Chemotherapeutische Untersuchungen an der experimentellen Zystizerkose der Ratte, hervorgerufen durch Strobilocercus *(Cysticercus fasciolaris).* Z. Tropenmed. Parasit. *12:* 430–437 (1961).

236 Hinz, E.: Chemotherapeutische Untersuchungen mit Endoxan an der experimentellen Finneninfektion der weissen Maus. Z. Tropenmed. Parasit. *15:* 332–336 (1964).

237 Hinz, E.: Zur Chemotherapie der Echinokokkose und Zysticerkose. Therapie Gegenw. *106:* 111–1121 (1967).

238 Hinz, E.: Zur Chemotherapie der experimentellen larvalen Echinococcose mit Fenbendazole. Zentbl. Bakt. ParasitKde *241:* 388–394 (1978).

239 Hörchner, F. et al.: Die Wirkung von Mebendazole und Praziquantel auf larvale Taenienstadien bei Maus, Kaninchen und Schwein. Tropenmed. Parasitol. *28:* 44–50 (1976).

240 Hörchner, F. et al.: Zur Bekämpfung und Diagnostik der Rinderfinnen. 1. Therapie und Reinfektion. Berl. Münch. tierärztl. Wschr. *92:* 107–111 (1979).

241 Hromatka, L. et al.: Versuche mit dem Bandwurmmitel Scolaban® beim Hund. Wien. tierärztl. Mschr. *53:* 616–617 (1966).

242 Hughes, H. C. et al.: Niclosamide as a treatment for *Hymenolepis nana* and *Hymenolepis diminuta* in rats. Lab. Anim. Sci. *23:* 72–73 (1973).

243 Ishida, K. et al.: The treatment with paromomycin, and serological studies of *Diphyllobothrium latum* infections. Jap. J. Parasit. *26:* 22 (1977).

244 Isaeva, K. B. et al.: Restrobilation of *Hymenolepis nana* after phenasal treatment. Medskaya Parazit. *44:* 662–666 (1975).

245 Isaeva, K. B. et al.: The causes of stubborn hymenolepiasis in children. Medskaya Parazit. *47:* 21–23 (1978).

246 James, M. P.: Mansonil toxicity in dogs. N. Z. vet. J. *23:* 18 (1975).

247 Jiménez-Quirós, O.: Difentano 70: tratamiento electivo en *Hymenolepis nana.* Revta Biol. trop. *7:* 75–80 (1961).

248 Jones, W. E.: Niclosamide as a treatment for *Hymenolepis diminuta* and *Dipylidium caninum* infections in man. Am. J. trop. Med. Hyg. *28:* 300–302 (1979).

249 Joppling, W. H. et al.: Treatment of tapeworm infections in man. Br. med. J. *ii:* 542–544 (1959).

250 Junod, C.: Sur la persistance du taeniasis rebelle *(T. saginata).* Etude statistique des facteurs favorisants. Bull. Soc. Path. exot. *60:* 272–281 (1967).

251 Kahra, A. et al.: Expelling the broad tapeworm with Yomesan. Suom. Lääk. *18:* 325–327 (1963).

252 Kalawski, K. et al.: Inwazje tasiemca nieuzbrojonego *(Taeniarhynchus saginatus)* na terenie miasta poznania w latach 1954–1968. Przegl. Epid. Rok. *24:* 377–380 (1970).

253 Kammerer, W. S. et al.: Estado actual de la quimioterapia de la hidatidosis. Boln Of. sanit. pan-am. *75:* 523–529 (1973).

254 Kammerer, W. S. et al.: Chemotherapy of experimental *Echinococcus granulosus* infection. Trials in CF_1 mice and birds *(Meriones unguiculatus)*. Am. J. trop. Med. Hyg. *24:* 90–95 (1975).

255 Kammerer, W. S. et al.: Chemotherapy of hydatid disease *(Echinococcus granulosus)* in mice with mebendazole and bithionol. Am. J. trop. Med. Hyg. *25:* 714–717 (1976).

256 Kanazawa, Y.: A case of fish tapeworm infections treated with paromomycin and observations on its mode of activity. J. Antibiot., Tokyo *24:* 143–145 (1971).

257 Karnaukhov, V. K.: The clinical picture and treatment of children with Taeniarhynchus infestation. Pediatriya *46:* 58–61 (1967).

258 Karnaukhov, V. K. et al.: On the treatment of patients with taeniarhynchiasis. Sov. Med. *29:* 144–146 (1966).

259 Karnaukhov, V. K. et al.: Phenasal in the treatment of patients with hymenolepiasis. Medskaya Parazit. *42:* 573–576 (1973).

260 Karnaukhov, V. K. et al.: Comparative efficiency and tolerance of various methods of phenasal treatment with hymenolepis infections. Medskaya Parazit. *46:* 182–186 (1977).

261 Kassai, T. et al.: Investigations on the efficiency of some anticestode compounds against *Echinococcus granulosus* in the dog. Parasitol. hung. *8:* 29–35 (1975).

262 Kassai, T. et al.: Az ebek echinococcosisának orvoslása bunamidin hidroxinaftóat hatóanyagtartalmú gyógyszeres pálcikával. Magy. Allatorv. Lap. *32:* 373–377 (1977).

263 Katz, N. et al.: Ensaio clínico com mebendazole nas teníasis. Rev. Soc. bras. Med. trop. *7:* 225–229 (1973).

264 Keeling, J. E. D.: The chemotherapy of cestode infections. Adv. Chemotherapy, vol. 3, pp. 109–152 (Academic Press, New York 1968).

265 Keeling, J. E. D.: Activity of some dialkylnaphthamidines against tapeworms. SCI Monogr., No. 33, pp. 56–71 (1969).

266 Kern, P. et al.: Chemotherapy of echinococcosis with mebendazole. Clinical observations of 7 patients. Tropenmed. Parasit. *30:* 65–72 (1979).

267 Khalil, H. M.: Treatment of cestode infections with Radevern. Trans. R. Soc. trop. Med. Hyg. *63:* 76–78 (1969).

268 Khodakova, V. I. et al.: The effect of dichlosal and phenasal on the development of the eggs of *Diphyllobothrium latum*. Medskaya Parazit. *37:* 541–543 (1968).

269 Kobulej, T. et al.: Efficacy of Droncit® against canine echinococcosis. Magy. Allatorv. Lap. *33:* 306–308 (1978).

270 Kobulej, T. et al.: Droncit – a milestone in the control of *Echinococcus granulosus* in dogs. Acta vet. hung. *26:* 351–355 (1978).

271 Kondo, K. et al.: Anthelmintic effect of bunamidine as a taeniacide for dogs and cats. J. Jap. vet. med. Ass. *22:* 247–250 (1969).

272 Kovalenko, F. P. et al.: Experimental treatment of hydatid disease. I. Laboratory model of hydatid disease and the effect of sarcolysinacridin, levamisole and mebendazole on the development of the cyst. Medskaya Parazit. *45:* 546–551 (1976).

273 Kovalev, N. E.: Treatment of *Taenia saginata* infection with Phenasal. Medskaya Parazit. *35:* 234–236 (1966).

274 Kovalev, N. E.: Dissemination of *Taenia saginata* oncospheres before and after anthelmintic treatment. Medskaya Parazit. *36:* 438–441 (1967).

275 Kovalev, N. E.: Treatment of resistant forms of *T. saginata* infections. Sov. Med., No. 5, pp. 147–148 (1973).

276 Kovchur, V. N.: Comparative efficiency of Trichlosal, Phenasal and Dichlosal in patients with diphyllobothriasis. Medskaya Parazit. *40:* 403–408 (1971).

277 Kozakiewicz, B. et al.: Skutecznosc niclosamidu i bunamidyny w zwalczaniu echinokokzy u psow. Medycyna wet. *1:* 460–462 (1975).

278 Kroidl, R. et al.: Ungewöhnliche klinische und morphologische Präsentation einer Lungenechinokokkose. Prax. Pneum. *32:* 200–203 (1978).

279 Krotov, A. I.: Experimental study of the effectiveness of a combination of amino-acrichin, yomesan and extract of male fern. I. Effect on the imago stage of *Hymenolepis nana* in white mice. Medskaya Parazit. *33:* 215–221 (1964).

280 Krotov, A. I. et al.: Experimental study of a combination of yomesan and acrichin. Medskaya Parazit. *32:* 193–196 (1963).

281 Krotov, A. I. et al.: A new combination of anthelmintics (phenasal and bithionol) for the treatment of cestodiasis. Communication 1. Efficiency of bithionol and its combination with phenasal in experimental hymenolepid infections of white mice. Medskaya Parazit. *37:* 672–675 (1968).

282 Krotov, A. I. et al.: Treatment of *Taenia saginata, Hymenolepis and Diphyllobothrium* infections with phenasal and dichlosal. 8th Int. Congr. Trop. Med., Malar (Teheran), pp. 1135–1137 (1968).

283 Krotov, A. I. et al.: Investigation of the effectiveness of a combination of 2,6-bis(2′oxy-5-chlorobenzyl)-4-chlorophenol with phenasal (Trichlosal) in mice infected with *Hymenolepis nana* and in man with taeniasis and diphyllobothriasis. Medskaya Parazit. *38:* 550–552 (1969).

284 Krotov, A. I. et al.: A study of the anthelmintic and molluscidal activity of the piperazine salt of phenasal in comparison with phenasal. Medskaya Parazit. *41:* 341–346 (1972).

285 Krotov, A. I. et al.: Experimental study of the efficiency of phenasal with cucurbitine and novocaine in hymenolepidid infections of white mice. Medskaya Parazit. *41:* 417–419 (1972).

286 Krotov, A. I. et al.: Effects of diurnal migration of *Hymenolepis nana* in the intestinal tract of white mice on the efficiency of worming. Medskaya Parazit. *42:* 565–567 (1973).

287 Krotov, A. I. et al.: Search for compounds effective against *Hymenolepis nana* larvae. Medskaya Parazit. *43:* 697–700 (1974).

288 Krotov, A. I. et al.: Experimental therapy of alveococcosis. II. Experimental anti-nematocidal substances against alveococcosis in laboratory animals. Medskaya Parazit. *43:* 314–319 (1974).

289 Krotov, A. I. et al.: Experimental therapy of alveococcosis. III. Influence of

thiabendazole, sarcolysin-acridin, levamisole and mebendazole on the development of alveococcus larvocysts in albino mice. Medskaya Parazit. *45:* 164–168 (1976).
290 Krotov, A. I. et al.: The efficacy of benzimidazole derivatives on the susceptibility of white mice to *Hymenolepis nana* infection. Medskaya Parazit. *46:* 186–187 (1977).
291 Krotov, A. I. et al.: Experimental therapy of alveococcosis. V. Effectiveness in laboratory animals of mebendazole given by different routes. Medskaya Parazit. *46:* 480–484 (1977).
292 Krotov, A. I. et al.: Experimental therapy of multilocular hydatidosis. Communication VI. The effect of the size of the mebendazole particles on its toxicity and its efficacy in laboratory animals at different modes of administration. Medskaya Parazit. *47:* 48–50 (1978).
293 Krotov, A. I. et al.: Experimental therapy of multilocular hydatidosis. Communication VII. Comparative study of the efficacy of a series of benzimidazole derivatives on laboratory animals. Medskaya Parazit. *48:* 29–32 (1979).
294 Kruglov, Y. V.: Results of the control of *Taenia saginata* in the Volgograd region. Medskaya Parazit. *36:* 491–492 (1967).
295 Kunkle, D. W. et al.: Activity of parbendazole against cestodes in mice. J. Parasit. *57:* 319 (1971).
296 Kurelec, B. et al.: O mogucnosti lijecenja trakavicavosti pasa i kokosi yomesanom. Vet. Glasn. *15:* 602–606 (1961).
297 Langes, A.: Zur Chemotherapie von *Cysticercus tenuicollis* und *C. pisiformis* bei Schwein und Kaninchen; vet. Diss. Berlin (1976), p. 42.
298 Lapshina, I. G.: Treatment of diphyllobothriasis using bithionol with phenasal. Medskaya Parazit. *38:* 548–549 (1969).
299 Lassance, M. et al.: Note sur un taeniafuge de masse nouveau, l'anthiphen. Annls Soc. belge Méd. trop. *37:* 627–630 (1957).
300 Laws, G. F.: Taeniid ovicides. Proc. Univ. Otago med. Sch. *43:* 11–12 (1965).
301 Laws, G. F.: Chemical ovacidal measures as applied to *Taenia hydatigena, Taenia ovis, Taenia pisiformis* and *Echinococcus granulosus.* Expl Parasit. *20:* 27–37 (1967).
302 Laws, G. F. et al.: Bunamidine hydrochloride: its effect in vitro on the tegument of *Taenia hydatigena.* Proc. Univ. Otago med. Sch. *48:* 42–44 (1970).
303 Leopold, G. et al.: Pharmakokinetik von Praziquantel. Tropenmed. Parasitol. *28:* 276 (1977).
304 Leopold, G. et al.: Clinical pharmacology in normal volunteers of praziquantel, a new drug against schistosomes and cestodes. Eur. J. clin. Pharmacol. *14:* 281–291 (1978).
305 Lerner, P. M.: Prerequisites for the rationalization of control measures against *Hymenolepis* infections. Trudy uzbek. nauch. issled. Inst. Eksperiment. Med. Parazit. gel'mint. *6:* 104–198 (1969).
306 Lerner, P. M. et al.: Two-years work on the control of hymenolepidiasis in the population of Samarkand. Medskaya Parazit. *39:* 559–564 (1970).
307 Lerner, P. M. et al.: Consideration of 'caecotrophagy' during experimental studies on intra-intestinal autosuperinfection with *Hymenolepis.* Medskaya Parazit. *40:* 239–240 (197)1.

308 Lerner, P. M. et al.: Effect of marked reduction in hymenolepid infections on the incidence of acute intestinal disease. Medskaya Parazit. *42:* 153–156 (1973).

309 Lerner, P. M. et al.: On the duration of follow-up observations after treatment of patients with hymenolepiasis. Medskaya Parazit. *42:* 713–716 (1973).

310 Leushin, N. V.: Anthelmintics tested against *Echinococcus* and *Multiceps* infections in dogs. Byull. nauchno-tekh inf. vses. Inst. gel'mint. K. I. Skryabina, No. 4, pp. 85–86 (1970).

311 Litvinov, S. K. et al.: Treatment of *Taenia saginata* with Yomesan. Medskaya Parazit. *34:* 460–481 (1965).

312 Lloyd, S. et al.: Effect of albendazole on the metacestodes of *Taenia saginata* in calves. Experientia *34:* 723–724 (1978).

313 Lobova, G. A. et al.: Dichlosal (Yomesan and dichlorophen mixture) in the treatment of *Taenia saginata* in man. Mater. nauch. Konf. vses. Obshch. gel' mint. Pt *4:* 181–183 (1966).

314 Lubinsky, G.: Attempts at chemotherapy of *Echinococcus multilocularis* infections in rodents. Can. J. Zool. *47:* 1001–1004 (1969).

315 Lubinsky, G. et al.: Attempts at chemotherapy of *Echinococcus multilocularis* infections in rodents. II. A study of some parasiticides and cytostatic agents. Can. J. Zool. *47:* 1301–1304 (1971).

316 Lüdin, C. E. et al.: Therapy of alveococcosis in man. J. Int. Med. Res. *5:* 367–368 (1977).

317 Lukashenko, N. P. et al.: Effect of several chemical compounds on viability and respiration of larval scolices of *Echinococcus multilocularis* (Leuckart, 1863). Acta vet. hung. *20:* 339–352 (1970).

318 Lukashenko, N. P. et al.: Effect of some chemical compounds on free and encapsulated scolices of *Alveococcus multilocularis* (Leuckart, 1863) Abuladze, 1959. Medskaya Parazit. *40:* 86–95 (1970).

319 Lurie, A. A. et al.: Study of the distribution and excretion of mebendazole in white mice with experimental hydatidosis. Medskaya Parazit. *47:* 59–62 (1978).

320 Machemer, L. et al.: Mutagenicity studies with praziquantel, a new anthelmintic drug, in mammalian systems. Archs Toxicol. *39:* 187–197 (1978).

321 Mackie, A. et al.: Some observations on taeniid ovicides: the effects of some organic compounds and pesticides on activity and hatching. J. Helminth. *41:* 167–210 (1967).

322 Markell, E. K.: Mebendazole and hydatid disease. Lancet *i:* 925 (1975).

323 Markin, A. V. et al.: Results obtained with Trichlosal outpatients treatment against *Taenia saginata* infections. Medskaya Parazit. *44:* 730–731 (1975).

324 Marsboom, R.: Toxicologic studies on mebendazole. Toxicol. appl. Pharmacol. *24:* 371–377 (1973).

325 Martinez Báez, M. et al.: Estudio histologico de proglotides de *Taenia solium* expulsados despues de la administracion de Yomesan. Revta Invest. Salud Publica *31:* 152–162 (1972).

326 Matchanov, N. M. et al.: Tests of phenasal and dichlorophen against cestodes in dogs. Trudy uzbek. nauchno-issled. Inst. vet. *20:* 84–86 (1973).

327 Mazzotti, L. et al.: El difentano-70 en el tratamiento de las teniasis humanas. Revta Inst. Salubr. Enferm. trop. Méx. *16:* 9–14 (1956).

328 McConnell, J. D. et al.: The control of hydatid disease in Tasmania. Aust. vet. J. *55:* 140–145 (1979).

329 McNair, A. L.: Mebendazole and hydatid disease. Br. med. J. *i:* 1055 (1980).

330 Menrath, R. L. E. et al.: Toxicity of bunamidine. 2. Metabolic effects. N. Z. vet. J. *21:* 212–215 (1973).

331 Merdivenci, A. et al.: Investigation on the treatment of hymenolepiasis with mebendazole in rural areas. 1st Med. Conf. Parasit., Izmir, Turkey, pp. 114–116 (1977).

332 Meymerian, E. et al.: Host-parasite relationships in echinococcosis. VII. Resistance of the ova of *Echinococcus granulosus* to germicides. Am. J. trop. Med. Hyg. *11:* 360–364 (1962).

333 Meymerian, E. et al.: Host-parasite relationships in echinococcosis. X. Laboratory evaluation of chemical scolicides as adjuncts to hydatid surgery. Ann. Surg. *158:* 211–215 (1963).

334 Monisov, A. A. et al.: Treatment of patients with *Taenia saginata* with phenasal in combination with dichlorophen or acrichin. Medskaya Parazit. *35:* 603–604 (1966).

335 Mosbech, J.: Forsøg på behandling af mepacrin og dichloropen *Taenia saginata* med. Ugeskr. Laeg. *120:* 703–704 (1958).

336 Most, H. et al.: Yomesan (niclosamide) therapy of *Hymenolepis nana* infections. Am. J. trop. Med. Hyg. *20:* 206–208 (1971).

337 Mürmann, P. et al.: Notes on the tolerance of Droncit®. Vet. Med. Rev. *ii:* 142–153 (1976).

338 Murray-Lion, I. M. et al.: Complications of mebendazole treatment for hydatid disease. Br. med. J. *ii:* 1111–1112 (1979).

339 Nadzhafov, I. G.: Yomesan treatment of patients with persistent *Taenia saginata* infections. Trudy azerb. nauchno-issled. Inst. Med. Parazit. trop. S. M. Kirova *7:* 32–34 (1969).

340 Nadzhofov, I. G. et al.: Trichlorophen and trichlosal treatment of patients with normal and resistant *Taenia saginata* infestations. Medskaya Parazit. *43:* 491 (1974).

341 Nagahana, M. et al.: Treatment of *Taenia saginata* and *Diphyllobothrium latum* infections with bithionol. Am. J. trop. Med. Hyg. *15:* 351–354 (1966).

342 Nagaty, H. F. et al.: Clinical trials with 'Yomesan' in *Hymenolepis nana* infection. J. trop. Med. Hyg. *65:* 128–129 (1962).

343 Neumann, J. et al.: Mansonil – přípravek, k terapii taeniasis u psu a koček. Veterinárštvi (Czechoslovakia) *21:* 281–282 (1971).

344 Nikitin, V. F. et al.: Efficiency of bunamidine oxynaphthoate against experimental infections in dogs with *Echinococcus* and *Multiceps*. Byull. nauchno-tekh. inf. vses. Inst. gel'mint. K. I. Skryabina *12:* 55–57 (1974).

345 Nosik, A. F.: Resistance of oncospheres of *Echinococcus granulosus* to the influence of some physical and chemical factors. Proc. Kharkov Vet. Inst. *21:* 304–311 (1952).

346 Novak, M.: Efficacy of a new cestocide, Praziquantel, against larval *Mesocestoides corti* and *Taenia crassiceps* in mice. J. Parasit. *63:* 949–950 (1977).

347 Novak, M. et al.: The effect of mebendazole on different developmental stages of *Hymenolepis diminuta* cysticercoids. Can. J. Zool. *56:* 604–607 (1978).

348 Nurtaeva, K. S.: Experimental study with kamala and its combination with phenasal. Medskaya Parazit. *41:* 741–745 (1972).

349 Nurtaeva, K. S.: Experimental study of combinations of the piperazine and sodium salts of phenasal with bithionol, Trichlorophen and Kamala in Hymenolepis infections. Medskaya Parazit. *42:* 560–565 (1973).

350 Obermeier, J. et al.: Mutogenicity studies with praziquantel, a new anthelmintic drug: tissue-, host-, and urine-mediated mutagenicity assays. Archs Toxicol. *38:* 149–161 (1977).

351 Oguz, T.: The treatment of experimental cysticercosis *(Cysticercus tenuicollis).* Vet. Fak. Derg. Ankara Univ. *23:* 385–395 (1976).

352 Okoshi, S. et al.: Anthelmintic effect of dicestal tablets by oral administration on the canine tapeworm *Dipylidium caninum.* J. Jap. vet. med. Ass. *13:* 59–61 (1960).

353 Osborne, D. R.: Mebendazole and hydatid disease. Br. med. J. *i:* 796 (1980).

354 Pagani, G. L. et al.: Il sale della piperazina *N*-(2′-cloro-4′nitrofenil)-5-clorosalicilamide nella terapia delle teniasi del cane. Boll. Ass. ital. vet. pic. anim. *8:* No. 2 (1969).

355 Palva, I. P.: The effectiveness of certain drugs in the expulsion of the fish tapeworm. Annls Med. intern. Penn. *52:* 89–92 (1963).

356 Park Davis & Co.: Biomedical Sciences Division Medical Summary C1-358. Humatin® in Taeniasis (Ann Arbor, Michigan 1968).

357 Parmanova, S. K.: The effect of dichlorophen and phenasal on dogs. Samarkand. Koop. Inst. V. V. Kuibysheva, pp. 112–113 (1972).

358 Parmanova, S. K.: Experimental study of the effect of phenasal and dichlorophen on pre-imaginal *Echinococcus granulosus* and *Multiceps* in dogs. Samarkand. Koop. Inst. V. V. Kuibysheva, pp. 138–139 (1972).

359 Parnell, I. W.: Some observations on taeniid ovicides: screening techniques, and the effect of some inorganic compounds. J. Helminth. *39:* 257–272 (1965).

360 Pawlowski, Z.: Inorganic tin compounds as the alternative drug in human taeniarhynchosis. J. Parasit. *56:* 261 (1970).

361 Pawlowski, Z. et al.: Taeniasis and cysticercosis *(Taenia saginata).* Adv. Parasitol. *10:* 269–343 (1972).

362 Pawlowski, Z. et al.: Effect of mebendazole on hydatid cysts in pigs. Vet. Parasitol. *2:* 299–302 (1976).

363 Pawlowski, Z. et al.: The efficacy of mebendazole and praziquantel against *Taenia saginata* cysticercosis in cattle. Vet. Sci. Commun. *2:* 137–139 (1978).

364 Paz, G.: Tratamiento de teniasis saginata con praziquantel (Embay 8440). Boln chil. Parasit. *32:* 14–16 (1977).

365 Peña Chavarria, A. et al.: Mebendazole in the treatment of Taeniasis solium and Taeniasis saginata. Am. J. trop. Med. Hyg. *26:* 118–120 (1977).

366 Perera, D. R. et al.: Niclosamide treatment of cestodiasis. Clinical trials in the United States. Am. J. trop. Med. Hyg. *19:* 610–612 (1970).

367 Perez-Esandi, M. V. et al.: The ovicidal effect of selected chemicals against eggs of *Echinococcus granulosus.* Bull. Wld Hlth Org. *51:* 550–551 (1974).

368 Petrosyan, N. A. et al.: Results of treatment of taeniasis with phenasal and dichlosal. Medskaya Parazit. *38:* 244–245 (1969).

369 Piazza, V. et al.: Risultati terapeutici in alcune cestodiasi con l'associazione paramomicina e *N*-(2'-cloro-4'-nitrofenil)-5-cloro-salicilamide. Clinica terap. *34:* 313–324 (1965).

370 Polydorou, K.: The anti-echinococcosis campaign in Cyprus. Trop. Anim. Health Prod. *9:* 141–146 (1977).

371 Poole, J. B. et al.: Efficacy of niclosamide for the removal of tapeworm *(Dipylidium caninum* and *Taenia pisiformis)* from dogs. J. Am. vet. med. Ass. *159:* 78–80 (1971).

372 Prokopenko, L. I.: Taeniasis and its control in the USSR. Medskaya Parazit. *35:* 652–661 (1966).

373 Prokopenko, L. I. et al.: On the control of diphyllobothriasis in the Volgograd region. Medskaya Parazit. *39:* 442–447 (1971).

374 Prokopenko, L. I. et al.: The current state and prospects of eradication of *Taenia saginata* in the USSR. Medskaya Parazit. *44:* 131–137 (1975).

375 Prokopenko, L. I. et al.: The problem of diphyllobothriasis and the task of science and practice in the control of this infection. Medskaya Parazit. *45:* 135–142 (1976).

376 Quilici, M. et al.: Hydatidose: traitement préopératoire par flurombendazole. Nouv. Presse méd. *8:* 524 (1979).

377 Rajkovic Janje, R. et al.: Djelovanje Echinona® na *Echinococcus granulosus* u pasa. Vet. Glasn. *32:* 225–229 (1978).

378 Razumova, E. P. et al.: Effectiveness of treatment of diphyllobothriasis with dichlosal and Phenasal. Medskaya Parazit. *6:* 159–161 (1967).

379 Redl, P.: Újabb eredmények a kutya-galandférgesség terápiájában. Magy. Allatorv. Lap. *30:* 276–277 (1975).

380 Redl, P. et al.: A bunamidinhidroinaftoát és a niklozamid *Echinococcus granulosus* ellenes Hatékonyságának vizsgálata kutyákban. Magy. Allatorv. Lap. *30:* 332–335 (1975).

381 Redzhapov, A. et al.: Dehelminthization of dogs with cestodiasis. Veterinariya, No. 3, pp. 75–76 (1971).

382 Reisin, I. L. et al.: The permeability of the membranes of experimental secondary cysts of *Echinococcus granulosus* to (C^{14}) mebendazole. Int. J. Parasitol. *7:* 189–194 (1977).

383 Rim, H. J. et al.: Anthelmintic effect of Embay 8440 (Praziquantel) against cestodiasis. Korean J. Parasit. *15:* 168 (1977).

384 Rim, J. J. et al.: Therapeutic effects of praziquantel (Embay 8440) against *Hymenolepis nana* infection. Korean J. Parasit. *16:* 82–87 (1978).

385 Roberson, E. L.: Comparative effects of Uredofos, Niclosamide and Bunamidine hydrochloride against tapeworm infections in dogs. Am. J. vet. Res. *37:* 1483–1484 (1976).

386 Roberson, E. L.: Anticestodal and antitrematodal drugs; in Jones, Booth, McDonald, Veterinary pharmacology and therapeutics; 4th ed., pp. 1052–1078 (Iowa State University Press, 1977).

387 Roberson, E. L. et al.: Uredofos: anthelmintic activity against nematodes and cestodes in dogs with naturally occurring infections. Am. J. vet. Res. *37:* 1479–1482 (1976).

388 Rommel, M. V. et al.: zur Wirksamkeit von Praziquantel gegen Bandwürmer

89: 255–257 (1976).
in experimentell infizierten Hunden und Katzen. Berl. Münch. tierärztl. Wschr.

389 Ronald, N. E. et al.: Treatment of *Hymenolepis nana* in hamsters with Yomesan® (niclosamide). Lab. Anim. Sci. *25:* 219–220 (1975).

390 Rusak, L. V. et al.: The effect of trichlorophen, phenasal, bithionol and their mixtures on the tegument of different parts of the strobilar of *Diphyllobothrium latum*. Medskaya Parazit. *40:* 419–422 (1971).

391 Sakamoto, T.: Studies on echinococcosis. XXV. Anthelmintic action of drugs on larval *Echinococcus multilocularis* in vitro. Jap. J. vet. Res. *21:* 73–91 (1973).

392 Sakamoto, T.: Evaluation of the results of in vitro anthelmintic tests using *Echinococcus* protoscolices. Jap. J. Parasit. *24:* 65–66 (1975).

393 Sakamoto, T.: Comparison between scolicidal action of drugs against *Echinococcus multilocularis* in vitro and their therapeutic effect upon experimental echinococcosis in mice. Jap. J. Parasit. *24:* 66 (1975).

394 Sakamoto, T.: The anthelmintic effect of Droncit® on adult tapeworms of *Hydatigera taeniaeformis, Mesocestoides corti, Echinococcus multilocularis, Diphyllobothrium erinacei* and *D. latum*. Vet. Med. Rev. *i:* 64–74 (1977).

395 Sakamoto, T.: The cestocidal effect of praziquantel on the larval stages of *Hydatigera taeniaeformis, Mesocestoides corti* and *Echinococcus multilocularis* in laboratory animals. Vet. Med. Rev. *ii:* 153–162 (1977).

396 Sakamoto, T.: Relationships between anthelmintic effects of drugs against *Echinococcus multilocularis* in vitro and in vivo. Mem. Fac. Agric. Kagoshima Univ. *15:* 115–123 (1979).

397 Sakamoto, T. et al.: Studies on echinococcosis. XVI. Effects of drugs upon scolices and daughter cysts of *Echinococcus multilocularis* in vitro. Jap. J. vet. Res. *13:* 127–136 (1965).

398 Sakamoto, T. et al.: Studies on pharmaco-therapy against larval and adult multiocular echinococcosis. 1. Anthelmintic and ovicidal effects of drugs against adult *Echinococcus multilocularis*. Jap. J. Parasit. *20:* 120–131 (1971).

399 Sakamoto, T. et al.: Studies on effects of drugs upon protoscoleces of *Echinococcus granulosus* in vitro. 1. Scolicidal effect of salicylanilide and bisphenol derivatives against *Echinococcus granulosus* in vitro. Jap. J. vet. Res. *23:* 81–94 (1975).

400 Sakamoto, T. et al.: Studies on effects of drugs upon protoscoleces of *Echinococcus granulosus* in vitro. II. Scolicidal effect of antibiotics, antineoplastic and other agents against *Echinococcus granulosus* in vitro. Mem. Fac. Agric. Kagoshima Univ. *15:* 125–130 (1979).

401 Sakamoto, T. et al.: Studies on anthelmintic effects of praziquantel against parasites in animals. 1. The efficacy of praziquantel against various cestodes in animals. Bull. Fac. Agric. Kagoshima Univ. *29:* 81–87 (1979).

402 Salas, C.: Vergleich der Wirksamkeit von 2 neuen Verbindungen bei der Behandlung der Hymenolepiasis; Diss. Universität Mexico (1962).

403 Salem, H. H. et al.: Paromomycin and *Taenia saginata*. Lancet *ii:* 1360 (1967).

404 Salem, H. H. et al. Treatment of *Taenia saginata* and *Hymenolepis nana* infections with paromomycin. Trans. R. Soc. trop. Med. Hyg. *63:* 833–836 (1969).

405 Schantz, P. M. et al.: The efficiency of divided doses of fospirate against im-

mature *Echinococcus granulosus* infections in dogs. Am. J. vet. Res. *37:* 619–620 (1976).

406 Schantz, P. M. et al.: Efficacy of divided doses of GS23654 against immature *Echinococcus granulosus* infections in dogs. Am. J. vet. Res. *37:* 621–622 (1976).

407 Schenone, H. et al.: Tratamiento de las infecciones por *Hymenolepis nana* en niños con una dosis oral única de praziquantel (Embay 8440). Boln chil. Parasit. *32:* 11–13 (1977).

408 Schneider, J.: Traitement du taeniasis par le 5-5′dichloro-2,2′-dihydroxydiphényl méthane. Thérapie *14:* 63–67 (1959).

409 Schneider, J.: Traitement du taeniasis a *T. saginata* par le niclosamide: 5-chloro-*N*-(2-chloro-4-nitrophényl) salicylamide. Bull. Soc. Path. exot. *56:* 451–461 (1963).

410 Schultz, M. G. et al.: An epizootic of bovine cysticercosis. J. Am. vet. Med. Ass. *155:* 1708–1717 (1969).

411 Schwabe, C. W. et al.: Host-parasite relationships in echinococcosis. IX. In vitro survival of hydatid scolices and the effects of drugs upon scolex respiration. Am. J. trop. Med. Hyg. *12:* 338–345 (1963).

412 Seaton, D. R.: A short way with *Taenia saginata.* Lancet *i:* 808–809 (1956).

413 Seaton, D. R.: On the use of dichlorophen as a taeniafuge for *Taenia saginata.* Ann. trop. Med. Parasit. *54:* 338–340 (1960).

414 Seaton, D. R.: Chemotherapy of intestinal helminthiasis. Practitioner *188:* 58–61 (1962).

415 Seftel, H. C. et al.: Treatment of human tapeworm infections with Yomesan. Single dose treatment in non-fasting subjects. S. Afr. med. J. *38:* 263 (1964).

416 Sen, A. B. et al.: Screening of cesticidal compounds on a tapeworm *Hymenolepis nana* in vitro. Br. J. Pharmacol. *15:* 436–439 (1960).

417 Seubert, J. et al.: Synthesis and properties of praziquantel, a novel broad spectrum anthelmintic with excellent activity against schistosomes and cestodes. Experientia *33:* 1036–1037 (1977).

418 Shafei, A. Z.: Clinical trials on a new taeniacidal drug 2,2′-dihydroxy-5,5′-dichloro-diphenyl methane. J. Egypt. med. Ass. *42:* 488–492 (1959).

419 Shafei, A. Z.: Ensaios sobre o efecto da *N*-2′-chloro-4′-nitrofenil-5-clorosalicilamida. Hospital *67:* 1308–1311 (1965).

420 Shafei, A. Z.: The treatment of pregnant women with *N*-(2-chloro-4-nitro-phenyl)-5-chloro-salicylamide: a new taeniacidal drug. Alex. med. J. *11:* 35–37 (1965).

421 Shafei, A. Z. et al.: *N*-(2′-chlor-4′nitrophenyl)-5-chlorsalicylamide in the treatment of *Taenia saginata* and *Hymenolepis nana* infections. Z. Tropenmed. Parasit. *13:* 194–198 (1962).

422 Shah, P. M. et al.: Observations on *Taenia saginata* infestation in children and measures for eradication. J. Indian med. Ass. *45:* 423–426 (1965).

423 Shah, P. M. et al.: Therapeutic trials in *Taenia saginata* infestation. Indian J. med. Sci. *19:* 399–406 (1965).

424 Sharp, M. L. et al.: A comparative critical assay on canine anthelmintics. Vet. Med. small Animal Clin. *68:* 131–132 (1973).

425 Shearer, G. C. et al.: The efficiency of bunamidine hydroxynaphthoate against *Echinococcus granulosus* in dogs. Res. vet. Sci. *10:* 296–299 (1969).

426 Siedel, M. C. et al.: A new broad-spectrum anthelmintic for dogs and cats. Proc. 20th Wld Vet. Congr., Thessaloniki 1975, p. 805.

427 Sirot, M.: Un nouveau traitement de *Taenia saginata:* le sulfate de Paromomycine. A propos de 20 observations personnelles; thèse médecine de Lyon No 217 (1965).

428 Standen, O.: Chemotherapy of helminthic infections; in Schnitzer, Hawking, Experimental chemotherapy, vol. 1, pp. 701–892 (Academic Press, New York 1963).

429 Steiner, K. et al.: The fate of praziquantel in the organism. I. Pharmacokinetics in animals. Eur. J. Drug Metab. Pharmacokinet. *2:* 85–95 (1976).

430 Steiner, K. et al.: The fate of praziquantel in the organism. II. Distribution in rats. Eur. J. Drug Metab. Pharmacokinet. *2:* 97–106 (1976).

431 Strufe, R. et al.: Experimentelle Untersuchungen mit *N*-(2′-Chlor-4′-Nitrophenyl)-5-Chlorsalicylamid, einem neuen Bandwurmmittel. Mitteilung 3: Studien über die Verteilung im Intestinaltrakt der Ratte. Arzneimittel-Forsch. *10:* 886–890 (1960).

432 Strufe, R. et al.: Über die Beeinflussung des Bandwurmstoffwechsels durch Arzneimittel. Z. Tropenmed. Parasit. *18:* 193–202 (1967).

433 Suvorov, V. Y. Treatment of *Taenia saginata* with dichlosal (Phenasal with dichlorophen) and Phenasal with acrichin. Medskaya Parazit. *35:* 233–234 (1966).

434 Szanto, J. et al.: Critical evaluation of taeniacidal antibiotic S15-1 (SQ21,704) for the removal of natural tapeworm infections in dogs and cats. Am. J. vet. Res. *40:* 673–675 (1979).

435 Taffs, L. F.: Continuous feed medication with thiabendazole for the removal of *Hymenolepis nana, Saphacia obvelata* and *Aspiculuris tetraptera* in naturally infected mice. J. Helminth. *49:* 173–177 (1975).

436 Taffs, L. F.: Further studies on the efficacy of triabendazole given in the diet of mice infected with *H. nana, S. obvelata* and *A. tetraptera.* Vet. Rec. *99:* 143–144 (1976).

437 Teichmann, P. et al.: Zur Taeniasis bei Hund und Katze und ihre Behandlung mit Vermitin. Mh. VetMed. *24:* 949–953 (1964).

438 Tetzlaff, R. D. et al.: Anthelmintic control of concurrent *Hymenolepis nana* and *Syphacia obvelata* infections in the mouse with Uredofos. Lab. Anim. Sci. *28:* 287–289 (1978).

439 Thakur, A. S. et al.: Efficacy of Droncit against *Echinococcus granulosus* in dogs. Am. J. vet. Res. *39:* 859–860 (1978).

440 Thakur, A. S. et al.: *Echinococcus granulosus:* ovicidal activity of praziquantel and bunamidine hydrochloride. Expl Parasit. *47:* 131–133 (1979).

441 Thakur, A. S. et al.: Empleo del praziquantel solo y en combinación con el bromhidrato de arecolina para el tratamiento contra *Echinococcus granulosus* en perros. Revta Med. vet. B. Aires *60:* 154–157 (1979).

442 Thienpont, D. et al.: Anthelmintic activity of mebendazole against *Cysticercus fasciolaris.* J. Parasit. *60:* 1052–1053 (1974).

443 Thomas, H.: Reinfektion und Rezidiv bei *Hymenolepis-nana*-Infektionen. Z. ParasitKde *26:* 25–33 (1975).

444 Thomas, H. et al.: A new compound against adult tapeworms. 7th Wld Ass. Adv. Vet. Parasit., Thessaloniki 1975.

445 Thomas, H. et al.: Investigations about treatment of larval cestodes. 7th Wld Adv. Vet. Parasit., Thessaloniki 1975.

446 Thomas, H. et al.: Praziquantel – a new cestocide. Pestic. Sci. *8:* 556–560 (1977).

447 Thomas, H. et al.: The efficacy of praziquantel against cestodes in animals. Z. ParasitKde *52:* 117–127 (1977).

448 Thomas, H. et al.: The efficacy of praziquantel against cestodes in cats, dogs and sheep. Res. vet. Sci. *24:* 20–25 (1978).

449 Thomas, H. et al.: Zur Wirksamkeit von Praziquantel bei der experimentellen Cysticercose und Hydatidose. Z. ParasitKde *55:* 165–179 (1978).

450 Thompson, C. D. et al.: Human infection with a tapeworm *Bertiella* sp., probably of African origin. Br. med. J. *iii:* 659–660 (1967).

451 Thomson, R. L.: Obstructive jaundice due to hydatid cyst of the liver. Med. J. Aust. *i:* 664–666 (1978).

452 Tinar, R. et al.: The efficacy of praziquantel (Droncit, Embay 8440) against *Hymenolepis nana* in mice. Vet. Fak. Derg. Ankara Üniv. *25:* 366–371 (1978).

453 Todd, K. S. et al.: Activity of uredofos, niclosamide, bunamidine, hydrochloride and arecoline hydrobromide against *Mesocestoides corti* in experimentally infected dogs. Am. J. vet. Res. *39:* 315–316 (1978).

454 Todorov, R.: Our experience in the treatment of taeniasis. Savremenna Med. *24:* 22–24 (1973).

455 Trejos, A. et al.: Comparative value of arecoline hydrobromide and bunamidine hydrochloride for the treatment of *Echinococcus granulosus* in dogs. Res. vet. Sci. *19:* 212–213 (1975).

456 Tsai, C. S. et al.: The mass treatment of *Taenia saginata* with bithionol. Jap. J. Parasit. *20:* 177–180 (1971).

457 Tumol'skaya, N. I. et al.: Mebendazole in the treatment of acute and chronic states of helminthiasis. Communication 2. Mebendazole (Vermox) in the treatment of unilocular and multilocular hydatidosis. Medskaya Parazit. *48:* 17–24 (1979).

458 Ulivelli, A.: Terapia antibiotica della teniasi (primi favorevoli risultati del trattamento con paromomicina). Riv. Clin. pediat. *72:* 371–383 (1963).

459 Ulvelli, A.: A proposito della terapia antibiotica (con paromycina) in alcune cestodiasi. Mal. infett. parassit. *19:* 308–310 (1967).

460 Vakil, B. J. et al.: Clinical trials with mebendazole, a new broad spectrum anthelmintic. J. trop. Med. Hyg. *78:* 154–158 (1975).

461 Van den Bossche, H.: Biochemical effects of the anthelmintic drug mebendazole; in Van den Bossche, Comparative biochemistry of parasites, pp. 139–157 (Academic Press, New York 1972).

462 Vanparijs, O. et al.: Anthelminthische Wirkung des Mebendazols gegen Nematoden und Zestoden bei Hunden. Dt. tierärztl. Wschr. *80:* 320–322 (1973).

463 Verheyen, A. et al.: The effects of mebendazole on the ultrastructure of cestodes; in Van den Bossche, Biochemistry of parasites and host parasite relationships, pp. 605–618 (Elsevier, North-Holland Biomedical Press, Amsterdam 1976).

464 Verheyen, A. et al.: Scanning electron microscopic observations of *Cysticercus fasciolaris (Taenia taeniaeformis)* after treatment of mice with mebendazole. J. Parasit. *64:* 411–425 (1978).

465 Virji, A. S. et al.: Bunamidine uptake and distribution in rats and dogs. Aust. J. exp. Biol. med. Sci. *50:* 209–215 (1972).

466 Waitz, J. A. et al.: Effects of paromomycin on tapeworms of mice, rats and cats. J. Parasit. *52:* 830–831 (1966).

467 Walther, M. et al.: Zur Wirksamkeit von Praziquantel bei der experimentellen Saginata-Zystizerkose des Rindes. Zentbl. VetMed. B *26:* 828–834 (1979).

468 Walther, M. et al.: The efficacy of praziquantel against *Taenia saginata* cysticercosis in naturally infected calves. Tropenmed. Parasitol. *30:* 401–403 (1979).

469 Waris, E.: Dichlorophen in the treatment of diphyllobothriasis. Annls Med. intern. Fenn. *49:* 225–234 (1960).

470 Watkins, T. I.: The chemotherapy of helminthiasis. J. Pharm. Pharmac. *10:* 209–227 (1958).

471 Webbe, G.: The hatching and activation of taeniid ova in relation to the development of cysticercosis in man. Tropenmed. Parasitol. *18:* 354–369 (1967).

472 Weinmann, C. J.: Cestodes and Acanthocephala; in Jackson, Herman, Singer, Immunity to parasitic animals, vol. 2, pp. 1021–1059 (Appleton-Century-Crofts, New York 1970).

473 Werczberger, A. et al.: Disseminated echinococcosis with repeated anaphylactic shock. Treated with mebendazole. Chest *76:* 482–484 (1979).

474 Westcott, R. B.: Efficacy of niclosamide in the treatment of *Taenia taeniaeformis* infections in cats. Am. J. vet. Res. *28:* 1475–1477 (1967).

475 White, J. B. et al.: Ovine cysticercosis in the Albany region of Western Australia. Aust. vet. J. *52:* 73–79 (1976).

476 Whitten, L. K.: The treatment of tapeworm infestations in man and animals. Vet. Revs Annot. *2:* 1–24 (1956).

477 Wikerhauser, T. et al.: The efficiency of praziquantel against immature stages of *Echinococcus granulosus* in the dog. Acta parasitol. iugosl. *7:* 33–36 (1976).

478 Wikerhauser, T. et al.: A study of the effect of mebendazole and praziquantel on secondary *Echinococcus granulosus* in mice. Acta parasitol. iugosl. *9:* 57–63 (1978).

479 Williams, J. F. et al.: The influence of gelatin capsules upon the activity of bunamidine hydrochloride against *Echinococcus granulosus* in dogs. Res. vet. Sci. *11:* 392–394 (1970).

480 Williams, J. F. et al.: The effect of bunamidine hydrochloride on the infectivity of taeniid ova. J. Parasit. *59:* 1141–1144 (1973).

481 Williams, J. F. et al.: Sudden death associated with treatment of three dogs with bunamidine hydrochloride. J. Am. vet. med. Ass. *168:* 689–691 (1976).

482 Williams, R. J.: Determination of the value of formalin and boiling water as taeniid ovicides. Res. vet. Sci. *4:* 550–555 (1963).

483 Wilson, J. F. et al.: A clinical trial of mebendazole in the treatment of alveolar hydatid disease. Am. Rev. resp. Dis. *118:* 747–757 (1978).

484 Wittner, M. et al.: Paromomycin therapy of human cestodiasis with special reference to hymenolepiasis. Am. J. trop. Med. Hyg. *20:* 433–435 (1971).

485 Yagudaev, M. S.: The influence of a protein diet on the efficacy of Phenasal and other anthemintics in white mice infected with *Hymenolepis nana.* Medskaya Parazit. *43:* 305–307 (1974).

486 Yamashita, J. et al.: The use of drugs against larval stages of *Echinococcus*. Bull. Wld Hlth Org. *39:* 130–131 (1968).
487 Zhuravets, A. K.: Tests on the worming of dogs infected with *Echinococcus*. Sb. nauch. Rab. Severo-Kavk. Zonal. Nauchno-issled. Vet. Inst. *15:* 199–205 (1972).
488 Zhuravets, A. K. et al.: Bunamidine oxynaphthoate as an effective anthelmintic against *Echinococcus* and *Multiceps* in dogs. Byull. nauchno-tekh. inf. vses. Inst. gel'mint. K. I. Skryabina *14:* 22–23 (1974).
489 Zhuravets, A. K. et al.: A field trial of bunamidine oxynaphthoate against cestodes in dogs. Byull. nauchno-tekh. inf. vses. Inst. gel'mint. K. I. Skryabina *14:* 24–25 (1974).
490 Zukovic, M. et al.: Istraživanja anthelmintičkog djelovanja scolbana na trakavicu *E. granulosus* u psa. Vet. Arh. *37:* 163–166 (1967).
491 Zukovic, M. et al.: Djelovanje praziquantela (Droncita) na trakavicu *Echinococcus granulosus* u psa. Acta parasitol. iugosl. *7:* 75–77 (1976).

M. A. Gemmell, Hydatid Research Unit, Research Division,
Ministry of Agriculture and Fisheries, University of Otago Medical School,
PO Box 913, Dunedin (New Zealand)

Antibiotics Chemother., vol. 30, pp. 115–134 (Karger, Basel 1981)

Chagas' Disease

Ricardo Ribeiro-dos-Santos[a], *Anis Rassi*[b], *Fritz Köberle*[a]

[a] Faculty of Medicine of Ribeirão Preto, University of São Paulo, Brazil;
[b] Faculty of Medicine, Federal University of Goiás, Brazil

Introduction

Chagas' disease is the most frequent and treacherous plague on the American continent and occupies an exclusive and unique position amongst all existing morbid entities because of the extraordinary way it was discovered. It is perhaps the only illness that really deserves to be called by the name of the man who discovered it because *Chagas* described both the etiologic agent and the disease simultaneously.

It is fascinating that *Chagas,* 28 years old, living in an old railroad car at a construction site in the interior of Brazil (Minas Gerais) and having only the simplest medical instruments, managed to identify an unknown illness among a jumble of diseases, such as malaria, dysentery, verminosis, subnutrition, chronic alcoholism and others. *Chagas* had successfully resolved the antimalaria campaign in Santos, and in 1908 was appointed to supervise a similar program in the state of Minas Gerais (Lassance), where the company building a new railway was desperately fighting against malaria. While engaged in this very demanding and responsible job, *Chagas* discovered that the primitive huts in this area were infected with innumerous blood-sucking bugs (Triatominae), which lived in the countless clefts of the mud walls and came out at night to suck the blood of the inhabitants. By examining these bugs, he discovered as yet unidentified trypanosomes in their intestines. He immediately suspected that these flagellates could be transmitted to vertebrates and man, eventually producing disease. Following this idea, he soon found the same flagellates in the blood of a house cat and later in the blood of a feverish child in the same house.

In 1909 *Chagas* [11] reported to the National Academy of Medicine in Rio de Janeiro his discovery of the new trypanosomiasis caused by *Schizotrypanum cruzi,* which was named in honor of his teacher *Oswaldo Cruz,* and is known today as *Trypanosoma cruzi.*

Parasitology and Life Cycle

T. cruzi [11] is a flagellate protozoan belonging to the class Mastigophora and the family Trypanosomatidae. In the blood stream of vertebrate hosts, which include man, cats, dogs, monkeys and opossums, the parasite takes the tripomastigote form. It is approximately 25 μm in length and 2 μm in width and exhibits a large subterminal blepharoplast. In contrast to all other trypanosomes, *T. cruzi* does not multiply in the blood stream. It penetrates the host cells, where it changes to the amastigote forms and then divides by successive binary fission. Multiplication of the amastigotes leads to the formation of a pseudocyst that distends the cell, and the amastigotes then differentiate to tripomastigotes (flagellate forms). When the pseudocyst is formed, the actively moving tripomastigotes rupture the cell membrane and disperse, returning to the blood or entering a new cell. The fact that *T. cruzi* division in the host occurs intracellularly makes the treatment of Chagas' disease particularly difficult.

In addition to the cycle in the certebrate host, *T. cruzi* also undergoes changes in invertebrate vectors. The vectors are the strictly hematophagous Hemiptera insects belonging to the family Reduviidae, subfamily Triatominae, which ingest trypanosomes while feeding on infected vertebrates. The most important species in South America are *Triatoma infestans, Panstrongylus megistus* and *Rhodnius prolixus.* The typical trypanosome form (tripomastigote) found in the blood of vertebrates may be ingested by the transmitting insect and pass through various developmental stages in its intestinal tract, evolving into the metacyclic trypanosome (infective form) only when the rectum is reached. Reproduction is by binary fission of the epimastigote forms in the midgut. This stage lasts 8–10 days.

The metacyclic trypanosomes (tripomastigotes), found in feces, are infectious to both men and animals. They penetrate the interior of the cells through the normal mucosa or through a skin lesion. They lose their flagella and undulating membrane at the site of inoculation, thus becoming the amastigote forms.

Epidemiology

American trypanosomiasis or Chagas' disease affects a wide variety of human and animal populations throughout the American continent, from the Southern United States to the Argentine. Approximately 10 million people have been estimated to be infected in Brazil alone. The American trypanosomiasis was probably originally an invertebrate parasitosis. After inclusion of various vertebrates in the life cycle and adaptation of several vector species to human habitation, it took on the character of a typical zoonosis [13].

The infection is transmitted from man to man or from animal to man by a triatomine bug. About 100 species have been found on the American continent. Outside the American continent, approximately 10 species have been reported, though none of them is naturally infected by *T. cruzi.*

The triatomine insects adapted to human dwellings are generally found in mud huts where they live in the cracks of the walls and behind pictures. They come out after dark and usually bite uncovered parts of the body. Their bite is painless and does not awake the victim. These insects are exclusively hematophagous and more active in summer. In endemic areas the percentage of infected triatomine insects varies from 20 to 40%. Transmission of *T. cruzi* usually occurs by rubbing the faeces of the triatomine insects, which are rich in metacycle (tripomastigotes) trypanosomes, on skin abrasions caused by scratching or by the bite. The mucosa is a frequent site of entrance for the parasite but transmission through normal skin is not possible.

Congenital transmission, suspected by *Chagas* [12], has been observed in animals by *Mayer and Rocha-Lima* [27], *Nathan-Larrier* [29] and *Mazza* [28] and was demonstrated in man by *Dao* [16], *Howard* [19] and *Lisboa-Bittencourt* [25]. Transmission to humans by blood transfusion was proved by *Freitas* et al. [17], and today this represents the only mechanism of transmission outside endemic areas.

The most suitable animals for laboratory studies are the dog, cat, mouse, rat and guinea pig, which are most sensitive to the infection, especially when young. Birds, reptiles, and batrachians are refractory to this infection.

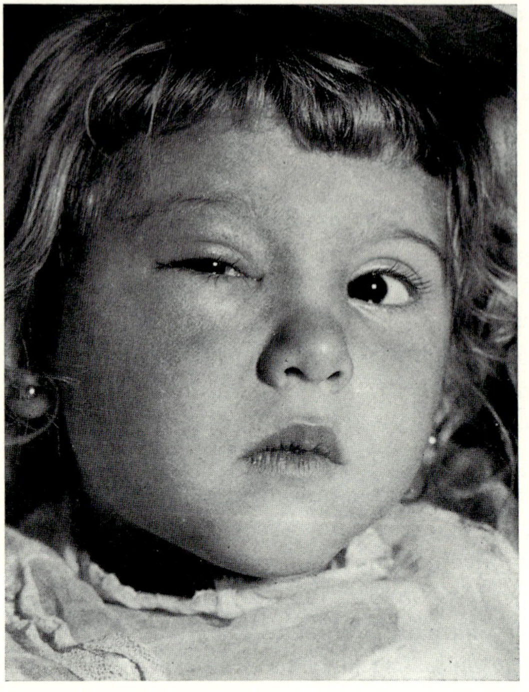

Fig. 1. Sign of portal entry in Chagas' disease (ophthalmic complex and chagoma).

Acute Phase

This form occurs mainly in young children generally after an incubation period of 1–2 weeks. It is characterized by fever, slight generalized lymph node enlargement, moderate hepatosplenomegaly, and facial or generalized edema. Tachycardia is often present owing to acute myocarditis. The acute phase can only be characterized by the demonstration of *T. cruzi* in the blood stream. In about 50% of the cases, the site of entry is indicated by unilateral bipalpebral edema with satellite preauricular lymph node enlargement (fig. 1). In others, the site of entry is indicated by ulcerative and nodular skin lesions (chagoma), followed by regional lymph node enlargement. In the remaining 25% of cases it is impossible to demonstrate the site of entry.

After binary division of the parasites (amastigote forms) inside the cells of the portal of entry, flagellate forms (tripomastigotes) begin to ap-

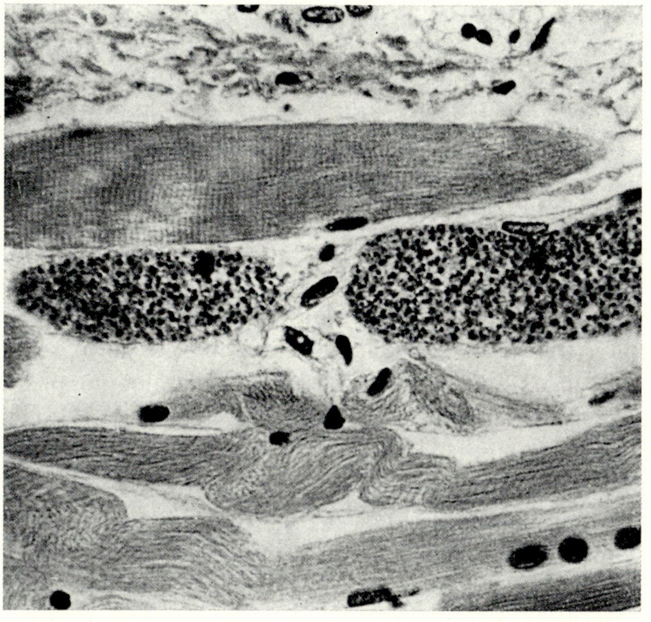

Fig. 2. Pseudocyst of amastigote forms in striated muscle fibers of the esophagus.

pear in the blood stream, and a generalized infection occurs. During dissemination of the infection, the parasites (tripomastigotes) may penetrate any tissue but preferentially muscle (smooth, striated or cardiac fiber) glia and fat cells.

Although clinical manifestations of cardiac involvement are not always conspicuous in the acute phase, moderate heart enlargement, accompanied by electrocardiographic changes, which include sinus tachycardia, low voltage, prolonged P-R interval and primary T wave change. Hematological study reveals leukocytosis due to marked lymphocytosis with relative neutropenia.

The histologic alterations found in chagoma are: proliferation of reticular endothelial cells as well as fibroblasts; presence of amastigote parasites in reticular endothelial cells or in macrophages; hyperemia and localized edema. Parasites are found in almost all organs where they divide and differentiate inside the cells (about 5 days) (fig. 2). The parasite-infected cells, rupture and tripomastigote forms are again disseminated through the blood stream. Two kinds or tissue reactions appear around the ruptured pseudocyst: a degenerative reaction with eventual lysis of some cells (mainly neurons and cardiac muscle cells), followed by inflammatory mononuclear infiltration. The mechanism of these alterations will be discussed later.

Chronic Phase

As the symptomatology of the acute phase disappears (4–6 weeks), the chronic phase arises, generally without any important manifestations but with very low parasitemia, demonstrable only by means of xenodiagnosis. Only in rare cases does a suspicious symptomatology appear soon after the acute phase. In the overwhelming majority of cases, symptoms arise only after an asymptomatic or apparently asymptomatic period of 10–20 years or even after a much longer interval. However, the diagnosis may still be confirmed by xenodiagnosis or by highly specific serological tests. These so-called 'late manifestations' in the chronic phase have been attributed to a subliminal, pauciparasitemic infection developing over many years mainly in the heart muscle, where it finally produces the most frequent and impressive chronic chagasic cardiopathy.

Chagas' Syndromes

When *Chagas* asked his collaborator *Vianna* for an anatomopathological and histological study he requested a special examination of the nervous system. This strange solicitation indicates that *Chagas* suspected an important lesion of the nervous system, which was actually found by *Vianna* [40]. Quantitative studies on biopsy and necropsy material from man and animals with natural and experimental infections showed a reduction in the number of ganglion cells in different areas of the central and/or peripheral nervous system [20].

The destruction of nervous cells occurs exclusively or principally during the acute phase of the disease and represents the indispensable causal factor of the numerous Chagas' syndromes. After these quantitative investigations of the nervous system, the initial pathogenetic concept of American trypanosomiasis was modified. Chagas' disease is essentially like most other diseases caused by trypanosomes, a disease of the nervous system and, according to *Chagas* [14]: 'one that, in human pathology, provokes the largest number of organic changes in the central nervous system'. Today we know that this affirmation is also valid for the peripheral autonomous system [21, 22].

We wish to emphasize that denervation is the absolutely indispensable element for the appearance of the numerous Chagas' syndromes, but its development depends on the conjoint action of many other factors, among which are localization and intensity of denervation, sensitivity of the affected organ to denervation, solicitation and overloading of the damaged structure. To determine the intensity and evolution of the syndrome, the contribution of each of these factors must be evaluated and whenever possible, quantitatively.

Concerning localization, it is evident that the clinical manifestation depends on the damage to the corresponding part of the nervous system, be it situated in the organ itself, in its vicinity, or in the central nervous system.

The intensity of denervation has real value only when related to the sensitivity of the affected organ. We have established the limits of tolerance for denervation to heart (20%), colon (50%), bronchi (75%) and esophagus ($>$ 90%) for the appearance of morphological alterations in these organs. It is obvious that the intensity of denervation needed for functional alterations to appear is much lower [23].

It is easy to understand that functional disturbances become more evident, and occur sooner, the more frequently, the more intensely and the longer the organs are requested or overloaded. Thus, some syndromes appear immediately after ganglion cell destruction, whereas others become manifest only after an asymptomatic or latent period of many years.

Furthermore, we must consider that in all parts of the central and peripheral nervous system a sometimes considerable physiological denervation occurs which increases with age. For the normal human esophagus and colon there is approximately 50% reduction in the number of ganglion cells in the myenteric plexus between the ages of 20 and 75 years. In addition to this physiological denervation, another type occurs which is caused by overloading and which plays a significant role in chagasic organs by markedly reducing the number of nervous cells.

To summarize, we can state that the absolutely indispensable prerequisite for the appearance of functional or morphological manifestations of chagasic syndromes is composed of three elements: the original chagasic denervation, the increasing physiological denervation and finally the neuronal destruction in consequence of the overloading and exhaustion of

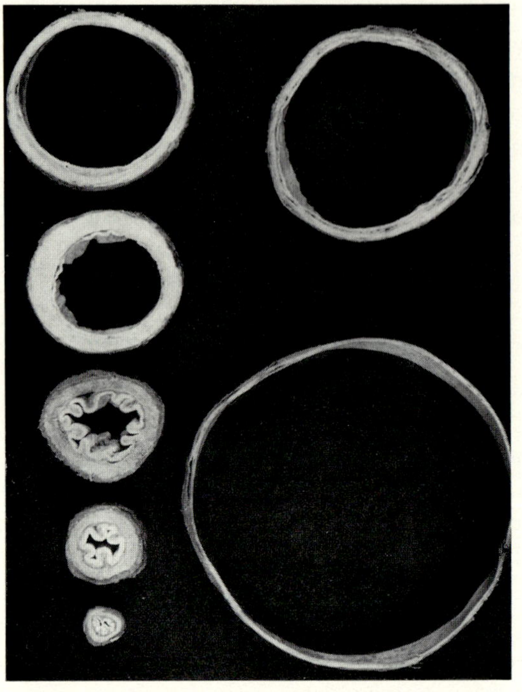

Fig. 3. Evolution of chagasic megaesophagus.

still existing ganglion cells. The sum of these three mechanisms of neuronal destruction explains the appearance of the 'late manifestations' many years after the acute infection, when total denervation reaches the limit of tolerance to denervation of the organ.

Quantitative investigations on organs of chagasic patients with and without morphological lesions have shown denervation in all organs, but the morphologically altered ones exhibited considerably more marked neuronal reduction than the apparently normal organs [24]. This study shows that the verification of the presence of chagasic symptoms or syndromes depends essentially on the method used.

It is impossible to discuss all the central or peripheral chagasic neuropathies in a short review, therefore we will concentrate our discussion on two manifestations: megas and cardiopathy.

The evolution of megaesophagus is shown in figure 3. The first alteration caused by the disturbed peristalsis is an insignificant dilatation of the organ which is only temporary and soon compensated for by hypertrophy of the musculature. Through a vicious circle of dilatation and hypertrophy the muscle layer may increase up to 25 times its normal weight. However, insufficient irrigation of this megaesophagus finally leads to muscle atrophy and wall atony with enormous dilatation and elongation of the organ (mega-dolicho-esophagus). The same pathogenetic mechanism leads to the same alterations in all the hollow muscular organs.

Obviously denervation is not the only causative factor determining the megas syndromes, in addition to peripheral neuronal destruction, many other factors may enhance the intensity of dilation and the time of appearance.

Chagas' cardiomyopathy is by far the most frequent and serious late manifestation of American trypanosomiasis. *Chagas* considered the principal abnormality seen in this form of cardiomyopathy to be an 'alteration in the formation and conduction of the excitatory impulse', an observation subsequently confirmed by others. A large number of patients die from heart block or ventricular fibrillation as a consequence of altered heart function. Alternatively, enormous cardiomegaly may be found with severe damage to the myocardium in patients who never have suffered from any symptoms of heart disease and who have died from other causes. Diagnosing Chagas' cardiomyopathy can therefore be difficult both clinically and pathologically. Macroscopically, the great majority of hearts in Chagas' cardiomyopathy show alteration in size and frequently in shape. Every degree of heart enlargement occurs, though usually enlargement of the right heart predominates. The mean weight is between 500 and 600 g and weights greater than 800 g are rare.

The majority of chagasic hearts show a greater or lesser degree of muscular hypertrophy and considerable dilatation of the chambers. A more typical and pathognomonic change is seen in the apices in more than half of all cases (fig. 4). This consists of a thinning and bulging of the apical region of the left ventricle and less frequently of the right ventricle or of both. Very rarely they may rupture, but thrombosis within them is very common. Thrombosis also occurs in the apical part of the ventricles in the absence of an aneurysm, a common occurrence in any chronically failing dilated ventricle. The presence of these thrombi explains the frequency of pulmonary and systemic emboli. The valves are never involved and the coronary arteries are often dilated.

Histological examination rarely reveals parasitic pseudocysts or granulomas, which explains why the parasite was not considered to be an

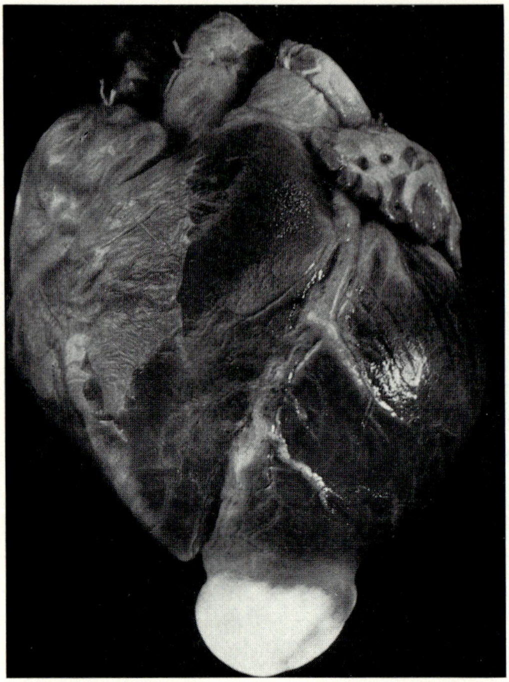

Fig. 4. Chronic chagasic cardiopathy with left apical aneurism.

etiological cause for chronic cardiomyopathy. Some degree of muscle hypertrophy is present, but in areas where muscle fibers are atrophied there may be focal interstitial fibrosis. Multiple foci of myocytolysis are frequently found, especially in the ventricular myocardium near the apex. Another important histological finding is the presence of many foci of mononuclear inflammatory cells frequently around the myocardial fibers. Parasites or their remains are never seen in these infiltrates which are probably not directly related to the presence of parasites.

The interpretation of the functional and morphological alterations seen in Chagas' cardiopathy is still very controversial. Many suggestions have been made to explain the peculiar clinical and structural changes found. They have been attributed to inflammation, hypoxemia, neurogenic, allergic, autoimmune and mechanical factors. All the mechanisms mentioned may play some part in the pathogenesis of this cardiomyopathy.

As we have stated before, we do believe that denervation, chiefly of the parasympathetic system, is the paramount event on the pathogenesis of Chagas' syndrome. The heart involvement is not an exception, though it is still the most disputed concept in the pathogenesis of Chaga's disease. Ganglion cell countings in the heart give support to this view. In addition, *Oliveira* [30] was able to reproduce experimentally the very picture of Chagas' heart disease by causing a pharmacological imbalance of the vegetative system of the heart.

Immunopathology

Although the pathological findings in Chagas' disease have been well described the mechanism of pathogenesis has not been fully elucidated. One of the most significant features of this disease was first described by *Vianna* [40]. He observed that when a parasite pseudocyst ruptured and released *T. cruzi* organisms, many of the surrounding uninfected cells were affected by degeneration, necrosis or lysis. *Magarinos-Torres* [26] and *Chagas* [15] suggested that this may be due to a hypersensitivity reaction which, although elicited by *T. cruzi* products, involved uninfected cells by an unexplained mechanism. Later experimental evidence provided support for the notion that mammalian cells might share common antigens with *T. cruzi* [35] and so an antiparasite response could give rise to an autoimmune reaction involving uninfected host cells. We believe that an alternative explanation may be provided by the demonstration that *T. cruzi* antigens can bind to mammalian cell surfaces [33] thereby rendering them potential targets for the host's immune response against the parasite (fig. 5).

The immunological consequences of this membrane modification may provide an explanation for the widespread destruction of nonparasited cells in the acute phase of Chaga's disease. *Ribeiro-dos-Santos and Hudson* [34] investigated the in vitro participation of the immune response to *T. cruzi* against syngenic and halogenic cell lines infected or previously sensitized with *T. cruzi* antigen and they suggested that parasite antigens are released following the disruption of infected cells or due to the destruction of parasites by the immune response. Parasite antigens could bind to host cells and thus render them susceptible to the host's own immune response against the infection. If parasite antigen production and subsequent host cell death is sustained over sufficiently long intervals,

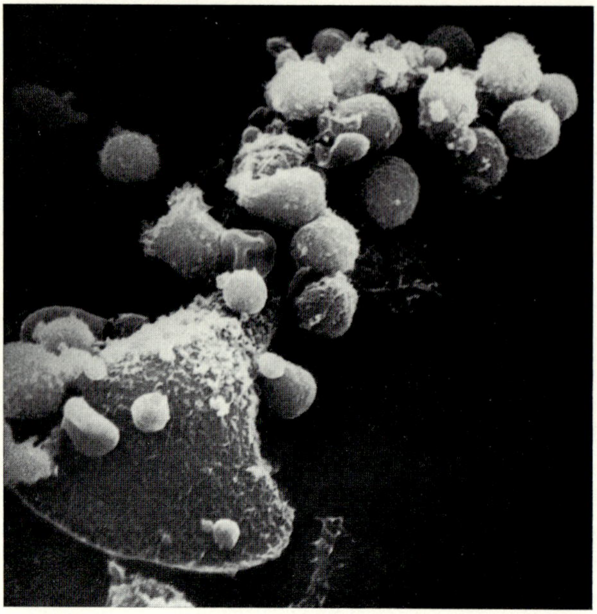

Fig. 5. Scanning electron microscopy of a neuron sensitized with *T. cruzi* antigens and incubated with singenic lymphocytes from a chronic chagasic mouse.

chronic release of self cell components might elicit an autoimmune response. The observation that pathological changes indicative of autoimmunity are only observed in a low percentage of patiens with *T. cruzi* infection suggests that a genetic predisposition might be required for the development of a self-sustaining autoimmune response which could perpetuate tissue damage.

Chemotherapy

The etiological treatment of Chagas' disease has been attempted since the discovery of the disease. A large number of drugs have been evaluated in vitro, on experimental animals and on man: bismuth salts, iodine compounds, emetine, acridine, arsenic and antimony compounds, kinolein derivatives, diamidines, sulfamides, sulfa-arsenobenzolic drugs, antibiotics, phenantridine compounds, semicarbazone compounds, nitrofurans, *p*-aminosalicylic acid, imidazole derivatives, piperazine and purine derivatives [6, 18, 32]. Some of these drugs were used in random trials, others because they had been recently added to the chemotherapeutic arsenal, or because of their effectiveness in the treatment of other trypanosomiasis or protozooses having an etiologic agent similar to *T. cruzi.*

On the basis of the pertinent literature, it can be concluded that most of the drugs assayed proved to be totally ineffective, although some (kinolein derivatives, sulfa-arsenobenzolic drugs, phenantridine derivatives, nitrofuran compounds, stylomycin, piperazine derivatives, and imidazole compounds) showed a clear antiparasitic activity of varying intensity.

It should be pointed out that until 1960 the methodology used for chemotherapeutic assays left much to be desired, mainly because of the absence of standardized criteria regarding dosage and evaluation of the therapeutic effects. Today we would consider the duration of treatment of most of these studies to be inadequate, often lasting no more than a few days, with results limited to reduced parasitemia, shorter duration of the acute phase, and decreased mortality index for the animals inoculated. The consensus of the investigators involved in these trials was that the drugs, though active against *T. cruzi,* were unable to cure the infection, since their antiparasitic effect was only on the trypomastigote forms, while the amastigote forms were unaffected.

A new phase in the attempts at the etiological treatment of Chagas' disease started in 1961 because of two significant contributions. The first was made by *Brener* [7] and concerned prolonged administration of drugs recognized to be active on the circulating forms. According to *Brener,* the use of these drugs for a sufficiently long period of time would theoretically permit eradication of the infection by parasite exhaustion, since, with continuous destruction of blood forms, no tissue forms could appear owing to a disruption in the 'parasite location in the cell–blood–new location in the cell' cycle. Thus, the well-known obstacle to treatment represented by the ineffectiveness of drugs on the tissue forms could be bypassed, since the tissue forms would be reached indirectly. To test this hypothesis, *Brener* administered nitrofurazone, the whole suppressive effect on *T. cruzi* had already been shown by *Packchanian* [31], to infected mice, at a dose of 100 mg/kg/day for 20 or 53 days. The longer period of treatment was more effective.

The second contribution consisted of the creation of a study group for the treatment of Chagas' disease in Brazil in 1962. The participants agreed to the standardization of working methods by establishing criteria for drug screening, selection of patients for treatment, treatment programs, and evaluation of results.

During this new period of attempted etiologic treatment of Chagas' disease, when long-lasting treatment programs were combined with newly-established rules for trials, many studies were performed on man, both on acute and chronic infection, with nitrofurazone (Eaton), levo-furaltadone (Eaton), furazolidone (Eaton), nifurtimox (Bayer), and benzonidal (Roche), and some studies with the kinolein compound BW 349.C.59 (Wellcome), metronidazole (Rhodia), and the piperazine compound CL 7.366 (Lederle). The results of these trials identified two drugs that deserved the attention of researchers in terms of the binomium tolerance and effectiveness: nifurtimox and benzonidazole, both commercially available, but still under careful scrutiny with respect to their curative ability.

The evaluation of these drugs is based mainly on xenodiagnosis (parasitologic criterion) and serum diagnostic tests (serologic criterion). In view of the peculiarities of the natural history of Chagas' disease, the clinical criterion is of quite limited value, both during the chronic and the acute phase. During the acute phase, because of the spontaneous regression of clinical manifestations, which occurs after a few weeks or a few months in most cases. The cases with intense manifestations or poor prognosis, such as meningoencephalitis and heart failure, might perhaps provide a satisfactory testing system. During the chronic phase, the value of the clinical criterion is even more limited if we consider that visceral damage is normally irreversible and that regression of some alterations can occur spontaneously in a few cases or simply after symptomatic treatment. Not even the follow-up of treated cases could provide the opportunity for full evaluation, since infected individuals may not show evidence for evolution of the disease, even when left untreated, after a few decades from the initial observation. A specific therapeutic treatment can be evaluated in absolute terms only when the disease evolves after treatment, thus demonstrating the ineffectiveness of the drug used. Some aspects of the parasitologic criterion (direct examination and hemoculture) can also be criticized. A direct blood test will show the presence of *T. cruzi* only during the acute phase, usually up to the end of the first month after infection. Thus, it cannot be used as a criterion for cure, even at this stage. However, on the basis of the results obtained, it can be useful to indicate whether or not more sensitive tests should be made. Hemoculture deserves further study in order to increase its sensitivity. When compared to xenodiagnosis, it is less cumbersome and often gives earlier results, though its sensitivity is lower.

Argentina, Brazil and Chile are the countries where both drugs have been more intensively used in clinical trials, both during the acute and the chronic phase, with comparable approaches used after the phase of experimental treatment. Several dosage programs have been tried, with the objective of reconciling effectiveness with tolerance.

Nifurtimox (3-methyl-4-(5′-nitrofurfurylidene-amine)-tetrahydro-4H-1,4-thiazine-1,1-dioxide), originally named Bayer 2502, was synthetized by Bayer and is sold under the name Lampit in pills containing 120 mg of the basic substance. An active series of clinical trials with nifurtimox was started in 1965, with results that can be considered discrepant when those obtained in Argentina and Chile are compared with those obtained in Brazil. In Argentina and Chile, the drug was shown to have a marked antiparasitic activity, demonstrated by the fact that a significant number of repeatedly negative xenodiagnoses were obtained after treatment in most cases, while in Brazil this result was obtained in a much smaller number of patients. The only exception is the results obtained in Rio Grande do Sul (a Brazilian state bordering with Argentina), which were similar to those reported for Argentina and Chile [4]. In view of the sharp differences in susceptibility to nifurtimox demonstrated by *Andrade* et al. [1] and *Brener* et al. [8] for different *T. cruzi* strains, the discrepancy of the results could be explained by the existence of different strains in the areas in question.

Benzonidazole (N-benzyl-2-nitro-1-imidazoleacetamide), originally called Ro 7-1051, was synthetized by Roche and is sold under the name of Rochagan in pills containing 100 mg of the active substance. Clinical trials with benzonidazole were started in 1971, and the results, in contrast to those obtained with nifurtimox, were consistent in all three countries. Benzonidazole also shows appreciable antiparasitic activity, since a large number of patients show a significant number of repeatedly negative xenodiagnoses after treatment [4].

At present, nifurtimox is used at a dose of 8–10 mg/kg body weight per day for adults, and 15 mg/kg body weight per day for children, for 60, 80 or 120 days, as tolerated. Among the side effects of the drug are hyporexia, weight loss, nausea and/or vomiting, and peripheral neuropathy, all of them reversible.

Benzonidazole is used at a dose of 5 mg/kg body weight per day for adults, and 10 mg/kg body weight per day for children, for 60 days. Its main side effects are skin allergy (generally of the polymorphous, nonbullous erythematous type) and peripheral neuropathy, both reversible.

It should be pointed out that, although specific treatment has a considerable effect on parasitemia, as shown by the negative xenodiagnoses both during the acute and the chronic phase of infection, in the experience of every investigator the behavior of the serum diagnostic tests has not been the same for both phases when compared to xenodiagnosis. During the acute phase the results of the serum diagnostic tests agree with those of xenodiagnosis, i. e. both tests are negative (demonstrating cure of the infection), or both continue to be positive (showing unsuccessful treatment). During the chronic phase, however, the serum diagnostic tests are persistently positive in parallel with a significant number of repeatedly negative xenodiagnoses. An exception of this rule is represented by recent chronic cases, i. e. the cases in which the initial period of infection occurred a few years before, whose behavior is similar to that observed during the acute phase. It was for this reason that we indicated earlier that the curative ability of the drugs under study remains partially under scrutiny.

It should be expected that, once the antigen *(T. cruzi)* is eliminated, no antibodies should be detected, and consequently the serum diagnostic tests should give negative results. Or it could be that, as proposed by *Schenone* et al. [36] and *Cerisola* et al. [10], serologic memory occurs, a mechanism by which the serum tests would remain positive for a long period of time or even for ever, even after the infection was eradicated?

Despite all the limitations indicated, it can be said that recently the specific treatment of Chagas' disease has given more encouraging results than a few years ago. We know that nifurtimox and benzonidazole are also active against the tissue forms, which they destroy [2, 5, 9], and the same has been observed for nitrofurazone [3] after the hypothesis raised by *Brener* [7]. However, treatment programs of prolonged duration are still being used, because they are needed even when the drugs in question are used. More active and less toxic compounds will have to be prepared.

Immunoprophylaxis

The progression of *T. cruzi* infection from an acute to a chronic stage and its recrudescence during immunosuppression in the chronic stage indicate that the immune response is able to control infection, but, since sterile immunity is rarely, if ever, achieved, the response is not totally effective. Thus potential immunoprophylactic regimes must improve upon adaptive immunity acquired by infection. Any candidate vaccine must therefore either be more immunogenic than the natural infection, using, for example, adjuvants or improved antigen presentation, or by analogy to the experimental protection achieved against tumors, must be able to immunize selectively avoiding either antigenic competition from nonprotective antigens or the induction of undesirable elements of the immune response such as 'blocking antibodies' or circulating immune complexes.

The observation of *Teixeira* et al. [39] and *Teixeira and Santos-Buch* [38] on the pathology of experimental Chagas' disease indicated the importance of determining the antigenic composition of vaccines. These investigators showed that the pathology associated with *T. cruzi* infection in rabbits could be reproduced using long-term immunization with killed parasites on their subfractions. This suggested that there might be cross-reactive antigens common to both the parasite and host tissue.

Although attempts have been made to analyze and characterize protective and cross-reactive antigens, the inherent complexity of the protozoan life cycle makes it difficult to formulate a rational basis upon which to proceed. Several investigators have used immune sera from patients and animals in immunoelectrophoresis as a means of limiting the spectrum of antigens. Arguably, however, these might well be the very antigens that one wished to avoid, those producing a vigorous but ineffective in vivo immune response.

A more compelling approach is to search for major antigens common to each of the mammalian life cycle stages. The identification of a single (or highly restricted) cell surface glycoprotein [37] that could be isolated by affinity chromatography was a significant contribution to this approach.

When one considers protection on a purely immunological basis, the most useful antigens must be those associated with the infected host cell, as shown in other virus, bacterial or protozoan infections. If one could detect and isolate parasite-associated antigens from amastigote-infected cells then the problem of immune elimination during the chronic phase might be solvable.

Ribeiro-dos-Santos and Hudson [33] using *T. cruzi*-infected human and murine cell lines, have used cell surface immunofluorescence to follow the expression of parasite antigens on infected host cells. Up to 72 h after infection, heavily infected muscle cells showed no evidence of parasite antigens on their membranes. At later times, corresponding to the appearance of extracellular parasites, large quantities of parasite antigens were detected on both infected and uninfected cells. In other experiments, they showed that these parasite-derived antigens had released into the medium and, even at concentrations as low as 10 $\mu g \cdot ml^{-1}$, were avidly adsorbed to the mammalian cells. This adsorption was not nonspecific; lymphocytes and erythrocytes, for example, did not adsorb these antigens.

The acquisition of parasite antigens renders even uninfected cells susceptible to the anti-parasite immune response in vitro. On this basis, the autoreactivity seen in association with *T. cruzi* infection would be a secondary phenomenon consequent upon the release of 'self' antigen after immune destruction of parasite-modified host cells. This model might provide one basis on which to screen candidate vaccines to avoid inducing an immunopathogenesis. The sensitizing antigens will either have to be characterized and removed or, more simply, be rendered biologically inactive but still immunogenic. Unfortunately, until now all experiments with *T. cruzi* vaccines have provided only partial protection.

References

1 Andrade, S. G.; Figueira, R. M.; Carvalho, M. L.; Gorini, D. F.: Influência da cepa do *Trypanosoma cruzi* na resposta à terapêutica experimental pelo Bay 2502. Resultados de tratamento a longo prazo. Rev. Inst. Med. trop. S. Paulo *17:* 380–389 (1975).

2 Andrade, S. G.; Figueira, R. M.: Estudo experimental sobre a ação terapêutica da droga Ro 7-1051 na infecção por diferentes cepas do *Trypanosoma cruzi.* Rev. Inst. Med. trop. S. Paulo *19:* 335–341 (1977).

3 Andrade, Z. A.; Brener, Z.: Ação da nitrofurazona (5-nitro-2-furaldeído-semicarbazona) sobre as formas intracelulares do *Trypanosoma cruzi* na doença de Chagas experimental. Rev. Inst. Med. trop. S. Paulo *11:* 222–228 (1969).

4 Boainain, E.; Rassi, A.: Terapêutica etiológica da doença de Chagas. Arq. bras. Cardiol. *32:* 395–399 (1979).

5 Bock, M.; Gönnert, R.; Haberkorn, A.: Studies with Bay 2502 on animals. Boln chil. Parasit *24:* 13–19 (1969).

6 Brener, Z.: Contribuição ao estudo da terapêutica experimental da doença de Chagas; tese Univ. Minas Gerais, Belo Horizonte (1961).

7 Brener, Z.: Atividade terapêutica do 5-nitro-furaldeído-semicarbazona (nitrofurazona) em esquemas de duração prolongada na infecção experimental do camundongo pelo *Trypanosoma cruzi.* Rev. Inst. Med. trop. S. Paulo *3:* 43–49 (1961).

8 Brener, Z.; Costa, C. A. G.; Chiari, C.: Differences in the susceptibility of *Trypanosoma cruzi* strains to active chemotherapeutic agents. Rev. Inst. Med. trop. S. Paulo *18:* 450–455 (1976).

9 Brener, Z.; Tafuri, W. L.; Almeida, M. T.: An electron microscope study of *Trypanosoma cruzi* intracellular forms in mice treated with an active nitrofuran compound. Rev. Inst. Med. trop. S. Paulo *11:* 245–249 (1969).

10 Cerisola, J. A.; Lugones, H.; Rabinovich, L. B.: Tratamiento de la enfermedad de Chagas (Talleres Gráficos Elias Porter, Buenos Aires 1972).

11 Chagas, C.: Nova tripanosomiase humana. Estudos sobre a morfologia e o ciclo evolutivo do *Schizotrypanum cruzi* n. g., n. sp., agente etiológico de nova entidade mórbida no homem. Mem. Inst. Oswaldo Cruz *1:* 159–218 (1909).

12 Chagas, C.: Nova entidade mórbida do homem. Resumo geral de estudos etiológicos e clínicos. Mem. Inst. Oswaldo Cruz *3:* 219–275 (1911).

13 Chagas, C.: O mal de Chagas. Arq. Soc. Med. Cirurg. S. Paulo *3:* 34–66 (1912).

14 Chagas, C.: Les formes nerveuses d'une nouvelle trypanosomiase *(Trypanosoma cruzi,* inoculé par *Triatoma megista).* Nouv. Iconogr. Salpêtr. *26:* 1–19 (1913).

15 Chagas, C.: Estado actual da trypanosomiase americana. Rev. Biol. Hyg. S. Paulo *5:* 58–64 (1934).

16 Dao, L.: Otros casos de enfermedad de Chagas en el Estado de Guarico (Venezuela). Formas agudas y crónicas. Observación sobre enfermedad de Chagas congénita. Rev. Policlín., Caracas *17:* 17–32 (1948).

17 Freitas, J. L.; Amato, V.; Sonntag, R.; Biancalana, A.; Nussenzweig, B.; Barreto, J. G.: Primeiras verificaçoes de transmissão acidental da moléstia de Chagas ao homem por transfusão de sangue. Rev. paul. Med. *40:* 36–40 (1952).

18 Goble, F. C.: Tratamiento de la enfermedad de Chagas. Bol. Of. sanit. panamer. *51:* 439–449 (1961).

19 Howard, J. E.: Clinical aspects of congenital Chagas' disease. New approaches in American trypanosomiasis. PAHO Sc. Publ. *318:* 212–215 (1975).

20 Köberle, F.: Chagaskrankheit: eine Erkrankung der neurovegetativen Peripherie. Wien. klin. Wschr. *68:* 333–339 (1956).

21 Köberle, F.: Megaesophagus. Gastroenterology *34:* 460–466 (1958).

22 Köberle, F.: Enteromegaly and cardiomegaly in Chagas' disease. Gut *4:* 339–405 (1963).

23 Köberle, F.: Chagas' disease and Chagas' syndromes. The pathology of American trypanosomiasis. Adv. Parasitol. *6:* 63–116 (1968).

24 Köberle, F.: Pathogenesis of Chagas' disease; in Trypanosomiasis and leishmaniasis with special reference to Chagas' disease. Ciba Found. Symp. 20 (new series), pp. 137–158 (Elsevier-Excerpta Medica-North-Holland, Amsterdam 1974).

25 Lisboa-Bittencourt, A.: Congenital Chagas' disease. Am. J. Dis. Child. *130:* 97–103 (1976).

26 Magarinos-Torres, C. B.: Patogénia de la miocarditis crónica en la enfermedad de Chagas. 5 Reunion Soc. Argent. Patol. Reg. Norte, vol. 2, pp. 902–916 (1929).

27 Mayer, M.; Rocha-Lima, H.: Zum Verhalten von *Schizotrypanum cruzi* in Warmblütern und Arthropoden. Arch. Schiffs-TropenHyg. *18:* 101–136 (1914).

28 Mazza, S.: Frecuencia y importancia de la infección natural de perros y gatos por *S. cruzi* y la cuestión de la herencia del mismo en los primeiros animales. Novena Reunión Soc. Argent. Patol., vol. 1, pp. 412–417 (1935).

29 Nathan-Larrier, L.: Heredité des infections expérimentales à *Schizotrypanum cruzi.* Bull. Soc. Path. exot. *14:* 232–238 (1921).

30 Oliveira, J. S. M.: Cardiopatia 'chagásica' experimental. Rev. goiana Med. *15:* 77–133 (1969).

31 Packchanian, A.: Chemotherapy of experimental Chagas' disease with nitrofuran compounds. Antibiotics Chemother. *7:* 13–23 (1957).

32 Prata, A.: Estado atual de terapêutica específica da doença de Chagas; revisão dos medicamentos até hoje utilizados. Rev. goiana Med. *9:* suppl., pp. 109–124 (1963).

33 Ribeiro-dos-Santos, R.; Hudson, L.: *Trypanosoma cruzi:* binding of parasite antigens to mammalian cell membranes. Parasite Immunol. *2:* 1–10 (1980).

34 Ribeiro-dos-Santos, R.; Hudson, L.: *Trypanosoma cruzi:* immunological consequences of parasite modification of host cells. Clin. exp. Immunol. *40:* 36–41 (1980).

35 Santos-Buch, C. A.; Teixeira, A. R. L.: The immunology of experimental Chagas' disease. III. Rejection of allogenic heart cells in vitro. J. exp. Med. *140:* 38–53 (1974).

36 Schenone, H.; Concha, L.; Aranda, R.; Rojas, A.; Alfaro, E.: Experiência terapéutica con el Bay 2502 en la infección chagásica crónica del adulto. Importancia del uso adecuado del xenodiagnóstico. Bol. chil. Parasit. *24:* 66–69 (1969).

37 Snary, D.; Hudson, L.: *Trypanosoma cruzi* cell surface proteins: identification of one major glycoprotein. FEBS Lett. *100:* 166–170 (1979).

38 Teixeira, A. R. L.; Santos-Buch, C. A.: The immunology of experimental Chagas' disease. II. Delayed hypersensitivity to *Trypanosoma cruzi* antigens. Immunology *28:* 401–410 (1975).

39 Teixeira, A. R. L.; Teixeira, M. L.; Santos-Buch, C. A.: The immunology of experimental Chagas' disease. IV. Production of lesions in rabbits similar to those of chronic Chagas' disease in man. Am. J. Path. *80:* 163–180 (1975).

40 Vianna, G.: Contribuição para o estudo da anatomia patologica da moléstia de Carlos Chagas. Mem. Inst. Oswaldo Cruz *3:* 276–294 (1911).

R. Ribeiro-dos-Santos, MD, Faculty of Medicine of Ribeirão Preto,
Department of Parasitology, Microbiology and Immunology,
University of São Paulo, 14100 Ribeirão Preto, SP (Brazil)

Antibiotics Chemother., vol. 30, pp. 135–162 (Karger, Basel 1981)

Chemotherapy of Filariasis

Frank Hawking

Commonwealth Institute of Helminthology, St. Albans, Herts., England

General Introduction

Filariasis is an infection with nematode worms which live in the tissues of the body. The female worm produces millions of larvae or microfilariae which disseminate themselves throughout the blood or the skin. These must be picked up by a blood-sucking arthropod vector and conveyed to a new host before they can grow further. In the new host the larvae develop and become mature. The sexes mate and the female produces the next generation of microfilariae. The adult worms live about 10 years and the microfilariae about 6–12 months. One cycle of development commonly takes most of a year.

Human Filarial Worms

(i) *Wuchereria bancrofti* which is transmitted by mosquitoes especially *Culex fatigans*. It infects millions of people in India, Indonesia and southern China, many in Africa and fewer in tropical America and the Pacific islands. It probably originated in the Malaysian region and spread from thence to the Pacific, India and Africa. It was conveyed to America by the slave trade.

(ii) *Brugia malayi,* which resembles *W. bancrofti* but is transmitted by *Mansonia* mosquitoes and is limited to India, China and Southeast Asia. *B. timori* is a similar species found in Timor.

(iii) *Loa loa* which is transmitted by *Chrysops* and which occurs in the rain forests of West and Central Africa.

(iv) *Onchocerca volvulus*. The adult worms live in subcutaneous nodules and the microfilariae collect in the superficial layers of the skin. This parasite occurs in Africa south of the Sahara and in Central America and is transmitted by *Simulium*. It often causes blindness and on that account an enormous control programme, the Onchocerciasis Control Project, has been organized in West Africa under the auspices of WHO.

(v) *Dipetalonema perstans,* which is widespread in Africa but is non-pathogenic.

(vi) *Mansonella ozzardi,* which is widespread in Central and South America, but it also is non-pathogenic.

(vii) In addition to these, it is appropriate to mention *Dracunculus medinensis* or Guinea worm. The adult female grows under the skin of the legs and pours out millions of larvae. Some of these fall into water where they develop inside *Cyclops,* etc. Man becomes infected by drinking contaminated water. The infection is common in semi-arid areas of West Africa, the Middle East and western India, and it causes much crippling.

Pathology. In endemic areas of *W. bancrofti, B. malayi* or *O. volvulus* almost everyone becomes infected, many people with numerous worms. Most of these people experience no ill effects but a certain proportion develop serious chronic lesions, probably due to allergic reactions between the host and the parasite. With *W. bancrofti* and *B. malayi,* there are often acute attacks of severe lymphangitis and if these are repeated they may lead on to elephantiasis and hydrocoele. With *L. loa* there may be allergic swellings in the skin. With *O. volvulus* the microfilariae often cause chronic thickening and other cutaneous lesions; more important, microfilariae in the skin of the head invade the eyes and cause many lesions going on to blindness. In heavily infected villages in West Africa, 10 or 20% of the inhabitants may be blinded by these worms – the so-called 'river blindness'.

Laboratory Infections

(i) *Litomosoides carinii* in *Sigmodon hispidus* and more recently in *Mastomys natalensis* which is a smaller and more convenient host. This is the most widely used chemotherapeutic model. The chemotherapeutic reactions of the microfilariae are similar to those of *W. bancrofti* but the adult worms are resistant to diethylcarbamazine.

(ii) *Dipetalonema viteae* in jirds *(Meriones).* Although this provides a second level of comparison it is not particularly useful or reliable since the chemotherapeutic reactions differ from those of human infections.

(iii) *B. malayi* (or *B. pahangi* or *B. patei*) in cats or in *Meriones un-*

guiculatus. Theoretically this should provide the ideal model since *B. malayi* is a human parasite. In actual practice the results with diethylcarbamazine in cats seem to be somewhat different from those in man, and its employment is relatively limited.

(iv) Many other parasites have been used in special circumstances by various investigators including *Dirofilaria immitis* in dogs, *Breinlia sergenti* [61], *Setaria labiatopapillosa* transplanted from slaughtered cattle to rats, *O. volvulus* in chimpanzees [15–17] and *O. gibsoni* or *O. gutturosa* in cattle.

In vitro Tests for Chemotherapeutic Compounds

These have little value for screening new compounds whether they are conducted on microfilariae or adult worms, and almost all tests should be made in vivo.

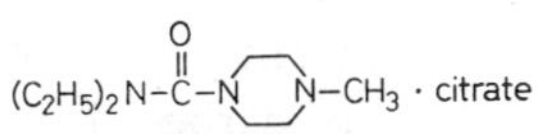

Diethylcarbamazine

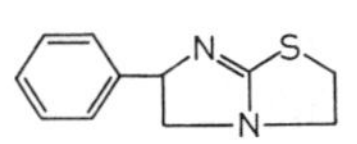

Levamisole (Laevo isomer)

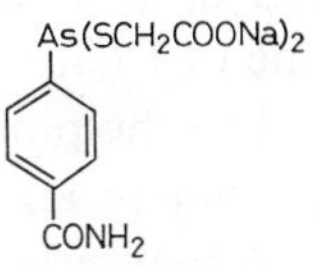

Arsenamide
(Thiacetarsamide sodium)

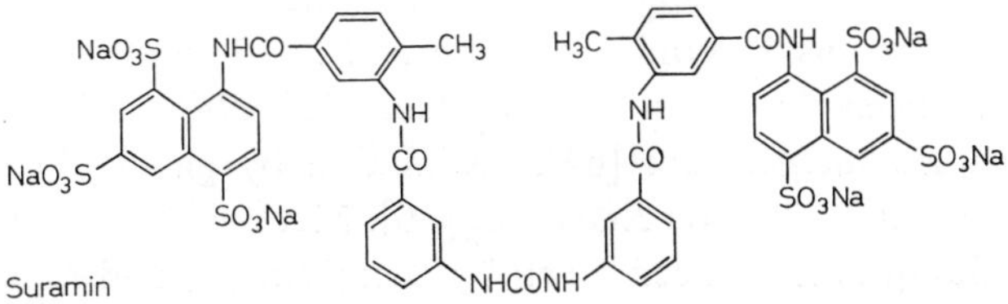

Suramin

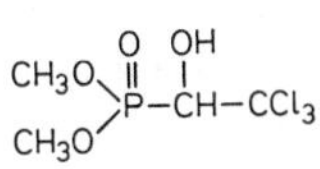

Metriphonate

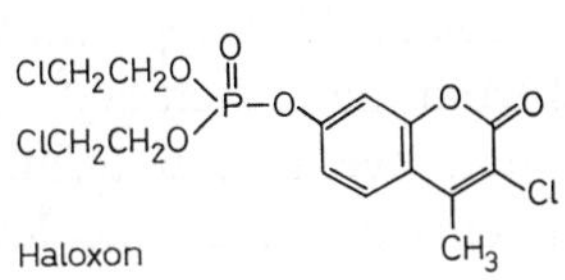

Haloxon

For the practical treatment of human infections there are only two compounds in general use, viz. diethylcarbamazine for all infections and suramin limited to onchocerciasis. Other compounds which are under trial will be considered in the final section.

Diethylcarbamazine

Diethylcarbamazine (DEC; hetrazan, banocide, notezine, etc.) was discovered by *Hewitt* et al. [36] and it has been reviewed in detail by *Hawking* [34].

Chemical Structure. Chemically it is 1-diethylcarbamyl-4-methyl-piperazine. It is freely soluble in water and is stable to autoclaving and to ordinary conditions of handling and storage. For its activity the piperazine ring is of fundamental importance. Apparently there must be two aliphatic amines connected by a saturated carbon framework; one amine must be basic and the other must be modified by some type of carbonyl function. The spatial separation of these amines in DEC is optimal and compounds with a wider separation are less active. A modification of this structure has been described by *Saxena* et al. [72] under the name of Centperazine. In this, the side chain has been bent round and attached to the piperazine ring, making the molecular structure rigid and approximately all in one plane. This compound is under investigation in India. Apparently its activity is closely similar to that of DEC.

Estimation. DEC can be estimated in blood and urine by a colorimetric method using bromthymol blue described by *Lubran* [53]. Amounts can be measured as low as 1 μg/ml for serum and 3–10 μg/ml for urine. Modifications have been described by *Hujimaki* [37], *Rao and Subrahmanyam* [65] and *Ramachandram* [64]. Estimation by gas-liquid chromatography has been described by *Rée* et al. [66]. Methods for estimation by radioactive techniques have been given by *Bangham* [6] and *Faulkner and Smith* [25].

Absorption, Excretion and Metabolism. When DEC is given by mouth, it is rapidly absorbed from the alimentary canal. One dose of 10 mg base/kg produces a peak blood level of 4–5 μg/ml in 3 h (when any toxic symptoms are most prominent) and then the level gradually falls to zero in about 48 h. The compound is rapidly distributed to all the tissues [69]. Most of the excretion in the urine occurs in the first 24 h during which time 10–26% of the dose may be recovered as DEC. When 3 mg base/kg is taken twice daily for 4½ days the blood concentration reaches 4–5 μg/ml by the 3rd day. There is no tendency to accumulate [30, 53]. According to *Hujimaki* [37], if 0.5 mg citrate/kg was given three times daily the blood concentration over most of the day was over 1.0 μg/ml and this was the minimum amount required for the extermination of microfilariae of *W. bancrofti.*

When radioactive DEC 20 mg/kg was given by mouth to rats, 10–20% of the dose was excreted in the urine unchanged, 50% appeared in the urine as diethylcarbamazine-N-oxide, 25% as 1-ethylcarbamyl-4-methylpiperazine (i. e. one ethyl group split off) and the remainder as various products with loss of alkyl groups and side chains [25]. The antifilarial activity is due to the intact molecules and not to metabolites. When solutions of DEC are applied to the eye or to the skin they are readily absorbed and these methods have been used for the local destruction of microfilariae of *O. volvulus* in such positions (see below).

Pharmacology. In non-infected persons or animals, DEC is relatively inactive. In large doses it may cause headache, or sleepiness, or vomiting (probably due to direct action on the vomiting centre). Apparently it has no harmful effects on the pregnant uterus. *Fraser* [26] gave large doses (100–200 mg/kg) by mouth daily to pregnant rats and mice and found no abortifacient action or harmful effect on the fetuses.

Various anti-inflammatory actions have been described but these are difficult to define and they are often controversial [for review see 34]. Apparently DEC has a general tendency to inhibit the release of SRS-A which takes place following antigen-antibody reaction or during inflammation. There have been many reports that a daily dose of 10 mg/kg is effective in the treatment of bronchial asthma but this has not been found by other workers. According to *Koivikko* [42], good reports tend to come from geographical areas where human parasites are common and this may explain the differences.

Antifilarial Activity

The action on microfilariae and that on adult worms must be described separately. Also the effectiveness differs with different species of filaria.

Action on Microfilariae. In vitro, therapeutic concentrations of DEC have no significant action on any kind of microfilariae. In vivo, however, DEC causes microfilariae rapidly to disappear from the circulation. If 60 mg/kg is injected intravenously into a cotton-rat infected with *L. carinii,* 80 % of the microfilariae disappear within 1 min, and the same occurs with *W. bancrofti* if suitable doses are injected into man. On the other hand, even if large doses are given to cotton-rats or to man a few microfilariae often persist in the peripheral circulation. In heavily treated rats large numbers of living microfilariae may still be found in the pleural cavities; and similarly in man, living microfilariae of *W. bancrofti* may persist in hydrocoele fluid apparently unharmed. Accordingly the residue of microfilariae which often persists in the blood after adequate treatment, may be due to leakage from reservoirs in the tissues or body cavities back into the general circulation. Alternatively, or additionally, a small fraction of the microfilariae may be different from the others either biologically or immunologically. Microfilariae of *W. bancrofti* which persist in the blood after DEC are still capable of developing in mosquitoes [8].

As regards the different species of microfilariae, those of *L. carinii, W. bancrofti, L. loa, O. volvulus* and *Dipetalonema streptocerca* are all very sensitive to DEC. Microfilariae of *B. malayi* are very sensitive in man, but in cats some microfilariae still persisted in the blood after doses which had killed all the adult worms [22]. The reaction of *M. ozzardi* microfilariae seems to be uncertain. *Bartholomew* et al. [7] found that DEC has no action on the microfilariae or adults of *M. ozzardi* in Trinidad. The compound has little or no action on microfilariae of *D. perstans, D. viteae, Edesonfilaria malayensis* or *Dirofilaria repens.* It has only moderate action on those of *D. immitis.*

Mode of Action on Microfilariae. When a search is made for the microfilariae of *L. carinii* that have disappeared from the circulation of cotton-rats after DEC treatment, they can be found in the liver and to a lesser extent in the spleen and bone marrow. Within an hour phagocytes congregate round these microfilariae which have been trapped by the large fixed macrophages and within 18 h most of them have been destroyed. According to *Kobayashi* et al. [41] this seizure and destruction by phagocytes does not occur if antimicrofilarial antibodies are absent – i. e. if the microfilariae have just been transfused into a clean animal which is then subjected to treatment. In the ordinary animal or man, however, who has been infected for many weeks, many antibodies are present which lead to the reactions just described. Apparently before treatment with DEC, the microfilariae circulate safely through the host which does not recognise them as foreign bodies. Immediately DEC is given, their disguise is stripped off. The microfilariae are recognized as antigenically foreign bodies and they are destroyed by the usual immunological processes. The whole phenomenon is remarkable and it is still not well understood. Other papers on this subject are given by *Zahner* et al. [84] and *Tanaka* et al. [76].

In man infected with *W. bancrofti* the microfilariae are normally accumulated during the daytime in the small arterioles of the lungs. If DEC is given some of these microfilariae lose their grip in the lungs, presumably due to the action of the drug on their neuromuscular system, and they are swept out into the peripheral circulation, causing a rise in the microfilarial count there which subsides after 30–90 min. The number in the blood may rise as high as 7–30% of that at midnight. This phenomenon has been extensively used by many investigators in the field so as to detect microfilariae carriers by daytime blood examinations, instead of having to collect the blood samples after 10 p. m. *Russel* et al. [68] recommend that in *W. bancrofti* areas 4–6 mg/kg should be given by mouth and the blood should be examined 30–60 min later; in *B. malayi* areas the dose should be 2 mg/kg and the blood should be taken 90 min later. They claim that up to 60 or 93% of the night positives can be detected by this daytime sampling. A similar phenomenon occurs with the microfilariae of *O. volvulus* which appear to be mobilized when DEC is first given. Small numbers of microfilariae appear in the blood, urine and sputum [21]; these are interesting but not of practical importance. Mobilization into the cerebrospinal fluid is more dangerous and if the initial number of onchocercal microfilariae in the fluid exceeds 3 Mf/ml DEC treatment may provoke vertigo and other neurological symptoms [21]. With both species of microfilariae this early provocative action of DEC may be interpreted as a disturbance of the muscular mechanisms which normally hold them in their preferred position in the body.

Adult Worms. The action of DEC varies greatly according to the species. Briefly, it kills the adults of *L. loa, W. bancrofti* (most of them), *B. malayi, B. pahangi, D. streptocerca* and *Setaria digitata,* but not those of *O. volvulus, D. immitis, D. repens, L. carinii* or *D. viteae.* There is possibly a slight lethal or sterilizing action on *D. perstans* [56]. With animal infections, the death of adult worms can be verified by autopsy and with *L. loa* the adult worms can be found in wheals under the skin. With *W. bancrofti* the evidence is less direct, consisting of the occurrence of small areas of acute inflammation persisting for a week in the groin or other parts where adult worms are probably situated; moreover, after adequate treatment the microfilariae of most patients disappear and do not reappear even after 12 months. In cats infected with *B. malayi* or *B. pahangi,* adequate doses of DEC killed all the adult worms [22] but curiously some microfilariae still persisted in the blood; in man the microfilariae of *B. malayi* disappear quickly when DEC is given. The mechanism by which DEC kills adult worms is not clear.

Forms in Arthropod Vector. Apparently DEC has no action upon the larval forms developing in the arthropod vectors of *W. bancrofti* and *D. immitis* [39] or of *D. repens* or *L. carinii.*

Infective Larvae and Immature Worms. Infective larvae of *L. carinii* are killed by DEC in vivo and so are the fifth-stage larvae (25–32 days after infection). The early forms of *L. loa* are destroyed by doses greater than 5 mg/kg daily for at least 3 days. This is effective up to 1 month after infection [14]. The effect on immature worms of *W. bancrofti* is not known, but with *B. malayi* in cats, 25 mg/kg daily for 7 days after infection seem to destroy almost all the early worms [23]. DEC prevents the development of immature forms of *D. immitis* in dogs (even though it has no action on the adult worms); 5.5 mg/kg daily all through the mosquito season has been completely effective in protecting dogs from infection in Japan [44]. Apparently DEC has no chemoprophylactic action on *O. volvulus* judging by two experiments on chimpanzees [17].

Toxicity

In uninfected persons the toxicity of DEC is very low, but large oral doses of 10–20 mg base/kg may cause anorexia, nausea and vomiting which comes on in 2–4 h and also headache and sleepiness. With infected persons, however, different and more severe reactions may occur which are most marked with *O. volvulus* and much less with *W. bancrofti.* In patients with moderate infections of *O. volvulus* there is usually a strong reaction beginning after a few hours and which is well marked in 16 h. There is swelling and oedema of the skin, especially round the hips (where there are most microfilariae), intense pruritus, tenderness of lymph nodes, hyperpyrexia up to 39 °C, tachycardia and headache. The patient may be completely prostrated. These symptoms persist for 3–7 days and then subside after which high doses can be tolerated without further reaction. The severity of the reaction is proportional to the number of microfilariae in the skin rather than to the size of the initial dose. This reaction is so constant that the administration of 50 mg is widely used as a diagnostic test for onchocerciasis (Mazzotti's reaction). The symptoms are obviously due to some kind of allergic reaction to microfilariae being destroyed in the skin but the exact mechanism is still not clear. It is not counteracted by drug antagonists of histamine or serotonin but it can be diminished by previous treatment with corticosteroids especially beta-methasone. These symptoms are not specific for DEC but they tend to be caused by any compound which is effective in destroying microfilariae.

In patients infected with *B. malayi* or *L. loa* there are often similar but milder general symptoms without the local inflammation of the skin. In patients with *W. bancrofti* symptoms are often absent but some patients (25%) may suffer from headache, nausea, vomiting, cough and pain in the chest, pains in muscles and joints, general malaise and pyrexia. The reactions are proportional to the number of microfilariae in the blood. After a few days these symptoms subside and then higher doses can be given without any reaction. With bancroftian filariasis these symptoms are never so severe as to be dangerous but they are of great practical importance because they often render mass administration of the compound unpopular and inacceptable. In addition to these general symptoms, small foci of pain and inflammation sometimes develop in the groins and thighs which are probably a local reaction round dying adult worms. They subside in a few days.

Clinical Use

In discussing treatment, a distinction must be made as to whether it is designed to improve the condition of single patients or to suppress the infection in a whole community.

Single Patients. In the case of individual patients, microfilariae and adult worms of *W. bancrofti, B. malayi,* and *L. loa* can certainly be destroyed by adequate treatment. After the worms have been removed, further damage due to them will cease but the damage already caused, e. g. lymph stasis or elephantiasis, is not reversed. In the case of onchocerciasis the microfilariae can be destroyed but not the adult worms, so that after a few months the microfilariae will gradually reaccumulate in the skin.

Patients with *W. bancrofti.* A patient of average weight (60–70 kg) should be given 100 mg citrate salt by mouth 3 times a day for 10 days. The course may be extended to 21 days but it is better to check the result by examination of the blood at night; then if the microfilariae have not completely disappeared, a second course can be given a few weeks later. The drug can also be given as a single daily dose of 200–300 mg; this is simpler to administer but more likely to cause gastrointestinal disturbances. Patients may be classified into several categories: (a) The symptomless carrier with microfilariae in his blood. Although the worms seem to be causing no harm, they are certainly doing no good and they are a source of infection. Therefore, he should be treated. (b) The patient with lymphangitis with or without microfilariae. He should be treated, preferably in a quiescent period between attacks. (c) The patient with advanced hydrocoele, elephantiasis, chyluria, etc. Unless microfilariae are present, treatment is hardly worthwhile since it cannot reverse these chronic lesions. (d) Patients with tropical eosinophilia which is probably a hypersensitive state due to infection with a filarial worm, usually *W. bancrofti.* This should be treated with 6 mg/kg 3 times daily for 5 days [11]. Marked improvement should occur in 2–4 days and cure should be completed in 2 weeks. In 10% of *Danaraj*'s [11] patients severe bronchospasm occurred which was treated with antispasmodics. If microfilariae are present in the blood, smaller doses (3–4 mg/kg) should be given. In the rare cases which do not respond, arsenicals may be tried as for syphilis.

Patients with *B. malayi,* and with *L. loa.* They should be treated in the same way as those with *W. bancrofti.* Treatment is usually very effective but 'allergic' reactions are often greater. Accordingly the dose should be reduced to 50 mg citrate 3 times a day for 3 days and then 100 mg 3 times a day for 7 days. In patients with *L. loa* wheals may appear under the skin which mark the sites of dying worms.

Patients with *O. volvulus. Duke and Anderson* [20] recommend that light or moderate infections should be treated first with DEC to remove the microfilariae. Patients over 40 kg should be given 50 mg citrate on the 1st day, 100 mg twice on the 2nd day and 200 mg twice daily on the next 5 days. If the reaction is expected to be very severe, 1 mg beta-methasone 3 times daily should be given by mouth from 1 day before the DEC and continued for 3–5 days. After that the dose is gradually reduced to zero in the next 4 days. Later a course of suramin should be given to kill the adult worms (see below). If suramin is not acceptable, treatment with DEC may be repeated at 3–6 monthly intervals or 100 mg be taken weekly to suppress the microfilariae. During these subsequent treatments the allergic reactions will probably be much smaller. In heavily infected cases with ocular involvement, DEC may cause severe reactions and it should be given cautiously with doses as above and with beta-methasone. Its main use would be as an emergency drug in acute onchocerciasis of the anterior segment or to reduce the microfilariae in the eye before giving suramin. It may also be given (200 mg twice daily for 3 days) 3 weeks after a course of suramin to remove remaining microfilariae; but if severe ocular onchocerciasis is present, this is better omitted [2].

Local Application. Ocular onchocerciasis has also been treated by local applications of 3 or 5 % DEC neutralized to pH 7 – 2 drops into the conjunctival sac 4 times daily for 9 days [1]. This temporarily reduced the number of microfilariae in the anterior chamber but it provoked severe anterior uveitis in 3 of 6 patients. A device known as an 'ocuset' has been employed to give prolonged liberation of drug under the eyelid [3]. The whole subject of local application of DEC to the eye requires further investigation.

Local application of DEC has also been used to administer the compound for cutaneous onchocerciasis. An oil-water emulsion containing 1–2 % DEC has been applied to the whole body once daily for 4–12 days. The mean microfilaria count gradually fell to a low level, but it is not clear that the treatment had any advantages over oral administration which is simpler [49, 77].

Mass Therapy. DEC is very effective and satisfactory for individual patients, but the most valuable use lies in its administration to all the infected persons in a district so as to suppress the infection on a public health basis. The procedure is simple in theory, but in practice it has encountered many difficulties which are proportional to the size of the population to be treated. These difficulties are due to the minor toxic and allergic reactions described above which have often made the treatment unpopular and inacceptable to the population who have to be treated. Four main types of dosage schedule have been employed. In the first three, the compound is given to all the population without blood examination: (a) One dose (4 mg citrate/kg) daily for 5–7 days. This is the easiest schedule to administer and it is the minimum likely to be effective. It has been given in India, Japan, Africa and Brazil. (b) An interrupted dose of 5 mg/kg monthly or weekly for 6–12 doses. The total dose should be 72 mg/kg for *W. bancrofti* and 40 mg/kg for *B. malayi*. This schedule is more effective than the other schedule but more laborious to administer. It has been employed in the Pacific and Malaya. (c) A single large dose, e.g. 1.0–1.5 g given at night. Some patients vomit but this heroic dosage has been successfully employed on a large scale against Malayan filariasis in China [86]. Sometimes this was followed by a second dose some months or 1 year later. (d) Treatment restricted to microfilariae carriers who are detected by systematic surveys, e. g. 100 mg/person 3 times daily for 7 days. This is usually acceptable but is laborious to carry out and many carriers of light infections are missed. It has been used in Sri Lanka and in northeast Brazil.

In summary, mass therapy has been successful in small populations but less so in large ones. It has reduced lymphatic filariasis to a low level over most of the Pacific area, Malay peninsula and Japan. In Sri Lanka there has been great reduction followed recently by recrudescence. In Brazil there has been reduction in many parts but this is an area of low intensity. The success of mass therapy depends on how far the goodwill and co-operation of the population can be obtained. A people cannot be freed from filariasis or any other disease unless they themselves really wish to be freed.

Medicated Salt

Since most of the difficulties of mass administration of DEC are due to the difficulties of persuasion, it has been suggested that these might be circumvented by incorporation of the compound into cooking salt, e. g. 0.2 % or 0.3 % for some months. Several small-scale trials have been successful but larger ones have been more difficult [24, 35, 43, 73]. Cooking salt medicated with 0.3–0.4 % DEC has been given for periods of 4–6 months to relatively large populations in China and the results seem to have been good [86]. Other filarial infections are not very suitable for mass therapy.

Suramin

Suramin was first introduced by Bayer in 1921 as a cure for African sleeping sickness. During experiments on trypanosomiasis in volunteers in 1945, *Van Hoof* et al. discovered that it also acted on onchocerciasis [81].

It is the only clinically available compound which kills the adult worms of *O. volvulus* but its action on other human filariae is limited. Its use for the treatment of filariasis has been reviewed by *Hawking* [33].

Chemistry. Chemically it has a very complex structure, being the trisodium salt of 8,8′-[3″,3‴-ureylenebis(3⁗-benzamido-4⁗-methylbenzamido)]-bis-1,3,5-naphthalene trisulphonic acid. It has many synonyms, including Antrypol, Bayer 205, Germanin, etc. Physically it is highly soluble in water (more than 10% w/v) and solutions are stable to boiling. It can be estimated in body fluids by the method of *Dangerfield* et al. [12].

Absorption and Excretion. If given by mouth, suramin is poorly absorbed from the intestine. When injected subcutaneously or intramuscularly it causes intense local irritation. Consequently it is practically always given by intravenous injection. After injection it combines with serum proteins and much of it circulates in the blood for long periods (up to 6 months). Much is also deposited as granules in cells of the R-E-System. In man given a dose of 1 g intravenously, the mean plasma concentration after 1 day was 40 mg/l (i. e. 10% of the dose was still in the plasma); after 5 days it was 8–20 mg/l and after 10 days it was 8 mg/l [33]. When repeated doses of 1 g are given at 4- or 7-day intervals there is considerable accumulation in the plasma and concentrations as high as 340 mg/l may be reached. There are considerable variations between patients in the extent to which accumulation occurs and in some patients it may be almost absent leading to an impairment of the therapeutic action. Small amounts are excreted in the urine during the first few days after treatment but most of the compound cannot be traced. Apparently its catabolism in the body is slow.

Suramin inhibits many different enzymes. Most of these reactions are due to its non-specific combination as a large molecule with the enzyme; and non-active analogues of suramin combine with enzymes in the same manner. It forms complexes with serum proteins and is then taken up into lysosomes where it accumulates in the reticulo-endothelial cells all over the body, especially in the Kupffer cells of the liver and in the convoluted tubules of the kidney. It also accumulates in the placenta; and in pregnant rats it has a teratogenic action. It interferes with blood clotting.

Toxicity. Its toxicity in man is cumulative owing to the accumulation in the body following repeated doses. There may be immediate reactions (nausea and vomiting) immediately after intravenous injection but these are usually unimportant if the injection is given very slowly. In certain geographical areas (Sierra Leone and Venezuela) there has been cutaneous hyperaesthesia of the soles and palms beginning after 1 day and persisting for a week. The commonest toxic reaction is irritation of the kidney; and before each dose of suramin in the urine should be tested for albumin. Exfoliative dermatitis may occur as a late manifestation; it is rare but dangerous. Stomatitis may also occur; it is early and may be severe. Jaundice is rare but dangerous. During the treatment of onchocerciasis, weakness and debility are common and in rare cases this may develop into severe prostration accompanied by chronic diarrhoea which may terminate fatally. Perhaps suramin interferes with the multiplication of cells which normally have a high rate of division such as lymphocytes and the epithelium of the intestine.

Besides these toxic reactions due to direct action of the compound, there may also be allergic reactions due to the death of adult onchocercal worms and microfilariae. These usually come on after the 4th or 5th weekly dose. There may be mild manifestations such as (a) urticaria and swelling of the affected limb, (b) tenderness and swelling round nodules or worms and (c) itching, swelling and inflammation of the skin with papular or vesicular eruption and desquamation (due to the death of the microfilariae) or more severe reactions, such as (a) deep abscesses round worms dying between muscles and (b) painful immobilization of the hip joint due to the death of the worms near the hip joint capsule [20]. Such severe reactions can usually be controlled by stopping the drug and giving betamethasone 1 mg three times a day for a few days.

Although there is a formidable list of reactions, suramin is really quite a safe drug if administered carefully. It has been given in the field to 26,963 onchocerciasis patients in Venezuela with no deaths [10]. Nevertheless, it should not be given to patients in poor general condition or with evidence of allergy or of kidney or liver disease or to pregnant women (especially not in early pregnancy).

Antifilarial Action

Litomosoides Carinii. Suramin has no action upon filariae or trypanosomes in vitro. Nevertheless, its action in vivo is almost certainly due to the intact molecule and not to any activated metabolite. In the experimental filariasis of animals, no action of suramin on *L. carinii* could be seen if the animals are killed within 2 weeks of treatment, but when infected *Mastomys natalensis* were given 40 mg/kg s. c. on 5 successive days and were then observed for 6 weeks a remarkable delayed action was discovered [47]. During the first 28 days there was no change in the embryos or microfilariae of the uterus but after this time the production of microfilariae ceased and the embryos were deformed and degenerate. After 42 days all the adult worms were dead and were embedded in masses of fibrin. Apparently although the treatment had ceased after 5 days, the worms did not begin to die until 28 or 35 days later.

Onchocerca volvulus. When suramin is given in the usual dosage of 1 g/adult patient/week, the worms begin to die after the 4th or 5th week, at which time allergic reactions begin to appear. The female worms die first and the male worms stay alive and motile much longer. (This sex difference is seen with all antifilarial drugs.) Apparently a plasma concentration of suramin greater than 10 mg/100 ml should be maintained for about 2 weeks in order to ensure the death of all the adult female worms [16].

Other Filarial Worms. In Tahiti, *Thooris* [78] treated 20 patients infected with Pacific *W. bancrofti* and 1 year later the number of microfilariae was reduced to 5% of the original number, so that apparently suramin kills the adult worms and the microfilariae gradually die out. (Since *W. bancrofti* responds so well to DEC this result is not of practical importance but it is interesting theoretically.) There are no reports on other filariae.

Microfilariae. The natural life of microfilariae of *O. volvulus* is probably over 10 months, so that even when the adult worms are killed, many of the microfilariae might be expected to survive. This is not the case however and most of them seem to be killed about the 6th week after the beginning of treatment. Since microfilariae have no dividing cells, their death is difficult to explain on the hypothesis of suramin action described below. It may be that they are killed by immunological reaction set up by the death of the adult worms.

Immature Worms. Suramin has a pronounced effect upon all immature stages of *L. carinii* [45, 48]. With larvae of *O. volvulus* inoculated into man, *Duke* [17] found no evidence for prophylactic action but later in experiments with two chimpanzees, suramin prevented the development of infection [18].

Mode of Action. The in vivo actions of suramin on both filariae and on trypanosomes are remarkable in that they do not become manifest until after a considerable latent period – in onchocerciasis and animal filariasis until after 4–6 weeks, and in trypanosomiasis until after 4–7 cell divisions [*Hawking and Sen,* 1960]. It is postulated that suramin somehow interferes slightly with the DNA-RNA replication mechanism and that each replication becomes more imperfect until the mechanism is eventually brought to a halt by the accumulation of errors. In the case of filarial worms, the only actively multiplying cells are those of the gonads and the embryos in the uterus of the females, and it is upon these cells that suramin appears to act.

Clinical Treatment

Individual Patients. Suramin is always administered by slow intravenous injection of freshly prepared 10% solution. An initial dose of 0.1 g should be given to exclude a rare idiosyncrasy which may produce sudden collapse. If there is no reaction during the next 3 days, 1 g for adults of 60 kg body weight should be given weekly to a total dose of 6 g. Before each dose the urine should be tested for albuminuria. Light albuminuria can be disregarded but heavy albuminuria with many casts and/or an ill-looking patient indicate postponement or cessation of treatment. Severe allergic reactions can usually be controlled by stopping the drug and giving beta-methasone 1 mg 3 times a day for several days and then tailing off [20]. At the end of this treatment the adult female worms should be moribund but there will still be some live microfilariae in the skin. To destroy them, 3 weeks after the suramin DEC 200 mg twice daily should be given for 3 days. This usually produces a mild onchocercal reaction, in which case it should be repeated every 3 weeks until no reaction occurs. Great caution should be used in giving suramin treatment to patients with marked onchocercal infections of the eyes as severe reactions may be provoked.

Large-Scale Treatment. The employment of suramin on a wide scale in heavily infected areas is controversial. The early courses of treatment given 20 years ago were often too heavy and some deaths occurred but with revised modern schedules (4.5–6 g in 6 weeks) these should not occur. In Mexico it is still considered too dangerous. In Venezuela, where onchocercal infections are perhaps relatively light, it has been given to 27,000 cases [10] without any deaths or serious ill effects. It has also been used in Uganda but it requires medical supervision [9, 62]. In West Africa it has sometimes caused severe reactions in heavily infected patients. Probably it should be given to all heavily infected patients with considerable pruritus or with microfilariae in the skin of the head, but marked albuminuria, pregnancy, hypertension, anaemia or poor general condition are all counter-indications. The safety and acceptability depends largely on how well the field staff have been trained to select the patients and to administer the injections.

Other Antifilarial Drugs

Arsenicals

Phenyl arsenical compounds such as Arsenamide (*p*-carbamyl-phenyl-arsylene-dithio)diacetic acid) or Mel W (melarsenoxide potassium dimercaptosuccinate) possess a powerful and rapid lethal action on adult worms and a smaller one on microfilariae.

Mel W was given to 35 men infected with *W. bancrofti* as 1–5 doses of 10 mg/kg intramuscularly mostly within 3 days [27]. In 28 men the blood became free of microfilariae within 9 months and in the other 7 men the count was reduced to 1–37 % of its original value. Other clinical trials have been reported by *McCarthy* et al. [54], *van Dijk* [80] and *McFadzean and Hawking* [55]. Patients with onchocerciasis have been treated by *Friedheim* [28] and *Lartigue* [50]. The chief effect is exerted on the adult worms and microfilariae may survive in the skin for many months. Unfortunately these compounds have produced fatal complications (liver atrophy or encephalopathy) in a small number of cases (less than 1 %) often after quite small doses which have been well tolerated by 99 % of the subjects. Since filariasis is not a fatal infection, even a small number of deaths due to therapy cannot be tolerated and the compounds are usually regarded as too dangerous for general use. With dogs infected by *D. immitis* such occasional deaths are not so serious, and arsenicals are quite suitable for the treatment of heartworm. Arsenamide 0.45 mg/kg may be given intravenously daily for 15 days. *Aubrey* [4] reported that he treated 156 infected dogs in Northern Australia; 15 % died within 2 weeks but the rest showed clinical improvement.

Organophosphorus Compounds.

Metriphonate (Trichlorphor) (dimethyl-(2,2,2-trichloro-1-hydroxy ethyl)-phosphonate) was introduced by *Salazar Mallén* et al. [70] for human onchocerciasis being given by mouth as 10 mg/kg daily, 3–6 times on consecutive days or at varying intervals. The compound is highly effective against microfilariae (but not the adults) of *L. carinii* in *M. natalensis* [46, 47]. In experimental infections the effect seems to vary with the species of host concerned. In cats infected with *B. pahangi*, the principal effect seems to be on the adult worms [13]. Other series with onchocerciasis patients have been reported by *Fuglsang and Anderson* [29] and by *Awadzi and Gilles* [5]. The last-named treated 34 men daily with 10 mg/kg for 3 or 6 days, with belladonna to reduce the muscarinic effect of metriphonate. In spite of the belladonna, severe side effects were produced in 20 of the men and there were also allergic effects due to the destruction of microfilariae. About 72–83% of the microfilariae in the skin were destroyed but they gradually recovered their numbers. Metriphonate had no action on the adult worms of *O. volvulus* [82]. *Awadzi and Gilles* [5] considered that metriphonate was unlikely to replace DEC for the treatment of onchocerciasis. Other organophosphorus compounds with antifilarial action include fenthion, haloxon, tiguvon and dichlorvos but they are mostly too toxic for practical human therapy.

Broad-Action Anthelmintics

Various compounds of the mebendazole series are active against filariae as well as against other nematodes. The most promising one seems to be levamisole (L-2,3,5,6-tetrahydro-6-phenylimidazole[2,1*b*]thiazole HCl). This is active against the microfilariae of *L. carinii* in *M. natalensis* when given as 10–25 mg/kg orally for 5 days but the microfilariae soon return [46] and it is also active against the microfilariae and adult worms of *B. sergenti* in the slow loris [85] and those of *B. malayi* in cats [58].

10 patients infected with Pacific *W. bancrofti* in Tahiti were treated orally with 6 mg/kg daily for 3 days by *Merlin* et al. [59]. 1 man (who had previously reacted badly to DEC) reacted severely and could not complete the course, and 5 men reacted moderately. After 7 days the microfilariae had disappeared from the blood in 6 patients and were much reduced in the other 3. The microfilariae began to reappear, however, after 30 days and after 90 days they had returned to 52% of their original mean number. In another trial [52] levamisole 150 mg plus DEC 200 mg was given to 23 men in French Polynesia in a single dose. The microfilaria

count was much reduced but there were severe reactions. In another series, 54 Malayan patients infected with *B. malayi* or *W. bancrofti* have been treated with various doses of levamisole by *Mak and Zaman* [57]; they recommend an oral dose of 100 mg levamisole hydrochloride followed by 100 mg twice daily for 10 days. This dosage should not be exceeded and the patients should be kept under medical supervision. Such treatment removed microfilariae from the blood of all or most of the patients. Patients infected with *B. malayi* in China have been treated with levamisole 8 mg/kg daily for 3 days; 91–95 % became negative at the end of treatment and 49–51 % were still negative 4 months later [86]. 1 patient with onchocerciasis was treated with 2–2.5 mg/kg for 14 days but there was no discernible effect on microfilariae or adult worms [19].

After levamisole treatment many patients have shown fever and other allergic symptoms which are common after effective microfilaricidal treatment, but these reactions have usually been mild or transient. When treatment has been continued, the symptoms have subsided. On the other hand, 1 man who had received a single dose of 150 mg developed fits [57] and giddiness, dizziness and disorientation were seen in the onchocerciasis patient of *Duke* [19] after 2.5 mg/kg daily for 3 days. Possibly some of these neurological symptoms were due to the destruction of microfilariae inside the brain, but fits were also observed in 1 of 161 children given a single dose of 40–80 mg for the treatment of ascariasis in Sri Lanka [51], and neurological symptoms have been seen in cats treated with large doses [58]. Judging by all these results the use of levamisole for the treatment of human lymphatic filariasis is still under evaluation.

When used against *D. immitis* in dogs, the compound destroys microfilariae at doses of 11 mg/kg daily for 6–9 days but its action on adult worms is less complete [38, 79].

Mebendazole 25–100 mg/kg daily for 5 days has been injected intrathoracically into cotton-rats infected with *L. carinii;* it has a slow macrofilaricidal action manifested after 5 weeks like that of suramin [75].

Other Compounds

Various other compounds have been shown to have antifilarial action in experimental animals but for various reasons they have been unsuitable for practical use. These include antimonial compounds, cyanines, methylene violet and bis-isoquinolinium compounds. They have been reviewed by *Hawking* [31, 32]. Antifilarial action has also been observed in amodiaquin, azacrine 5-oxide, dithiazanine, nitrofurantoin, nifurtimox and 4-

isothiocyanato-4′-nitrodiphenylamine (C 9333-GO/CGP 4540) but none of these have yet been confirmed by clinical trial in man [for review see 34].

It has recently been shown by *Sänger* et al., 1980 [70a] that compound C 9333-GO (amoscanate) has strong action against both the microfilariae and the adult worms of *L. carinii, B. malayi* and *B. pahamgi* in *M. natalensis.*

Homidium (ethidium) is a trypanocidal compound which resembles suramin in its mode of action since it does not show its effect until after the delay of about 5 cell divisions. On *L. carinii* in cotton-rats homidium bromide 10 mg/kg on 5 successive days was as active as suramin (40 mg/kg × 5) and almost all the adult female worms were dead 48 days after treatment [83]. The action of homidium on species of *Onchocerca* has not yet been tested. Other similar trypanocidal compounds (quinapyramine, diminazene and isometamidium) seemed to be less active against *L. carinii.*

Treatment of Guinea Worm

It was reported by *Rousset* [67] from studies on infected villages that a course of DEC given prophylactically prevented the development of immature worms and killed the adults. Although this is interesting scientifically it is not really feasible in actual practice. Much can be done to cut down guinea worm infection by prophylaxis but it should be prophylaxis by organization of water supplies and other hygienic measures rather than by the administration of drugs. The therapeutic problem for drugs is the treatment of patients infected with one or three worms beginning to discharge larvae: how to extract the long fragile worm from the tissues as smoothly and quickly as possible without exciting inflammation and cellulitis. For this purpose the oral administration of thiabendazole (50–100 mg/kg daily for 1–3 days) or niridazole (30 mg/kg daily for 10 days) or metronidazole (800 mg thrice daily for 3–5 days) [63] have all been recommended. They all seem to produce expulsion or lysis of the worm within 3 weeks, with acceleration of healing. *Sastry* et al. [71] in India treated 400 cases of infection with thiabendazole (50–75 mg/kg); spontaneous extrusion of the worms and dramatic subsidence of inflammatory manifestations occurred in 314 cases (78.5 %), in 6 cases a second course was needed, and in 10 cases there was no response. Mebendazole (200 mg 4 times daily for 6 days) was given to 12 patients in Nigeria by *Shafei* [74] with very good results and it was also used by *Kane* [40].

The therapeutic value of all these compounds is well attested. On the other hand, according to *Muller* [60], who studied their action in experimentally infected rhesus monkeys, metronidazole, niridazole and thiabendazole have no lethal action on pre-emergent worms but they markedly reduce the tissue reactions of the host and thus allow easy extraction of the worms. Trimelarsan (Mel W) as a single intramuscular injection of 5 mg/kg (max. 200 mg) has also been recommended; it might indeed kill the adult worm but since it may cause occasional rare deaths from arsenical idiosyncrasy it is too dangerous to use for a non-fatal infection such as guinea worm.

Conclusion

At present the only compound for the practical treatment of human filariasis is DEC. This is effective against *W. bancrofti, B. malayi, L. loa* and the microfilariae of *O. volvulus.* It is non-toxic and it is cheap. For the adult worms of *O. volvulus* the only effective compound is suramin which is safe if administered with careful supervision but is only moderately suitable for mass therapy. There is great need for a new compound which would destroy the adult worms of *O. volvulus,* which would be safe and convenient for mass therapy and which would be reasonably cheap. It would also be advantageous to have a compound which killed the adult worms of *W. bancrofti* and *B. malayi,* which was simple and safe to use in mass therapy and which avoided the allergic reactions provoked by the death of microfilariae.

References

1 Anderson, J.; Fuglsang, H.: Topical diethylcarbamazine in ocular onchocerciasis. Trans. R. Soc. trop. Med. Hyg. *67:* 710–717 (1973).

2 Anderson, J.; Fuglsang, H.; Marshall, T. F. de C.: Effects of diethylcarbamazine on ocular onchocerciasis. Tropenmed. Parasitol. *27:* 263–278 (1976).

3 Anderson, J.; Jones, B.; Fuglsang, H.: WHO/ONCHO/77.137 (1977).

4 Aubrey, J. N.: Treatment of canine dirofilariasis in Northern Australia. Aust. vet. J. *40:* 161–162 (1964).

5 Awadzi, K.; Gilles, H. M.: The chemotherapy of onchocerciasis. IV. Further trials with metrifonate. Ann. trop. Med. Parasit. *74:* 355–362 (1980).

6 Bangham, D. R.: Metabolism and excretion of ^{14}C-labelled diethylcarbamazine (pp. 397–405). The mode of action of diethylcarbamazine investigated with ^{14}C-labelled drug (pp. 406–412). Br. J. Pharmac. Chemother. *10:* 397–405, 406–412 (1955).

7 Bartholomew, C. F.; Nathan, M. B.; Yikasingh, E. S.: The failure of diethylcarbamazine in the treatment of *Mansonella ozzardi* infections. Trans. R. Soc. trop. Hyg. *72:* 423–424 (1978).

8 Chen, C. C.; Fan, P. C.: The effect of diethylcarbamazine on the development of bancroftian microfilariae in *Culex p. fatigans*. Southeast Asian J. trop. Med. publ. Hlth *8:* 53–55 (1977).

9 Cherry, J. K.: The treatment of onchocerciasis. E. Afr. med. J. *37:* 550–558 (1960).

10 Convit, J.: in Research and Control of Onchocerciasis in the Western Hemispere. Pan. Am. Hlth Org. No. 298, p. 57 (1974).

11 Danaraj, T. J.: The treatment of eosinophilic lung (tropical eosinophilia) with diethylcarbamazine. Q. Jl Med. *27:* 243–263 (1958).

12 Dangerfield, W. G.; Gaunt, W. E.; Wormall, A.: Studies on Bayer 205 (Germanin) and Antrypol. I. The determination of small amounts of Bayer 205 (and Antrypol). The persistence of Bayer 205 in the bloodstream after injection into animals. Biochem. J. *32:* 59–70 (1938).

13 Denham, D. A.; Ponnudurai, T.; Nelson, G. S.; Guy, F.; Rodgers, R.: The effect of metrifonate on *Brugia pahangi* infections in domestic cats. Bull. Wld Hlth Org. *44:* 423–429 (1971).

14 Duke, B. O. L.: Studies on the chemoprophylaxis of loiasis. II. Observations on diethylcarbamazine citrate (Banocide) as a prophylactic in man. Ann. trop. Med. Parasit. *57:* 82–96 (1963).

15 Duke, B. O. L.: The effects of drugs on *Onchocerca volvulus*. I. Methods of assessment, population dynamics of the parasite and the effects of diethylcarbamazine. Bull. Wld Hlth Org. *39:* 137–146 (1968).

16 Duke, B. O. L.: The effects of drug on *Onchocerca volvulus*. 3. Trials of suramin at different dosages and a comparison of the brands Antrypol, Moranyl and Naganol. Bull. Wld Hlth Org. *39:* 157–167 (1968).

17 Duke, B. O. L.: Experiments on the chemoprophylaxis of *Onchocerca volvulus* infection. Bull. Wld Hlth Org. *39:* 179–186 (1968).

18 Duke, B. O. L.: The effect of suramin on the immature forms of *Onchocerca volvulus* in the vertebrate host. Tropenmed. Parasitol. *25:* 84–88 (1974).

19 Duke, B. O. L.: The effect of levamisole on *Onchocerca volvulus*. Trans. R. Soc. trop. Med. Hyg. *68:* 71 (1974).

20 Duke, B. O. L.; Anderson, J.: Onchocerciasis and its treatment. Trop. Doctor *2:* 107–114 (1972).

21 Duke, B. O. L.; Vincelette, J.; Moore, P. J.: Microfilariae in the cerebrospinal fluid and neurological complications during treatment of onchocerciasis with diethylcarbamazine. Tropenmed. Parasitol. *27:* 123–132 (1976).

22 Edeson, J. F. B.; Laing, A. B. G.: Studies on filariasis in Malaya: the effect of diethylcarbamazine on *Brugia malayi* and *B. pahangi* in domestic cats. Ann. trop. Med. Parasit. *53:* 394–399 (1959).

23 Ewert, A.; Emerson, G. A.: Effect of diethylcarbamazine on third stage *Brugia malayi* larvae in cats. Am. J. trop. Med. Hyg. *24:* 71–73 (1975).

24 Fan, P. C.; Wang, Y. C.; Liu, J. C.; Lo, H. S.; King, M. L.: Control of bancroftian filariasis by common salt medicated with diethylcarbamazine in Liehyu District (Little Kinmen), Kinmen (Quemoy) Islands, Republic of China. Ann. trop. Med. Parasit. *69:* 515–516 (1975).

25 Faulkner, J. K.; Smith, K. L.: Dealkylation and N-oxidation in the metabolism of 1-diethylcarbamyl-4-methyl piperazine in the rat. Xenobiotica *2:* 59–68 (1971).

26 Fraser, P. J.: Diethylcarbamazine: lack of teratogenic and abortifacient action in rats and rabbits. Indian J. med. Res. *60:* 1529–1532 (1972).

27 Friedheim, E. A. H.: Mel W in the treatment of filariasis due to *Wuchereria bancrofti:* results in 35 cases observed for 10–12 months after treatment. Ann. trop. Med. Parasitol. *56:* 337–342 (1962).

28 Friedheim, E. A. H.: Mel W in the treatment of onchocerciasis cases in leprosy patients: results in 12 cases observed for 20 months after treatment. Ann. trop. Med. Parasitol. *56:* 343–351 (1962).

29 Fuglsang, H.; Anderson, J.: WHO/ONCHO/77.139 (1977).

30 Hawking, F.: Some recent work on filariasis. Trans. R. Soc. trop. Med. Hyg. *44:* 153–186 (1950).

31 Hawking, F.: Chemotherapy of filariasis; in Schnitzer, Hawking, Experimental chemotherapy; 1st ed., pp. 893–912 (Academic Press, New York 1963).

32 Hawking, F.: Chemotherapy of tissue nematodes; in Cavier, Hawking, Chemotherapy of helminthiasis; 1st ed., vol. I, pp. 437–500 (Pergamon Press, Oxford 1973).

33 Hawking, F.: Suramin: with special reference to onchocerciasis. Adv. Pharmacol. Chemother., vol. 15, pp. 289–322 (Academic Press, New York 1978).

34 Hawking, F.: Diethylcarbamazine and new compounds for the treatment of filariasis. Adv. Pharmacol. Chemother., vol. 16, pp. 130–194 (Academic Press, New York 1979).

35 Hawking, F.; Marques, R. J.: Control of bancroftian filariasis by cooking salt medicated with diethylcarbamazine. Bull. Wld Hlth Org. *37:* 405–414 (1967).

36 Hewitt, R. I.; Kushner, S.; Stewart, H. W.; White, E.; Wallace, W. S.; Subbarow, Y.: Experimental chemotherapy of filariasis. III. Effect of 1-diethylcarbamyl-4 methyl-piperazine hydrochloride against naturally acquired filarial infections in cotton rats and dogs. J. Lab. clin. Med. *32:* 1314–1329 (1947).

37 Hujimaki H.: Nagasaki med. J. *33:* suppl., p. 156 (1958).

38 Jackson, R. F.: Some new chemotherapeutic agents for dirofilariasis. A preliminary report; in Bradley, Pacheco, 2nd Symp. Canine Heartworm Disease, pp. 129–134 (University of Florida Press, Gainesville 1972).

39 Kanda, T.; Tasaka, S.; Sasa, M.: The effects of diethylcarbamazine treatment on the viability of microfilariae ingested by intermediate hosts. Jap. J. exp. Med. *37:* 149–155 (1967).

40 Kane, O. O.: Mebendazole in the treatment of dracontiasis. Am. J. trop. Med. Hyg. *24:* 600–605 (1975).

41 Kobayashi, J.; Matsuda, H.; Fujita, K.; Sakai, T.; Shinoda, K.: Mode of action of diethylcarbamazine on cotton rat filaria. Jap. J. Parasit. *18:* 563–574 (1969).

42 Koivikko, A.: Diethylcarbamazine in bronchial asthma. Ann. Allergy *31:* 45–46 (1973).

43 Krishna Rao, C.; Sundaram, R. M.; Krishna Rao, P.; Das, M.; Koteswara Rao, N.; Rao, C. K.: Control of bancroftian filariasis with diethylcarbamazine medicated salt in open communities in rural and urban areas. J. commun. Dis. *8:* 193–203 (1976).

44 Kume, S.; Ohishi, I.; Kobayashi, S.: Prophylactic therapy against the developing stages of *Dirofilaria immitis*. Ann. J. vet. Res. *23:* 1257–1260 (1962).

45 Lämmler, G.; Hertzog, H.: Chemotherapeutic studies on *Litomosoides carinii* infection of *Mastomys natalensis*. 4. The prophylactic and suppressive activity of suramin. Tropenmed. Parasitol. *25:* 78–83 (1974).

46 Lämmler, G.; Hertzog, H.; Schütze, H. R.: Chemotherapeutic studies on *Litmosoides carinii* infection of *Mastomys natalensis*. II. The activity of drugs against microfilariae. Bull. Wld Hlth Org. *44:* 757–763 (1971).

47 Lämmler, G.; Hertzog, H.; Schütze, H. R.: Chemotherapeutic studies on *Litmosoides carinii* infection of *Mastomys natalensis*. 3. The activity of drugs against adult parasites. Bull. Wld Hlth Org. *44:* 765–770 (1971).

48 Lämmler, G.; Wolf, E.: Chemoprophylaktische Wirksamkeit filarizider Verbindungen bei der *Litmosoides carinii*-Infektion der *Mastomys natalensis*. Tropenmed. Parasitol. *28:* 205–225 (1977).

49 Langham, M. E.; Traub, Z. D.; Richardson, R.: A transepidermal chemotherapy of onchocerciasis. Tropenmed. Parasitol. *29:* 156–162 (1978).

50 Lartigue, J. J.: Le mélarsonyl potassique dans le traitement de l'onchocercose humaine. Note préliminaire. Constatations après dix mois d'observation. Bull. Soc. Path. exot. *37:* 536–546 (1964).

51 Lionel, N. D. W.; Mirando, E. H.; Nanayakkara, J. C.; Soysa, P. E.: Levamisole in the treatment of ascariasis in children. Br. med. J. *iv:* 340–341 (1969).

52 Louis, F. J.; Laigret, J.: Essai de l'ssociation diéthylcarbamazine (notézine) – levamisole (Solaskil) dans la lutte contre la filariose à *Wuchereria bancrofti* var. *pacifica,* en Polynésie française. Bull. Soc. Path. exot. *72:* 471–481 (1979).

53 Lubran, M.: Determination of Hetrazan in biological fluids. Br. J. Pharmac. Chemother. *5:* 210–216 (1950).

54 McCarthy, D. D.; Simpson, E.; Robati, P.: A new filaricidal agent. Report of trial using Mel W in the treatment of the nonperiodic type of *Wuchereria bancrofti* in Raratonga, Cook Islands. N. Z. med. J. *61:* 143–147 (1962).

55 McFadzean, J. A.; Hawking, F.: Arsenamide treatment of filariasis due to *W. bancrofti* and *A. perstans*. Br. med. J. *i:* 956–959 (1954).

56 McGregor, A. I.; Hawking, F.; Smith, D. A.: Control of filariasis with Hetrazan; field trial in rural village (Keneba) in Gambia. Br. med. J. *ii:* 908–911 (1952).

57 Mak, J. W.; Zaman, V.: Drug trials with levamisole hydrochloride and diethylcarbamazine citrate in Bancroftian and Malayan filariasis. Trans. R. Soc. trop. Med. Hyg. *74:* 285–291 (1980).

58 Mak, J. W.; Zaman, V.; Sivanandam, S.: Antifilarial activity of levamisole hydrochloride against subperiodic *Brugia malayi* infection of domestic cats. Am. J. trop. Med. Hyg. *23:* 369–374 (1974).

59 Merlin, M.; Carme, B.; Kauffer, H.; Laigret, J.: Activité du levamisole (Solaskil) dans la filariose lymphatique à *Wuchereria bancrofti* (variété *pacifique*). Bull. Soc. Path. exot. *69:* 257–265 (1977).

60 Muller, R.: The pathology of *Dracunculus medinensis* infection and its relevance to chemotherapy; in Soulsby, Pathophysiology of parasitic infection. Proc. 7th Int. Conf. Wld Ass. Adv. Vet. Parasit. Thessaloniki 1975, pp. 133–147 (Academic Press, New York 1976).

61 Natarajan, P. N.; Zaman, V.; Yeoh, T. S.: In vitro activity of diethylcarbama-

zine on the infective larvae, microfilariae and adult worms of *Breinlia sergenti.* Int. J. Parasitol. *3:* 803–807 (1973).

62 Nelson, G. S.: A preliminary report on the out-patient treatment of onchocerciasis with Antrypol in the West Nile District of Uganda. E. Afr. med. J. *32:* 413–429 (1955).

63 Padonou, K. O.: A controlled trial of metronidazole in the treatment of dracontiasis in Nigeria. Am. J. trop. Med. Hyg. *22:* 42–44 (1973).

64 Ramachandram, M.: Colorimetric determination of diethylcarbamazine (Hetrazan) with picric acid. Indian J. med. Res. *61:* 864–869 (1973).

65 Rao, K. N.; Subrahmanyam, D.: Estimation of diethylcarbamazine (Hetrazan). Indian J. med. Res. *58:* 746–752 (1970).

66 Rée, G. H.; Hall, A. P.; Hutchinson, D. B. A.; Weatherley, B. C.: Plasma levels of diethylcarbamazine in man. Trans. R. Soc. trop. Med. Hyg. *71:* 542–543 (1977).

67 Rousset, P.: Essai de prophylaxie et de traitement de la dracunculose par la notézine en Andrar. Bull. méd. A. O. F. *9:* 351–368 (1952).

68 Russel, S.; Sundaram, R. M.; Chandrasekharan, A.; Rao, C. K.: Provocative effect of daytime administration of diethylcarbamazine on microfilaraemia of *Wuchereria bancrofti* and *Brugia malayi.* J. commun. Dis. *7:* 59–64 (1975).

69 Sakuma, S.; Sakuma, M.; Sato, Y.; Sasa, M.; Kobayashi, J.: Studies on the distribution of tritium-labelled antifilarial drug ^{3}H-diethylcarbamazine by whole body autoradiography. Jap. J. Parasitol. *16:* 179–187 (1967).

70 Salazar Mallén, M.; Gonzalez Barranco, D.; Alvares Fuertes, G.: Onchocerca-

70a Sänger, I.; Lämmler, G.; Wegerhof, P. H.: The efficacy of amoscanate (C9333-Go/CGP 4540) on filarial infections of *Mastomys natalensis.* Acta Tropica *37:* 262–265 (1980).

Dermatose aus Mexiko und ihre Behandlung mit Metrifonate. Tropenmed. Parasitol. *21:* 213–219 (1970).

71 Sastry, S. C.; Kumar, K. J.; Lakshiminarayana, V.: The treatment of dracontiasis with thiabendazole. J. trop. Med. Hyg. *81:* 32–35 (1978).

72 Saxena, R.; Sharma, S.; Iyer, R. N.; Anand, N. I.: Studies in potential filaricides. 5. 3-Ethyl-8-methyl-1,3,8-triazabicyclo[4.4.o]-decan-2-one, a new antifilarial agent. J. med. Chem. *14:* 929–931 (1971).

73 Sen, A. B.; Chandra, R.; Katiyar, J. C.; Chandra, S.: Diethylcarbamazine medicated salt in the chemotherapeutic control of filariasis due to *Wuchereria bancrofti* in an open community. Indian J. med. Res. *62:* 1181–1189 (1974).

74 Shafei, A. Z.: Preliminary report on the therapeutic effect of mebendazole in guinea worm infection. J. trop. Med. Hyg. *79:* 197–200 (1976).

75 Shibuya, T.; Oikawa, Y.; Saito, M.; Tanaka, H.: Mebendazole – as low acting macro- and microfilaricide against *Litmosoides carinii* in cotton rat. Jap. J. exp. Med. *49:* 351–353 (1979).

76 Tanaka, H.; Eshita, Y.; Takaoka, M.; Fujii, G.: Suppression of microfilaricidal activity of diethylcarbamazine by anti-lymphocytic serum in cotton rat filariasis. Southeast Asian J. trop. Med. publ. Hlth *8:* 19–26 (1977).

77 Taylor, H. R.; Langham, M. E.; De Stahl, E. M.; Figueroa, L. N.; Beltranena, F.: Chemotherapy of onchocerciasis: a controlled clinical trial of topical diethylcarbamazine (DEC) in Guatemala. Tropenmed. Parasitol. *31:* 357–364 (1980).

78 Thooris, G. C.: Le traitement expérimental de la filariose à *Wuchereria bancrofti* en Océanie française par la suramine. Bull. Soc. Path. exot. *49:* 311–317 (1956).

79 Tulloch, G. S.; Anderson, R. A.: Tetramisole and canine dirofilariasis; in Bradley, Pacheco, 2nd Symp. Canine Heartworm Disease, pp. 101–104 (University of Florida Press, Gainesville 1972).

80 Van Dijk, W. J. O. M.: The action of Mel W against *Wuchereria bancrofti.* Trop. geogr. Med. *15:* 29–37 (1963).

81 Wanson, M.: Contribution à l'étude de l'onchocérose africaine humaine (Problèmes de prophylaxie à Léopoldville). Annls Soc. belge Méd. trop. *30:* 667–863 (1950).

82 Wolf, H.; Schulz-Key, H.; Albiez, E. J.; Geister, R.; Büttner, D. W.: Analysis of enzymatically isolated adults of *Onchocerca volvulus* after treatment of patients with suramin or metrifonate. Tropenmed. Parasitol. *31:* 143–148 (1980).

83 Worms, M. J.; Hawking, F.: Homidium bromide as a macrofilaricide. Trans. R. Soc. trop. Med. Hyg. *72:* 548–549 (1978).

84 Zahner, H.; Weidner, E.; Lämmler, G.; Soulsby, E. J. L.: Zur Wirkung von Diethylcarbamazin und Haloxon gegen Mikrofilarien von *Litomosoides carinii* in nicht immunen Wirten. Tropenmed. Parasitol. *28:* 273 (1977).

85 Zaman, V.; Natarajan, P. N.: Antifilarial activity of Levamisole on *Breinlia sergenti* and its comparison with diethylcarbamazine. J. trop. Med. Hyg. *76:* 126–130 (1973).

86 Zhong Chonghu; Zheng Huijun: Studies in control of malayan filariasis in China. Chin. med. J. *93:* 537–544 (1980).

Addendum

Chemotherapy of Filariasis Due to Dirofilaria immitis

The chemotherapy of infections of *Dirofilaria immitis* (heartworm) in dogs differs from that of human filariasis in many respects, due to the different susceptibility of the parasite and to the greater margin of possible toxicity which is permissible in a non-human patient.

Diethylcarbamazine (DEC)

The adult worm is not susceptible to DEC even when given in repeated high doses. The microfilariae are feebly susceptible and even doses of 12 mg/kg/day cause only a moderate diminution in the number [2]. Nonetheless it should not be given to dogs with microfilaraemia because it may cause severe reactions or even death. On the other hand, the infective larva entering the dog is highly susceptible. Dogs exposed to potentially infected mosquitoes can be protected against infection by the administration of 6.6 mg DEC citrate/kg/day incorporated into the diet. This has no harmful toxic effect and it has been used to prevent heartworm infection in military working dogs of the American Air Force during the mosquito season [3]. DEC does not kill the later immature worms.

Arsenical Compounds

Thiacetarsamide (also known as arsenamide or caparsolate) exerts a powerful and rapid lethal action on adult filarial worms and a smaller one on microfilariae. Unfortunately it cannot be used in human patients because a few of them show a fatal idiosyncrasy to these compounds. This contraindication however does not hold for dog filariasis and arsenicals have become the standard treatment for destroying the adult worms. The dose schedule recommended by the American Veterinary Medical Association [1] is 2.2 mg/kg i. v. twice daily for 2 days or, if desired, 3 days. In early trials carried out in 1963 on 24 infected dogs this killed all the worms in 23 dogs, and only three immature worms remained alive in 1 dog [6]. More recent experience has shown that some commercial preparations are less active than others and that it is important to use correctly formulated fresh preparations to obtain satisfactory results. Immature worms are less readily killed than mature adults and they may survive to cause infection later. When the adult worms have been killed they may cause fatal pulmonary embolisms. In 8 of 20 dogs, thiacetarsamide caused a sharp rise in SGPT level, indicating liver damage [4].

Dithiazanine Iodide
(3,3′-diethylthiadicarbocyanine iodide)

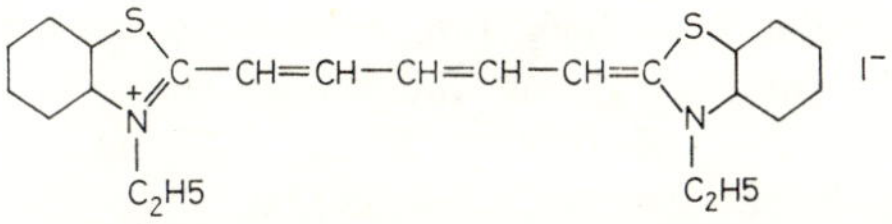

This compound is remarkable for its activity against *Trichuris trichiura* and *Strongyloides stercoralis.* Its absorption in the intestine is irregular and in human patients it may cause toxic effects. It is effective in dogs against the microfilariae of *D. immitis.* The recommended dose is 4.4 mg/kg/day for 7 days by mouth; if microfilariae are still present and there have been no reactions, the dose may be increased to 11 mg/kg/day for not more than 10 further days [1]. When this course was given to 10 infected dogs (in which the adult worms had previously been killed by thiacetarsamide) the microfilariae were all removed in 5 and greatly reduced in 5 [4]. It has no action on adult or immature worms. It is best given after previous treatment with thiacetarsamide.

Levamisole

In dogs, the chief use of levamisole is to kill microfilariae. The adult worms should first be killed by thiacetarsamide and then levamisole should be given as 11 mg/kg by mouth daily for not more than 15 days. When 130 dogs were treated in this way by *Jackson* [5] the microfilariae were all removed in 90 dogs, but in 11 dogs there were toxic reactions which required the treatment to be discontinued. On *adult* worms the action is incomplete and unpredictable even with high doses. As regards *infective larvae, Kume* [7] found that 5 mg/kg/day given for 30 days was the minimum required to prevent development. This treatment is too toxic in comparison with DEC to be practical. The toxic reactions in dogs consist mainly of vomiting (prevented by atropine) and central nervous system disturbances.

Fenthion (organophosphate) is active as a microfilaricide but it is not available commercially for this purpose. It has been applied to the back of the dog as 1 ml of a 20 % solution per 4.5 kg body weight once weekly for many months. This removes ticks and fleas and also microfilariae [8].

References

1 Anonymous: Recommended procedures for the management of canine heartworm disease; in Otto, Proc. Heartworm Symp., 1977, pp. 159–162 (Veterinary Medicine Publishing, Bonner Springs, Kans. 1978).

2 Burkhart, R. L.; Alford, B. T.: Pharmacology and mode of action of diethylcarbamazine; in Bradley, Pacheco, Canine heartworm disease: the current knowledge, pp. 17–26 (University of Florida Press, Gainesville 1972).

3 Casey, H. W.; Fineg, J.; Tulloch, G. S.; Davis, H. C.: Results of a two-year field evaluation of diethylcarbamazine as a heartworm prophylactic; in Bradley, Pacheco, Canine heartworm disease: the current knowledge, pp. 95–99 (University of Florida Press, Gainesville 1972).

4 Courtney, C. H.; Boring, J. G.: A comparison of the reaction to thiacetarsamide before and after the use of a microfilaricide; in Otto, Proc. Heartworm Symp., 1977, pp. 89–94 (Veterinary Medicine Publishing, Bonner Springs, Kans. 1978).

5 Jackson, R. F.: The activity of levamisole against the various stages of *Dirofilaria immitis* in the dog; in Otto, Proc. Heartworm Symp., 1977, pp. 111–116 (Veterinary Medicine Publishing, Bonner Springs, Kans. 1978).

6 Jackson, R. F.; Seymour, W. G.; Growney, P. J.: An evaluation of thiacetarsamide as an adulticide against *Dirofilaria immitis;* in Otto, Proc. Heartworm Symp., 1977, pp. 82–85 (Veterinary Medicine Publishing, Bonner Springs, Kans. 1978).

7 Kume, S.: Prophylactic therapy against *Dirofilaria immitis* with *DL*-tetramisole together with some observations on its microfilaricidal and adulticidal efficacy; in Proc. Heartworm Symp., 1974, pp. 68–72 (Veterinary Medicine Publishing, Bonner Springs, Kans. 1975).

8 Overcash, R.: in 7th Discussion Period; in Otto, Proc. Heartworm Symp., 1977, pp. 152–153 (Veterinary Medicine Publishing, Bonner Springs, Kans. 1978).

F. Hawking, MD, Commonwealth Institute of Helminthology,
103 St. Peter's Street, St. Albans, Herts. AL1 3EW (England)

Antibiotics Chemother., vol. 30, pp. 163–202 (Karger, Basel 1981)

Intestinal and Urogenital Flagellates

J. G. Meingassner, P. G. Heyworth
Sandoz Forschungsinstitut, Vienna, Austria

Although the human alimentary and urogenital tracts are parasitized by seven species of flagellate protozoa [115], only two, *Giardia lamblia* and *Trichomonas vaginalis,* are generally considered to be pathogens. This review, therefore, concentrates on these organisms and in particular on the experimental and clinical chemotherapy of trichomoniasis and giardiasis. Due to the limited space and the availability of excellent recently published reviews, topics such as life cycles, epidemiology, prevalence and pathology are only briefly discussed in the sections entitled 'Biological Aspects'. The reader seeking comprehensive reference lists and more information on *Trichomonas* and *Giardia* and the diseases they cause is referred to these reviews [22, 85, 94, 108, 152, 153, 219].

Urogenital Trichomoniasis

Biological Aspects

Although the urogenital trichomonad of man was discovered by *Donné* in 1836, it was not until 1916 that *Höhne* identified *Trichomonas vaginalis* as a pathogenic parasite [cited by 85]. Since then it has been shown that *T. vaginalis* is an extremely common pathogen in the female genitourinary tract. *T. vaginalis* exists only as the trophozoite which is usually ovoid or pyriform, approximately 7 × 10 μm in size and multiplies by binary fission. The morphology is variable depending upon the environment in the host or in culture. This variability has initiated many reports on 'abnormal forms' of *T. vaginalis* including multinuclear and multiflagellated cells, which probably merely reflect various degenerative stages of the parasite [95, 179]. *T. vaginalis* inhabits the female vagina, urethra, paraurethral glands and ducts, and occasionally the bladder. In the male the urethra and prostate gland are the most common sites but infections of the bladder, paraurethral glands, seminal vesicles, testes and epididymis have also been reported [for references see 94].

In nature *T. vaginalis* is confined to the human host and is typically transmitted during sexual intercourse [94], although nonvenereal routes of transmission cannot be excluded. However, as with other sexually transmitted diseases (STD), the incidence of trichomoniasis is directly related to sexual practices as confirmed by studies of the disease in promiscuous people and prostitutes [61, 228]. The incidence of urogenital trichomoniasis is relatively lower in men than in women and thus it is generally agreed that the infected female is the 'reservoir' of *T. vaginalis* and that the male is usually the 'vector' [85].

Viability outside the host is normally short-lived due to the trophozoites' low resistance to external factors, but certain conditions allow survival for several hours and hence for nonvenereal transmission [for details and references see 85, 94, 179, 206, 207]. There is no other explanation for trichomoniasis in newborn female infants, young girls or in adults denying sexual contacts [4, 215, 220]. Delivery by infected mothers, contact with contaminated toilet articles and clothing, as well as iatrogenic transmission have been implicated in these cases [179, 206, 220].

Although 'water-borne' transmission has not yet been proven, certain findings suggest that this route cannot be completely excluded. Viable, dividing organisms have been isolated from the water of swimming pools and baths [206, 207] and trichomonads have been shown to survive for hours in the water of thermal spas, in insufficiently chlorinated tap water [112, 206] and in medicinal baths [207]. Since the infective dose of trichomonads appears to be small [250], infections could theoretically occur in poorly chlorinated swimming pools, nonchlorinated spas or uncleaned baths [179]. An accurate assessment of the frequency of trichomoniasis is difficult as many infected people are asymptomatic. In addition, many reports on the subject [for references see 85, 94] provide a very wide range of figures depending on the group studied, diagnostic methods, and the experience of the investigator [61, 67, 179, 228].

In recent reports infection rates in women vary widely and include figures of 17.8% in symptomatic patients attending a VD clinic, 0.5% in a nonpromiscous family planning clinic group, 9.5% in unselected hospital patients in Sydney [228], and 1 and 1.2% in two Edinburgh surveys of women attending family planning clinics [73]. These figures are low compared to other studies. In Vienna, 56% of a group of prostitutes had vaginal trichomoniasis [61] and 32.7% of 400 women attending a VD clinic in Atlanta, Georgia, were infected [67]. Other reports from VD clinics in Colorado and Sweden quote figures of 7.5 and 5.6%, respectively [243, 255]. In Utrecht, 81% of a small selected group of women with cervicitis and colpitis harbored the organism [124]. According to various sources the prevalence of trichomoniasis in the US is 3–15% among healthy women, 10% in gynecology private practice, 30% in gynecology clinic practice and 38–56% in women attending VD clinics [247].

Most men infected with *Trichomonas* are thought to be asymptomatic. When symptoms occur, their mildness and the small number of parasites in male urethral secretions have made it difficult to assess the prevalence of trichomoniasis in men [1]. Recent papers report that *T. vaginalis* was found in 1.2–2.4% of patients with nongonococcal urethritis, but in less than 1% in equivalent control groups [35, 114, 190]. In another survey trichomonal urethritis was found in only 0.09% of unselected patients attending a VD clinic [255] but 22% of partners of *T. vaginalis*-infected women were shown to harbor the parasite [1]. *Wilson and Ackers* [250] were successful in isolating *T. vaginalis* from only 3 of 21 urine samples from known contacts of women with trichomoniasis. None of the urine samples from the remaining 227 males in the study group yielded a positive culture, giving a final prevalence rate of 3 out of 248 samples (1.2%). In another study involving 350 male consorts of infected women, 20.5% had trichomonal infections, approximately half of which were only detected by culturing urethroprostatic secretions obtained by massage. In the reverse situation a surprisingly low 28.6% of asymptomatic women, who were consorts of men with trichomonal urethritis, were identified as being infected. In approximately half of them the parasite was only observed in urethral cultures [215].

Detailed figures on the frequency of trichomoniasis are only available for England, Wales and Scotland. From annual reports, published since 1971, it can be seen that in 1977, 43.09 new cases were reported per 100,000 people seen at hospital clinics. The figure for men is 7.54 and for women 76.84 [52]. Provisional data from the 1978 survey show that 21,483 new cases of trichomoniasis were seen in clinics in a total number of > 447,000 patients [53]. These figures represent an increase compared to previous years. A similar trend is found in other countries [61, 62], so although treatment of the disease is effective in individuals, from an epidemiological point of view it is failing [215].

The large majority of patients infected with *T. vaginalis* is asymptomatic. The classical, acute form of trichomoniasis is seen only in about 10% of infected women, and the general course of the disease tends to be one of chronicity and acute relapses. In women exhibiting clinical patterns of acute trichomoniasis the main symptoms include malodorous discharge, itching, gross vulvovaginitis and dysuria. Gross tissue changes of the vulva are usually more prominent than changes of the vagina but neither the quality of the vaginal discharge nor objective gynecological findings allow a definite diagnosis. Petechiae in the vaginal mucosa or erythematous punctate lesions on the cervix ('strawberry vagina/cervix'), which are rarely seen, may be pathognomonic [67, 69]. In chronic cases of the disease the symptoms are few, vaginal discharge may only be scanty and leukorrhea may often only be identified by the examining physician.

Compared to noninfected persons, patients with trichomoniasis more frequently show marked inflammatory changes and dysplasia in the epithelial cells of the cervical smear, thus making a differentiation between reversible cellular abnormalities and neoplastic changes more difficult [9, 87]. Cytological findings return to normal within 2 weeks of effective treatment of vaginal trichomoniasis [19].

Trichomoniasis is not solely an infection of the vagina. *T. vaginalis* also occurs in the lower urinary tract and has been shown to be the only pathogen in cases of urethrocystitis [69]. In neither sex does the infestation tend to ascend the urinary tract to involve the urethers or kidneys and in females the organism does not appear above the level of the cervix [other infestations are the exception; 215, 226]. Infections in men are mostly latent or persist in a subclinical form. After a variable incubation period symptomatic patients develop urethritis, prostatic infection, balanitis and hemospermia [215].

Laboratory in vitro and in vivo Models

The susceptibility testing of trichomonads in vitro is basically identical to methods used for monitoring antibacterial therapy. Dilutions of the antitrichomonal agent are either made in a liquid culture medium (serial dilution test) or are added to filter paper discs which are placed on the plated medium containing the cells (agar disc diffusion test). Evaluation of the compound under test is based on the lowest concentration at which growth inhibition or death of the organism occurs, after incubation at 37 °C. Many variations of this principle exist [for details see 211] and therefore only basic information will be presented. The cultivation methods and a variety of undefined media suitable for *T. vaginalis* and *Tritrichomonas foetus* (the trichomonad of cattle which is also used in drug screening programmes) are described in previous reviews [34, 85, 94, 140, 229].

Most susceptibility tests are performed in serial dilution using tubes or more commonly multiwell trays, which are cheaper, easier to use and offer the possibility of automation [149, 167]. Agar disc diffusion tests have also been used for drug testing [123], bioautography [154] and the assay of antitrichomonal agents in serum or other body fluids. With this method, flooding of the culture with phenolphthalein monophosphate and alkali has been shown to facilitate reading of the plate, by differentiating by color between the zones of growth inhibition and uninhibited growth [154].

Trichomonads are cultivated axenically and are originally separated from contaminants by the use of antibiotics, which are then omitted from established pure cultures [94, 229]. As trichomonads may not have a stable drug sensitivity pattern [86], cryopreservation [127] is essential if various strains (or isolates) are used in comparative trials. The size of inocula used in tests depends on the assay conditions and the mode of evaluation [24, 88, 110]. Exposure times of 24–96 h are most frequently used [81, 110, 126, 185, 249] but evaluation based on shorter intervals has also been used [24, 88, 237].

Different workers base their evaluation of the efficacy of test compounds on different criteria. Some use minimal inhibitory concentration (MIC) to differentiate between the trichomonastatic concentration and the trichomonacidal concentration [88, 110, 238]. Trichomonastatic concentrations are based on the presence or absence of growth (i. e. increased cell numbers) in long-term experiments, and are determined by gross examination or by counting with a hemocytometer or electronic particle counter [24, 88, 110, 144]. Data on 90% end points or MIC_{50} and on the ratios of MIC_{50} to MIC and MLC to MIC have also been published [24, 88, 157, 158]. The trichomonacidal or minimal lethal concentration (MLC), defined as the smallest concentration of an agent causing subculture failure, is usually determined for trichomonads on the basis of morphological changes (lysis) and/or absence of motility, since subculture experiments after treatment with known antitrichomonal drugs have shown that confirmation by the transfer of grossly changed, round, immobile cells into new medium is not necessary [110]. (Admittedly, if compounds with unknown modes of action are handled, an exact evaluation, involving subculture, is required.)

It is clear then, that there are no standardized techniques and reference strains available for the in vitro testing of antitrichomonal agents. Not surprisingly, MIC and MLC data for such compounds show great variation, making it difficult to compare the figures from different laboratories. Strains, cell numbers, media, incubation atmosphere, exposure time and mode of evaluation are all factors likely to cause variability [88, 110, 126, 148]. A review of a few recently published papers will demonstrate this. When the antitrichomonal activity of tinidazole was compared with that of metronidazole its lethal activity was shown to be superior, whilst the inhibitory action of the drugs was equal [88]. This superiority has been confirmed by other workers using freshly isolated strains. Mean MLC values were 3.5 μg/ml for tinidazole and 8 μg/ml for metronidazole [126], but the strains in this study showed a wide range of sensitivities to both drugs, compared to other published studies [110, 144].

In contrast to the above findings another evaluation based on the MIC and using one laboratory strain and 10 isolates, demonstrated that metronidazole and secnidazole (MIC 0.6, 0.7 μg/ml, respectively) were superior to tinidazole (MIC 1.13 μg/ml). There was no significant difference between MLC values obtained in the same study [238]. In a study using 63 strains of *T. vaginalis* no difference could be detected between the potencies of metronidazole, tinidazole and nifuratel, at either static or cidal levels. The MICs ranged from 0.1 to 0.14 μg/ml with an inocula of 10^4 and from 0.1 to 1.1 with a tenfold inocula. The MLCs ranged from 0.5 to 0.7 and 2.8 to 4.0, respectively [110]. In other studies the MLC for nimorazole compared well with that of metronidazole [175]. In one study the MLC of ornidazole was shown to be 1 μg/ml, half of that of metronidazole [185], but in a comparative study involving 13 strains, 9 of them had MIC values for ornidazole of 0.63 μg/ml which compares well with the values for nimorazole, tinidazole and metronidazole. All of the isolates were inhibited by all the drugs at concentrations at 5.0 μg/ml [218].

Our own MLC data for metronidazole, tinidazole, nimorazole, ornidazole and nifuratel, obtained from an anaerobic assay [149] in modified TYM medium [84] with a laboratory strain, are 1.6, 1.6, 3.1, 0.8 and 12.5 μg/ml, respectively.

Experimental infections by *T. vaginalis* and *T. foetus* have been tried in a variety of laboratory animals. Most of these experiments, studying the host-parasite interactions, the pathogenic potential of the parasite, as well as the efficacy of antitrichomonal compounds were recently reviewed by *Honigberg* [85].

Table I. In vivo models used in testing antitrichomonal activity

Species	Mode of infection	Laboratory animal	Reference(s)
T. vaginalis	intravaginal	monkey	40
		rat	8, 31, 146, 157
		mouse	142
	intraperitoneal	mouse	15, 185
	subcutaneous	mouse	15, 142, 157, 235
	scrotal w/o simultaneous subcutaneous	mouse	235
	simultaneous i. p. and s. c.	mouse	144
T. vaginalis + *T. foetus* (double infection)	subcutaneous o i. p. and scrotal sac	mouse	235
T. foetus	intravaginal	rabbit	162
		guinea pig	130
		hamster	2, 157, 158
		mouse	249
	introperitoneal	mouse	88, 145, 235
	subcutaneous	mouse	157, 158
		hamster	158
	scrotal sac w/o simultaneous i. p.	mouse	235

i. p. = intraperitoneal
s. c. = subcutaneous

A number of experimental ectopical (unnatural tissue infection) and topical models used for chemotherapeutic testing are listed in table I [for additional references see 156, 211]. As with in vitro assays most workers prefer to use the strains, inocula size, route of infection, animals and treatment schedules which perform best in their own laboratories, and therefore no standard in vivo screen exists.

For extrapolation to the human disease, models using topical infection by *T. vaginalis* would be expected to give the most reliable results, but establishing vaginal infections, in particular with *T. vaginalis* in rats, has proved difficult. Workers have attempted to overcome these difficulties with various supporting measures [8, 27, 30, 142, 143, 156, 168, 249].

Table II. Efficacy of antitrichomonal drugs against *T. vaginalis* and *T. foetus* in different animal models

Compound	DC_{50}, mg/kg body weight[1]					
	T. foetus i. p./mouse	*T. foetus* s. c./mouse	*T. vaginalis* i. p./mouse	*T. vaginalis* s. c./mouse	*T. vaginalis* intravag./ mouse	*T. vaginalis* intravag./rat
Metronidazole	11.7	17.0	12.3	11.0	3.8	2.2
Tinidazole	3.5	6.9	21.8	7.5	1.4	2.6
Nimorazole	24.3	37.8	49.7	34.0	5.6	2.9
Ornidazole	6.5	10.1	17.6	11.0	4.6	1.4
Nifuratel	85.5	>300.0[2]	>300.0[2]	>300.0[2]	n. t.[3]	>200.0[2]

[1] Orally at 2, 18 and 24 h p. i.
[2] >300,0, >200 = highest doses used.
[3] Not tested.

Other workers have used *T. foetus,* which can be more easily introduced intravaginally [130, 158, 249], but in several respects, including drug sensitivity, is different from *T. vaginalis* [32, 158, 165]. Evaluation after either systemic or local treatment of the fatal intraperitoneal infection model is based on mean survival time and numbers of survivors. In other models curative power is verified microscopically by the presence or absence of motile trichomonads in peritoneal or vaginal washings and of caseous material at the site of injection. Cultures are also used.

Due to the variability of the models used, data on the efficacy of drugs differ widely, and comparisons of anti-infective activity of related drugs are notoriously misleading when they are based on results from different laboratories. Examples of the efficacy of antitrichomonal drugs in our models, using laboratory strains of *T. vaginalis* and *T. foetus,* are summarized in table II. Full details of these methods are published elsewhere [142, 143, 145, 146] but a brief outline is given here. For both i. p. and s. c. *T. foetus* infections an inoculum of 8×10^5 cells was used, whilst for i. p. and s. c. infections of *T. vaginalis,* inocula contained 1.2×10^6 and 8×10^5 cells, respectively. Topical infections were performed with 2.5×10^5 cells in mice and $5\text{–}8 \times 10^5$ cells in rats. Drugs were given in 3 peroral treatments at 2, 18 and 24 h after infection. Calculations of the DC_{50} (dose needed to cure 50% of infected animals) were either based on negative cultural findings with washings from the vagina or abdominal cavity taken at 4 and 6 days p. i. respectively, or on an absence of motile trichomonads in subcutaneous sites of injection on day 6 p. i.

It can be seen from table II that the nitroimidazole derivatives have similar efficacies, although slight differences within models do exist. In the topical assay nimorazole has a similar DC_{50} to other nitroimidazoles, whereas in the ectopical mouse model it is clearly less effective. The nitrofuran, nifuratel was shown to be weakly active only in intraperitoneal *T. foetus* infections of mice.

Susceptibility Testing of Isolates from Treatment Failures

Recent reports have shown that treatment failures can be caused by a decreased sensitivity of *T. vaginalis* to metronidazole [66, 81, 167, 233]. Susceptibility testing may therefore become increasingly important as an aid to diagnosing the cause of therapeutic failure. Isolates from cases of trichomoniasis refractory to normal treatment were found to be relatively resistant only when an aerobic method, using microtiter or multiwell-tissue culture plates with loose-fitting lids, or partly filled tubes were used for the determination of MLCs [66, 149, 167].

This technique was developed with a strain of *T. foetus* made resistant by increasing drug pressure [147], and has proved suitable in our laboratory using a variety of media [148], with all the resistant strains of *T. vaginalis* isolated so far. In anaerobic assays these strains showed normal sensitivity in terms of MLCs although a decreased sensitivity was also demonstrated in animal experiments. Comparative trials with test strains and normal sensitive strains both under aerobic and anaerobic conditions are recommended, since the activity of metronidazole is decreased under aerobic conditions [166], whilst MLC values for resistant strains are markedly increased. Strains of intermediate sensitivity to nitroimidazoles are best evaluated in animal experiments using the more successful subcutaneous route of infection [148]. In our experience using subcutaneous inocula of 4×10^5 cells in both flanks of mice, strains that cause infections not cured by 3 peroral doses of metronidazole at 35 mg/kg should be regarded as having decreased sensitivity [144].

Current Chemotherapy and Chemoprophylaxis

The permanent cure of trichomoniasis depends upon the eradication of every organism from all foci of infection in the urogenital tract of patients. Since locally applied medicaments do not reach all the trichomonal habitats, topical treatment, which is clearly impossible for male carriers of *T. vaginalis,* has also proved to be insufficient in most women. Relapses due to endogenous reinfection by extravaginal parasites are known to occur. The prescription of systemically active drugs is therefore the normal treatment of choice, unless other factors indicate local therapy. Treatment is necessary both in symptomatic patients and simultaneously in asymptomatic sexual consorts to prevent reinfection or possible spreading. Treatment is also indicated in asymptomatic females when the organism is associated with endocervicitis, cervicitis or cervical lesions, since there is evidence that the presence of trichomonads can interfere with the assessment of cytological smears [55].

The discovery in 1960 of the 5-nitroimidazole metronidazole as the first agent systemically active against trichomoniasis was a welcome innovation in the chemotherapy of this common venereal disease [48]. With the new drug, cure rates from 86–100% were reported [104, 191], instead of 10–20% using earlier treatments [69] and the prevalence of the disease decreased [69, 111]. Not surprisingly, metronidazole attracted attention from many drug companies, the more so as it proved to be valuable in the treatment of other diseases [10, 193]. Since 1969 the closely related 5-nitroimidazoles, nimorazole, tinidazole, ornidazole, secnidazole and carnidazole have been developed and introduced into clinical practice as antitrichomonal drugs. (Not all of them are available in every country; in the USA for instance only metronidazole is approved by the FDA for the treatment of trichomoniasis [51].)

A review of the data on the comparative trichomonacidal activity of the 5-nitroimidazoles does not reveal a clear advantage for any one compound over the others, but the results from different investigators are hard to compare, being based as they are on various treatment schedules and criteria of effectiveness, and frequently lacking any statistical analysis [6, 55, 60, 82, 103, 139, 170, 182, 203, 214, 234, 246]. To assess the efficacy of any drug used in the treatment of STDs one must differentiate between relapse (primary failure) and reinfection (secondary failure) due to sexual promiscuity of a portion of patients or failure to treat the consorts. The most reliable information is therefore gained from comparative studies in stationary patients, in whom the chances of reinfection and failure to take the drug can be excluded. In a study of 449 supervised patients treated with either 3 g of nimorazole in doses at 8-hour intervals, or with a single 2 or 3 g dose of tinidazole, or with a single 2 g dose of ornidazole, the data conclusively demonstrated that there was no significant difference in the efficacy of the three drugs [159]. These results agree with earlier data on multiple-dose treatment of female prisoners with metronidazole [105], which indicated that 5-nitroimidazoles are highly active when the avoidable reasons for failure are excluded. Cure rates for trichomoniasis reported in the reviewed literature mainly lie in the range 85–95 %. Symptoms are usually relieved within a few days.

In view of the good antitrichomonal activity and the satisfactory tolerability of the 5-nitroimidazoles, the original recommended regimens have been modified by various workers in an endeavor to shorten the course of treatment. Most of the currently used schedules are shown in table III. With the exception of pregnant patients, the 1-day course or single-dose treatments are now generally recommended [29]. The advantages of these schedules are numerous. A single supervised dose is indicated for those patients who are thought to be unreliable or where it is thought that a patient may stop the treatment once symptoms have subsided. The sexual partner is also more likely to take a single dose of tablets, particularly if he has no symptoms. From the epidemiological point of view, short-course therapy, which rapidly renders the patient noninfective, is especially valuable in the treatment of STDs. It also decreases the time during which patients are asked to abstain from sexual intercourse, but increases the possibility of reinfection if tracing and examination of the sexual contacts is not carried out rapidly.

Single-dose treatment is no less effective than multiple-dose treatment [39, 227, 231, 236, 253] and possibly superior with some nitroimidazoles. However, although cure rates are usually high with all the regimens listed, treatment failures do occur [203, 215, 242], other than those caused by reinfection, noncompliance or insufficient doses in children and overweight patients [49, 198, 220]. Primary failures were found to be due to low serum levels [100], or to possible inactivation of the drug by intestinal or vaginal microorganisms [57, 58, 89, 181]. As mentioned in the previous section, resistance has now been implicated as a further cause of treatment failure. Strains isolated from cases of trichomoniasis refractory to normal metronidazole treatment have been shown to be relatively insensitive to the other 5-nitroimidazoles [66, 81, 167, 233].

In cases of treatment failure cures have been obtained either by repeating courses of the drug [39, 65, 105, 215, 238] or by changing the chemotherapeutic approach. Changing from single-dose to multiple-dose treatment and vice versa [39, 160, 203] as well as increasing the dose and/or prolonging the treatment has produced cures [46, 77, 160, 167, 233].

Table III. Commonly used schedules in the treatment of urogenital trichomoniasis.

Drug	Long-term therapy	Reference(s)	Short-term therapy	Reference(s)	Single-dose treatment	Reference(s)
Metronidazole	200–250 mg t. i. d. × 7 days	51, 55, 171, 193	2 g in two doses × 2 days	77	2–2.5 g	29, 55, 193, 215, 231
			400 mg q. i. d. × 2 days	254		
	400–500 mg b. i. d. × 5 days	29, 69, 171, 231	1 g twice on 1 day	55		
	pediatric dose: 5 mg/kg t. i. d. × 7 days	51				
Nimorazole	250 mg b. i. d. × 6 days	25, 60, 234	2 g in two doses × 2 days	138	2 g	131, 171
			750 mg b. i. d. × 2 days	203		
			1 g three times at 12-h intervals	77		
Tinidazole	150 mg b. i. d. × 7 days	208			2 g	7, 208
	150 mg t. i. d. × 5 days	208	–		pediatric dose: 50 mg/kg	7
Ornidazole	1 g daily × 5 days	185	2–3 g in two doses on 1 day	185	1.5–2 g	82, 150, 218, 246
			or 1–3 g in two doses on 1 day combined with 500 mg to 1 g in a single dose intravag.	185		
Secnidazole	250 mg b. i. d. × 10 days	15	–		2 g	15, 238
Carnidazole	–		–		2 g	169

Alternative compounds have also been used, both at recommended and increased doses [6, 66, 139] and in combination with pessaries containing nitroimidazole derivatives or antiseptic compounds such as acetarsol, hydrargaphen and diiodohydroxyquinoline [46, 139]. Local pretreatment with antibiotic remedies may also be helpful [39]. Patients are normally cured by one or other of these therapeutic measures, but recently cases of trichomoniasis have been described which were [66, 81] refractory to all treatments.

The 5-nitroimidazoles, administered for trichomoniasis in total doses ranging from 2 to $>$ 20 g [167] are remarkably free from acute side effects. Even in patients receiving a high-dose short-duration treatment, in whom the incidence and severity of side effects are slightly higher than in patients taking lower doses over several days [29], the adverse effects are transient and relatively mild. The most common side effects are gastrointestinal, particularly nausea, anorexia and occasionally vomiting, diarrhea, epigastric distress and abdominal cramping. An unpleasant taste in the mouth is not unusual. Reported neurological disorders, occasionally dose-dependant with ornidazole [74, 136, 150], include headache, dizziness, vertigo, confusion, ataxia and tiredness. Nitroimidazoles are contraindicated in patients with active organic diseases of the central nervous system. Rare adverse reactions with some 5-nitroimidazoles, such as a disulfiram-like effect when alcohol is taken during treatment, exanthems and transient leucopenia may also be observed. Severe side effects after doses normally used in trichomoniasis are very rare and require prompt discontinuation [41, 71].

For several years it has been known that 5-nitroimidazoles and some of their human urinary metabolites are mutagenic in bacteria [118, 197, 241] and due to the possible correlation between genetic effects in prokaryotes and the ability to induce cancer in mammals [137], doubts have been raised about their continued use in humans for the treatment of protozoal and bacterial diseases. Most studies by independent laboratories on the carcinogenicity of the 5-nitroimidazoles have been performed with metronidazole. A very small number of studies have detected an increased incidence of tumors in mice and rats fed metronidazole for long periods at very high doses [200–202]. However, other animal studies have detected no increase in tumor incidence [36, 192]. Similarly, in mammalian test systems (unscheduled DNA synthesis and dominant lethal test) metronidazole was found to be free of mutagenic activity [21]. In a retrospective follow-up study of patients treated at least once with metronidazole there was no substantial increase in total cancer incidence compared to that expected in a normal population [14]. However, the follow-up periods ranged from only about 9 to 18 years, whereas the latency period for chemical carcinogenesis may be longer than 20 years.

It is clear that whilst the bulk of the evidence suggests that the 5-nitroimidazoles are safe drugs for use at the doses required for treating trichomoniasis, the evidence from the bacterial mutagenicity and tumor studies in mice and rats must be considered. At the moment there is no alternative effective treatment and the recommendation to initiate treatment with topical agents and to only use metronidazole in a single 2 g dose for nonresponders [109, 117] has not been generally accepted.

There have been no reported cases of damage to the fetus when metronidazole has been administered to pregnant women and teratogenic and embryotoxic studies in animals have generally proved negative [20]. Nevertheless, treatment with 5-nitroimidazoles is not recommended during the first 3 months of pregnancy or in nursing mothers [55]. During the first trimester, local antiseptic remedies are prescribed. For the later period of pregnancy some authors recommend only local 5-nitroimidazole treatment and others use systemic multiple-dose treatments [111, 183]. Local treatments may suppress symptoms but cure rates are poor [69, 116, 133, 210, 222].

Between 1966 and 1976, several papers [23, 25, 68, 79, 176] reported on the effectiveness of the nitrofuran derivative nifuratel in trichomonal, candidal and bacterial infections of the vagina. The usual treatment schedule combines oral treatment (200 mg t. i. d. for 7 days) with topical treatment (one vaginal pessary containing 250 mg/night for 10 nights) in the female and oral treatment only in male consorts. There is some controversy in the literature on the systemic efficacy of the drug [59, 78, 79], but when used solely as an oral treatment it proved less effective at increased doses[12] than the above combined treatment, thus reinforcing the recommendation of dual application.

There are no systemically active agents available as possible chemoprophylactics. The use of therapeutics is not recommended from the medical point of view. Topically applied chemical contraceptives may have trichomonacidal activity [216] but neither these or other preparations are widely used in the chemoprophylaxis of STDs [43].

New Advances and Future Needs

There have been no major advances in the last few years in the fields of trichomonal immunology and chemotherapy. Several workers have attempted to develop serological tests for use in the diagnosis of trichomoniasis but none of them have proved to be sensitive or specific enough [114, 134, 190]. Such a test would be especially useful in the diagnosis of asymptomatic male carriers, in whom microscopical diagnosis is often difficult.

In recent years, trichomonads have been the subject of many biochemical studies which have mainly concentrated on elucidating the pathways and subcellular organization of energy metabolism and on the activation and mechanism of action of the 5-nitroimidazoles. Relatively little is known about the biosynthetic capability of the organism, although studies have indicated that *T. vaginalis* is incapable of synthesizing de novo either the purine or pyrimidine ring and that it relies upon salvage pathways for the synthesis of nucleotides [80]. Tracer studies have also shown that the organism is unable to synthesize significant quantities of any of the major lipids [194].

The energy metabolism of trichomonads has been well reviewed in recent years [32, 85, 165] and therefore only a summary of current knowledge is given here, relating particularly to the activation of 5-nitroimidazoles by the organism. Whilst many of the recent studies have been performed with *T. foetus,* and whilst there are clear differences between the organisms with respect to energy metabolism, the main pathways appear to be qualitatively the same.

Trichomonads are aerotolerant anaerobes, lacking mitochondria, a functional tricarboxylic acid cycle and detectable cytochromes [125]. Endogenous glycogen reserves and exogenous carbohydrates serve as sources of energy and the initial stages of catabolism proceed via a typical glycolytic system, the enzymes of which, in *T. foetus* at least, are located in the cytosol [230]. Some phosphoenolpyruvate (PEP) formed by glycolysis is carboxylated in a GDP-dependant carboxykinase reaction to oxalacetate, then reduced to malate in both trichomonads and further reduced via fumarate to succinate in *T. foetus.*

The balance of the PEP, approximately half under anaerobic conditions but more in aerobiosis, is converted to pyruvate. Pyruvate is also formed from malate by the action of a decarboxylating malate dehydrogenase [122]. In *T. vaginalis* but not *T. foetus* pyruvate can be reduced by a cytoplasmic lactate dehydrogenase to lactate, a metabolic end product. In both organisms pyruvate undergoes oxidative decarboxylation to form acetyl CoA, with the electrons being transferred, via a ferredoxin-type protein, as yet not characterized [165], to form molecular hydrogen under anaerobic conditions. This reaction is similar to that occurring in *Clostridia* and other strictly anaerobic bacteria. Under aerobiosis oxygen can act as the terminal electron acceptor. Acetyl CoA is converted to acetate with the simultaneous formation of ATP (or GTP), thus conserving the energy of the thioester bond.

The enzymes involved in the conversion of pyruvate to acetate, a pyruvate: ferredoxin oxidoreductase and hydrogenase in the first step and acetate-succinate CoA transferase, succinate thiokinase and adenylate kinase in the second, are localized in a membrane-bound organelle, termed the hydrogenosome by *Lindmark and Müller* [122]. It should be pointed out that although acetate is a metabolic end product of both *T. foetus* and *T. vaginalis,* the enzymic steps involved in its formation from acetyl CoA have only been identified in *T. foetus* [165].

The reduction of the nitro group of 5-nitroimidazoles, a process which is essential for their antimicrobial activity, is intimately connected with the functioning of the hydrogenosome of trichomonads and the analogous enzyme systems of *Giardia, Entamoeba* and anaerobic bacteria. Thus, in *Trichomonas,* once metronidazole has entered the cell by diffusion, the nitro group is reduced in a nonenzymic reaction by electrons generated during hydrogenosomal pyruvate oxidation, and donated to the drug by the low redox potential ferredoxin-type protein. Oxygen competes for these electrons and it has been shown that under aerobic conditions, the trichomonacidal activity of metronidazole is diminished [166]. Reduction of metronidazole decreases its intracellular concentration and thus forms a concentration gradient and increases its uptake [164].

The active reduction product or products of 5-nitroimidazoles, which due to their instability have not been isolated, appear to act primarily on the DNA of the target cell. The drug, reduced in the presence of DNA, has been shown to bind to the nucleic acid causing strand breakage and destabilization of the helix. It has also been postulated that metronidazole inhibits the mechanisms which normally repair strand breakage in DNA, thus exerting a double attack [56].

The biochemical basis (or bases) of reduced sensitivity in *T. vaginalis* are not yet known, but a laboratory strain of *T. foetus* made resistant to metronidazole by growth under increasing drug pressure, was found to have no oxidative pyruvate metabolism and no anaerobic hydrogen production, both typical hydrogenosomal activities [33]. A decrease or absence of hydrogenosomal activity would clearly affect the ability of the organism to reduce and therefore activate metronidazole. However, it is clear that other factors are also involved because strains of *T. vaginalis* and *T. foetus,* resistant only under aerobic conditions, do not have reduced hydrogenosomal enzyme activities [*M. Müller,* pers. commun.].

Although the 5-nitroimidazoles are universally used and highly successful in the treatment of trichomoniasis, the almost total reliance on these compounds, the possible risks associated with them and the likelihood of further resistant strains appearing, emphasize the need for new antitrichomonal agents. Further biochemical studies, covering all aspects of trichomonal metabolism, may indicate possible chemotherapeutic targets and thus aid the development of new drugs.

In view of the contradictory data from tumorigenicity studies in animals, it is likely that only long-term follow-up studies in patients treated with 5-nitroimidazoles will solve the question of carcinogenicity. In cases of treatment failure with normal doses of 5-nitroimidazoles, there is a need for a standardized susceptibility test using reference strains of the organism, and for clinically tested alternative treatment schedules.

Giardiasis

Biological Aspects

It is peculiar that *Giardia* organisms, which are believed to have been first seen by *Antony von Leeuwenhoek* in 1681 in his own diarrheic stools and described in 1859 in detail by *Lambl* [cited by 221] in 'geleeartigem Schleimexkret' of children, should for many years be regarded as commensals. There is now no controversy regarding their pathogenicity; the organisms are causally associated with intestinal dysfunction.

Giardia lamblia, Giardia intestinalis and *Lamblia intestinalis* are common synonyms for the protozoa found in humans. However, the speciation needs further evaluation since morphologically identical organisms, defined as *G. duodenalis*-group organisms by *Filice* [64], are also found in a variety of other mammals including dogs, cats, rabbits and rodents.

The flagellated, binucleate trophozoite of *Giardia* bears a large ventral disc for attachment to the microvillous surface of the duodenum and jejunum. A cyst wall forms around them when they become detached and although it is the encysted parasite which is normally excreted, trophozoites may also be found in diarrheic feces. Infection occurs when mature, quadrinucleate cysts are ingested, which on excystation release quadrinucleate trophozoites, dividing to form two binucleate organisms [17,

153]. Under experimental conditions a dose of 100 or more cysts is 100% infective in humans [184].

The infection is spread either by direct fecal-oral contamination or by indirect transmission of cysts in food or water. Hand-to-mouth transmission is a likely mechanism in children, and direct person-to-person transmission may also occur in homosexuals [155]. In contrast to the above patterns in the endemic situation, water-borne transmission has been implicated in large-scale outbreaks [37]. Some data supports the view that animals can also act as reservoir hosts for *Giardia* infective to man [45].

Giardiasis is not an exotic disease. Endemic infections with *Giardia* are found in every country of the world but the incidence of infection differs widely from one area to another. Average prevalences generally range from 1.1 to 12.5% [152]. *G. lamblia* is the most frequently identified intestinal parasite in the USA and Britain [54, 199]. In the USA survey 3.8% of the fecal samples examined contained *Giardia* organisms. The incidence rate tends to be higher in tropical and subtropical areas, but increased prevalence and transmission as well as infection of epidemic proportions have also recently been found in nontropical countries [38, 44, 106, 212]. In these areas, besides local outbreaks, imported cases by tourists ('traveller's diarrhea') returning from areas with an endemic or epidemic pattern of infection are of considerable importance [for references see 152].

Giardiasis occurs more commonly in children than in adults, with the incidence rate decreasing with age [180]. The prevalence of infection is highest in children living in institutions where sanitary practices are substandard. Figures of 20–40% have been reported among 2- to 3-year-old children in day-care nurseries and kindergarten [3, 92, 106].

Individuals vary in their response to *Giardia* infections. Many are asymptomatic, others experience either short-lived intestinal disorders or suffer from persistent symptoms for months or years. Whether this is due to factors inherent in the parasite, such as differences in the virulence of strains or species and the parasite load or due to host-related factors, is a matter for conjecture. Factors which are considered to predispose towards clinical manifestation include childhood, malnutrition, intestinal disorders, bacterial overgrowth in the intestinal lumen und immune deficiency disorders [for references see 153].

Manifestation of giardiasis can result in a number of symptoms, depending on the duration of the infection. The main complaints are the onset of severe, watery, foul diarrhea free of blood or pus, marked abdominal distension, midepigastric cramps, flatulence, nausea and anorexia, after an incubation period of 1–3 weeks. Extreme lassitude is also a common symptom. The acute stage normally lasts for only 3–4 days but episodes may be prolonged for some months. The most common symptom, diarrhea, can be associated in chronic cases with severe weight loss and the syndrome of 'failure to thrive' in children. Steatorrhea and malabsorption may develop with the chronicity of infection.

A spectrum of pathomorphological and pathophysiological changes in the parasitized small intestine has been described. Findings range from normal intestinal villi and mucosa, to epithelial cell damage, marked inflammation, changes in the villus-crypt architecture and tissue invasion [for references see 26, 108, 219, 258]. Reduction in activities of brush border enzymes, resulting in maldigestion and malabsorption have also been reported [76, 258].

A correlation between duration and severeness of symptoms and histological damage and functional impairments has been demonstrated [256]. The abnormalities are more common in patients with underlying immune deficiencies than in persons with a normal immune system [76].

Laboratory in vitro and in vivo Infection Models

The in vitro evaluation of compounds active against *Giardia* has been hampered in the past by the inability to culture the organism. Many attempts to subculture established isolates failed until *Karapetyan*'s [101] report in 1960. Modifications of this monoxenic technique for the long-term culture of *Giardia* trophozoites with *Candida guilliermondii* led to the development of axenic cultures of *G. duodenalis*-type organisms [151, 239] and hence to valid in vitro screens. For monoxenically grown *G. duodenalis* the minimum lethal concentrations (MLC) of quinacrine and metronidazole were reported by *Mayer* et al. [cited by 153] to be 0.5 μg and 5.0 μg/ml, respectively. Quinacrine was also the most active compound against axenically grown cells with an MLC of 0.1 μg/ml whilst metronidazole and furazolidone had MLCs of 6.4 μg/ml under identical conditions. The antigiardial effect of metronidazole and tinidazole was tested by *Jokipii and Jokipii* [99] in a microculture system in an anaerobic assay recently.

Using *Diamond*'s [47] trichomonas medium, tinidazole was found to be more active than metronidazole against all but one tested isolate of *G. lamblia*. The single exception was an isolate equally sensitive to both drugs. It is interesting to note that there was a great variation in sensitivity.

The minimal immobilizing concentration of metronidazole, read after 24 h incubation, varied between strains from 1.6 to 50 μg/ml, and that of tinidazole from 0.2 to 12.5 μg/ml.

Successful infections of rats with *G. lamblia* are known [213], but probably owing to the poor reproducibility with the rat model, most workers have tested chemotherapeutic agents in mice, using *G. muris*-type organisms, which may differ significantly from human *Giardia*. As many mouse colonies host latent infections, spontaneously infected animals have been used. In such models metronidazole and secnidazole have been shown to be active [15, 18, 132]. Other workers have used experimental infections of *G. muris*-free mice, involving the intraesophageal administration of a defined number of trophozoites or cysts isolated from infected donor animals. The evaluation of compounds was based on the counting of trophozoites in the intestinal washings, or scrapings from the mucosa of the upper part of the small intestine and on a decrease or cessation of cyst output.

With an analogous system based on the eradication of trophozoites from the upper part of the small intestine 2 days after the third daily oral application, the authors calculated CD_{50} and CD_{95} values for metronidazole of 3 × 19 and 3 ×60 mg/kg, respectively [unpubl. report]. Similar published data showed that secnidazole is twice as active as metronidazole after two oral treatments [15]. The animal models of experimental giardiasis are described in detail elsewhere [28, 186, 188, 189, 224].

Current Chemotherapy and Chemoprophylaxis

The current therapy of giardiasis depends on the oral application of 5-nitroimidazole derivatives (metronidazole, tinidazole, nimorazole, ornidazole), the acridine dye mepacrine or the nitrofuran, furazolidone. The clinical effectiveness of these drugs has been demonstrated by many workers but there is some controversy regarding the drug of choice. For instance, in the United States, mepacrine is the most commonly used drug [219], whereas in many other countries the 5-nitroimidazoles are preferred [221]. Furazolidone is not widely used except as a suspension given orally, particularly to young children [219].

It is generally accepted that mepacrine and nitroimidazole derivatives are more active than furazolidone [13, 120, 217], but comparisons between mepacrine and metronidazole have given conflicting results [13, 102, 232]. A similar situation exists for the different 5-nitroimidazoles. This is especially true for the newly introduced derivatives used in single-dose or short-term regimens [11, 70, 97, 98, 129] since optimal dosages have not yet been defined and adequate data for comparison are not available yet. The cure rates reported are in the range 60–100 % depending on the drug used, treatment schedules and the criteria for successful cure. In most studies success is reported in 90–95 % of cases.

Failures or relapses which appear either clinically or parasitologically often later than a month after therapy, especially when a single-dose is used [75, 96–98] are often cured by a second or third course [26, 97, 107, 141], by the use of a higher dosage [50] or by changing the drug [135, 177]. The most promising results have been achieved by using chemically unrelated compounds for eradicating infections not cured by prior courses [178]. This observation, as well as reports of infected patients refractory to 2 or 3 courses of metronidazole or tinidazole [42, 177] suggests that drug-resistant strains of *Giardia* may exist. However, other factors which may mimic resistance, such as reinfection by asymptomatic passers or repeated exposure in endemic areas, have to be considered.

After successful therapy the resolution of symptoms and parasitological cure are observed within a few days [26]. Restoration of the morphological and functional abnormalities of the small intestinal mucosa occurs in most cases. A few reports describe clinical failure in patients who were cured by standard regimens parasitologically, probably due to persistent lactase deficiency. These patients got rid of the 'post-giardic syndrome' spontaneously 3–9 months after the first episode [98]. In addition to the immediate treatment of symptomatic giardiasis, it is also important, particularly within the family, to treat asymptomatic cyst passers in order to decrease the transmission of the organism and prevent the development of the parasites' potential pathogenicity in the carrier host. The specific treatment of asymptomatic and symptomatic infections is identical.

In pregnancy only women with severe symptoms definitely attributable to giardiasis should be treated, as little is known about the teratogenic risk of the available drugs [219].

Metronidazole has been used for the treatment of giardiasis since 1961 [209], but the original dosage of 500 mg daily for 5 days has been modified by many investigators. Total doses from 2.5 to 10 g, divided into 2–4 daily doses over 5–10 days [163, 209] were tested in an attempt to optimize the treatment. The most commonly used current regimens are tabulated (table IV).

In competition with the more recently introduced nitroimidazoles used as a single-dose, attempts were made to switch from the conventional

Table IV. Commonly used drugs for the treatment of giardiasis

Drug	Treatment schedule	Dose			
		adult dose	reference(s)	pediatric dose (age or weight)	reference(s)
Metronidazole	multiple-dose therapy	250 mg t. i. d. × 5–10 days	26, 51, 219, 221	5 mg/kg t. i. d. × 5–10 days	51, 219
				7 mg/kg t. i. d. × 10 days	26
		500 mg t. i. d. × 5–10 days	225	or	
				1–5 years: 125 mg t. i.d. × 5–10 days	
		2,000 mg once daily × 3 days	257	6–10 years: 250 mg b. i. d. × 5–10 days	221
		2,400 mg once daily × 2–3 days	98		
Tinidazole	single-dose therapy	2,000 mg	96, 98, 135, 178, 221	50 mg/kg	11
				or	
				1–5 years: 500–1,000 mg	
				6–10 years: 1,000–1,500 mg	221
	multiple-dose therapy	150 mg b. i. d. × 7 days	5, 120, 204	1–5 years: 75 mg b. i. d. × 5–10 days	
		150 mg t. i. d. × 5–10 days	221	6–10 years: 75 mg t. i. d. × 5–10 days	221
Nimorazole	single-dose therapy	2,000 mg	221	1–5 years: 500–1,000 mg	
				6–10 years: 1,000–1,500 mg	221
	multiple-dose therapy	250 mg t. i. d. × 5–10 days	221	1–5 years: 125 mg b. i. d. × 5–10 days	
		1,000 mg once daily × 5–6 days	174, 205	6–10 years: 125 mg t. i. d. × 5–10 days	221

Table IV (continued)

Drug	Treatment schedule	Dose			
		adult dose	reference(s)	pediatric dose (age or weight)	reference(s)
Ornidazole	single-dose therapy	2,000 mg	221	25–50 mg/kg or 1–5 years: 500–1,000 mg 6–10 years: 1,000–1,500 mg	90, 248 221
	multiple-dose therapy	500 mg b. i. d. × 5–10 days	221	< 1 year: 125 mg b. i. d. × 5–10 days 1–5 years: 250 mg b. i. d. × 5–10 days 6–10 years: 375 mg b. i. d. × 5–10 days	83 221
Mepacrine (quinacrine)	multiple-dose therapy	100 mg t. i. d. × 5–10 days	51, 108, 219, 225	2 mg/kg t. i.d. × 5–7 days (max. 300 mg/day) or < 1 year: 33 mg t. i. d. × 7 days 1–4 years: 50 mg b. i. d. × 7 days 4–8 years: 50 mg t. i. d. × 7 days > 8 years: 100 mg t. i. d. × 7 days	51, 219 26
Furazolidone	multiple-dose therapy	100 mg q. i. d. × 7 days	219	1.25–6 mg/kg q. i. d. × 7 days	51, 219

scheme for metronidazole of 600–750 mg daily for 7–10 days, to short-term dosages. The first attempts using single-doses were not encouraging [107, 113, 173] and several comparative experiments showed that metronidazole was inferior to tinidazole [11, 70, 98]. Satisfactory results were achieved with single-dose treatments on 2 or 3 successive days [98, 107, 257] and thus a compromise between patient compliance and efficacy of treatment was accomplished. Metronidazole, like the other available 5-nitroimidazoles, has amoebicidal activity and is therefore preferable to mepacrine in simultaneous infections. In these cases the drug should be given at higher concentrations or in combination with a luminal amoebicide [251]. Adverse effects of metronidazole and other 5-nitroimidazoles are mentioned in the section on trichomoniasis.

The efficacy of the 5-nitroimidazole tinidazole was first described by *Andersson* et al. [5] who treated 24 students infected with *Giardia* with 150 mg twice daily for 7 days. The antigiardial activity of the drug has been confirmed by many authors using multiple-dose treatments [96, 120, 204] but shortly after successful single-dose treatments of trichomoniasis had been reported the same schedule proved to be highly active in giardiasis [5]. The overall cure rates obtained with single-dose treatments range from 90 to 100% suggesting that the 'one-shot therapy' with tinidazole in the pediatric dose of 50 mg/kg or adult dose of 2 g is as good as, if not superior, to the conventional 7-day regimen [96, 204]. Superiority of single-dose tinidazole therapy in comparison with metronidazole was especially evident in children using 50 mg/kg [11, 70]. Tinidazole was also superior to metronidazole with respect to the time taken to relieve symptoms. In a comparative trial using-single doses of 2.0 and 2.4 g of tinidazole and metronidazole respectively, tinidazole had the greatest efficacy, matched only by 2 daily 2.4 g doses of metronidazole [98]. The authors thus favored tinidazole because it was more effective in adult symptomatic giardiasis and produced fewer side effects. Commonly used treatment schedules with nimorazole, another 5-nitroimidazole, are shown in table IV.

Ornidazole is a recently introduced 5-nitroimidazole which is also used in the treatment of giardiasis [63, 90]. Single-dose and multiple-dose therapies have been tried as shown in table IV [90, 119, 248].

Mepacrine (quinacrine) was introduced for malaria therapy in 1930 and later shown to be active against giardiasis and tapeworm infestations [195]. Advances in antiparasitic chemotherapy made mepacrine obsolete as an antimalarial and tenicidal drug, but it is still commonly used in symptomatic giardiasis of adults and older children [219]. Recommended doses are shown in table IV.

Mepacrine is generally well tolerated but transient toxic psychosis has been reported in 1.5% of adult patients [252] and is therefore contraindicated in patients with a history of psychosis. Other effects are mild and may include a deep yellow discoloration of the urine, nausea, vomiting, dizziness, abdominal cramping, diarrhea and headache. Yellow discoloration of the skin and sclera rarely occur with the dose required for giardiasis treatment. Mepacrine should not be given to patients with psoriasis as pronounced exacerbation is frequently produced and exfoliative lesions have sometimes developed. The drug should also not be given to pregnant women [195].

Furazolidone is especially recommended for use in children since (in the United States at least) it is the only antigiardial drug available as a pediatric preparation [219]. Dose regimens for the drug are given in table IV. Tolerance to furazolidone is lower than to other antigiardial compounds. Side effects are not uncommon. These include hypersensitivity, resulting in skin rash, fever, hypotension and gastrointestinal disturbances. Furazolidone may cause mild reversible hemolysis in glucose-6-phosphate dehydrogenase-deficient individuals. The urine may also become brownish. *Smith and Wolfe* [219] have reported that furazolidone induced mammary tumors in rats, but although the US FDA has questioned its safety in human beings it continues to be approved, with appropriate warnings, for giardiasis.

Prophylactic medication for giardiasis is a matter of some controversy. Although chemoprophylaxis is not generally recommended due to the lack of safe and effective drugs [219], courses of metronidazole were considered as being useful chemoprophylaxis for travellers [91, 180]. Good personal and environmental hygiene and the treatment of infected household animals are fundamental to prevention, and precautions regarding food and drink are the same as those advised for the prevention of any infectious gastrointestinal disease. Drinking water from possibly contaminated water supplies should be disinfected by adequate physical or chemical methods [93]. The cysts have been shown to remain viable for 2 months or longer in water at 8 °C [17].

New Advances and Future Needs

Recent developments have been made in research on *Giardia* and giardiasis stimulated by an increased interest in this disease. Axenic culture techniques for *G. duodenalis*-type organisms in liquid or semisolid media [72, 239], the cryopreservation [244] and the development of an excystation technique [17] enables cultures to be established and used for physiological, biochemical and immunological studies [16, 17, 121, 161, 196, 245], as well as for screening tests [99]. The development of a standard defined animal model [189] has facilitated the study of host-parasite interactions, elucidating possible mechanisms of resistance, pathogenicity and clearance [128, 172, 186–188, 223]. This model can also be used for the assessment of possible chemotherapeutic agents. Progress has also been made in human studies focusing on the pathogenesis of malabsorption and steatorrhea [76, 256] and on serologic diagnosis [240].

However, many problems remain, not least being that of nomenclature. The criteria used for the identification of *Giardia* species are insufficient and confusing. They do not allow an accurate speciation which would help epidemiologists to evaluate the reservoir of the human parasite, to identify species pathogenic to man and thus to elucidate the mechanism of transmission. More sophisticated criteria will be helpful in the characterization of genera, species and strains of *Giardia* organisms. Although animal experiments on the disease process are informative, extrapolation to the human host is always questionable; thus more studies in the human on predisposing factors, pathogenesis, pathogenic mechanisms and the immune response will be useful. From the clinician's point of view several developments would be welcomed, including a serologic test for diagnosis, the comparative evaluation of currently available drugs, the availability of a safe effective drug which is not absorbed intraintestinally, for the treatment of giardiasis in pregnancy and a prophylactic agent for travellers. A simple assay for drug sensitivity of isolated *Giardia* would also be helpful in case of treatment failure.

References

1 Ackers, J. P.; Catterall, R. D.; Lumsden, W. H. R.; McMillan, A.: Absence of detectable local antibody in genitourinary tract secretions of male contacts of women infected with *Trichomonas vaginalis*. Br. J. vener. Dis. *54:* 168–171 (1978).

2 Actor, P.; Ziv, D. S.; Pagano, J. F.: Resistance to metronidazole by *Trichomonas foetus* in hamsters infected intravaginally. Science *164:* 439–440 (1969).

3 Akimova, R. F.; Solovev, M. M.; Tolmazova, A. P.: Prevalence of intestinal protozoan infections in children of various ages in children's institutions of the Lenin district of Moscow. Medskaya Parazit. *46:* 466–472 (1977).

4 Al-Salihi, F. L.; Curran, J. P.; Wang, J. S.: Neonatal *Trichomonas vaginalis:* report of three cases and review of the literature. Pediatrics *53:* 196–200 (1974).

5 Andersson, T.; Forssel, J.; Sterner, G.: Outbreak of giardiasis: effect of a new antiflagellate drug, tinidazole. Br. med. J. *ii:* 449–451 (1972).

6 Anjaneyulu, R.; Gupte, S. A.; Desai, D. B.: Single-dose treatment of trichomonal vaginitis: a comparison of tinidazole and metronidazole. J. int. med. Res. *5:* 438–441 (1977).

7 Apte, V. V.; Packard, R. S.: Tinidazole in the treatment of trichomoniasis, giardiasis and amoebiasis. Report of a multicentre study. Drugs *15:* suppl. 1, pp. 43–48 (1978).

8 Asami, K.: Effects of metronidazole on *Trichomonas vaginalis* in culture and in an experimental host. Am. J. trop. Med. Hyg. *12:* 535–538 (1963).

9 Atia, W. A.; Thin, R. N.: Cervical cytology in genital infection. Br. J. vener. Dis. *51:* 331–332 (1975).

10 Baines, E. J.: Metronidazole: its past, present and future. J. antimicrob. Chemother. *4:* suppl. C, pp. 97–111 (1978).

11 Bakshi, J. S.; Ghiara, J. M.; Nanivadekar, A. S.: How does tinidazole compare with metronidazole? A summary report of Indian trials in amoebiasis and giardiasis. Drugs *15:* suppl. 1, pp. 33–42 (1978).

12 Baron, A.: Oral treatment of vaginal trichomoniasis; in Gasparri, The diagnosis and chemotherapy of urogenital, bacterial, protozoal and mycotic infections, pp. 163–167. Proc. Int. Symp., Florence 1971 (Edizioni Mediche P. Periti, Florence 1972).

13 Bassily, S.; Farid, Z.; Mikhail, J. W.; Kent, D. C.; Lehman, J. S., Jr.: The treatment of *Giardia lamblia* infection with mepacrine, metronidazole and furazolidone. J. trop. Med. Hyg. *73:* 15–18 (1970).

14 Beard, C. M.; Noller, K. L.; O'Fallon, W. M.; Kurland, L. T.; Dockerty, M. B.: Lack of evidence for cancer due to use of metronidazole. New Engl. J. Med. *301:* 519–522 (1979).

15 Benazet, F.; Guillaume, L.: Activités antiamibienne et trichomonacide du secnidazole au laboratoire. Bull. Soc. Path. exot. *69:* 309–319 (1976).

16 Bertram, M. A.; Jaroll, E. L.; Meyer, E. A.: Comparison of the electrophoretic mobility of enzymes of *Giardia* isolated from human, cat and guinea pig hosts. Abstr. 80th Annu. Meet. Am. Soc. Microbiol., Miami Beach 1980, p. 150, K 144.

17 Bingham, A. K.; Jaroll, E. L., Jr.; Meyer, E. A.; Radulescu, S.: *Giardia* sp.: physical factors of excystation in vitro, and excystation vs. eosin exclusion as determinants of viability. Expl Parasit. *47:* 284–291 (1979).

18 Bock, M.: Ergebnisse experimenteller Versuche mit 1-(Hydroxyaethyl)-2-methyl-5-nitroimidazol an *Trichomonas vaginalis* und *Entamoeba histolytica.* Arzneimittel-Forsch. *11:* 587–590 (1961).

19 Borten, M.; Friedman, E. A.: Duration of colposcopic changes associated with *Trichomonas vaginalis.* Obstet. Gynec. *51:* 111–113 (1978).

20 Bost, R. G.: Metronidazole: toxicology and teratology; in Finegold, Metronidazole, pp. 112–117. Proc. Int. Conf., Montreal 1976 (Excerpta Medica, Amsterdam 1977).

21 Bost, R. G.: Metronidazole: mammalian mutagenicity; in Finegold, Metroni-

dazole, pp. 126–131. Proc. Int. Conf., Montreal 1976 (Excerpta Medica, Amsterdam 1977).

22 Brandborg, L. L.; Owen, R.; Fogel, R.; Goldberg, H.; Garvie, J.; Grossman, S.: Giardiasis and traveler's diarrhea. Gastroenterology *78:* 1602–1614 (1980).

23 Brandl, E.: Lokale Salbenbehandlung der Vulvitis als Ergänzungstherapie der infektiösen Kolpitis. Therapiewoche *26:* 7251 (1976).

24 Brotherton, J.: Biological assay of potential trichomonacides in vitro using a counter apparatus. Arzneimittel-Forsch. *28:* 1665–1672 (1978).

25 Brown, M. T.: Trichomoniasis. Practitioner *209:* 639–644 (1972).

26 Burke, J. A.: The clinical and laboratory diagnosis of giardiasis. Crit. Rev. Clin. Lab. Sci. *7:* 373–391 (1977).

27 Cappuccinelli, P.; Lattes, C.; Cagliani, I.; Negro Ponzi, A.: Features of intravaginal *Trichomonas vaginalis* infection in the mouse and the effect of oestrogen treatment and immunodepression. G. Batt. Virol. Immun. *67:* 31–40 (1974).

28 Carneri, I. de; Trane, F.: Oral infection of mice with trophozoites of *Giardia muris.* Am. J. trop. Med. Hyg. *26:* 566–567 (1977).

29 Catterall, R. D.: Alternative dosage regimens in trichomoniasis; in Finegold, Metronidazole, pp. 79–82. Proc. Int. Conf., Montreal 1976 (Excerpta Medica, Amsterdam 1977).

30 Cavier, R.; Mossion, X.: Essais d'infestation expérimentale de la ratte par *Trichomonas vaginalis* (Donné, 1837). C. r. hebd. Séanc. Acad. Sci., Paris *242:* 2412–2414 (1956).

31 Cavier, R.; Savel, J.; Quemerais, M.-J.: Sur une technique d'essai in vivo des substances trichomonacides. C. r. hebd. Séanc. Acad. Sci., Paris *249:* 2641–2642 (1959).

32 Cerkasov, J.; Cerkasovova, A.; Kulda, J.: Carbohydrate metabolism of *Tritrichomonas foetus* with particular respect to enzyme reactions occurring in hydrogenosomes; in Federation of European Biochemical Societies, vol. 61 (trends in enzymology), industrial and clinical enzymology, pp. 257–275 (Pergamon Press, Oxford 1980).

33 Cerkasovova, A.; Cerkasov, J.; Kulda, J.; Dohnalova, M.: Metabolic properties of *Trichomonas foetus* resistant to metronidazole. 4th Int. Congr. Parasitol., Warsaw, 1978, section F, p. 43.

34 Chatterjee, D. K.; Ray, D. K.: A simple medium for in vitro culture of *Trichomonas vaginalis.* J. Parasit. *65:* 815–816 (1979).

35 Chintana, T.; Sucharit, P.; Chongsuphajaisiddhi, T.; Tongprasoeth, N.; Suphadtanaphongs, W.: Prevalence of *Trichomonas vaginalis* in selected groups of the population in Bangkok. Southeast Asian J. trop. Med. Publ. Hlth *10:* 162–163 (1979).

36 Cohen, S. M.; Ertürk, E.; Von Esch, A. M.; Crovetti, A. J.; Bryan, G. T.: Carcinogenicity of 5-nitrofurans, 5-nitroimidazoles, 4-nitrobenzenes, and related compounds. J. natn. Cancer Inst. *51:* 403–417 (1973).

37 Craun, G. F.: Water-borne outbreaks of giardiasis; in Jakubowski, Hoff, Waterborne transmission of giardiasis, pp. 127–147. Proc. Symp. 1978 (US Environmental Protection Agency, Cincinnati 1979).

38 Croll, N. A.; Gyorkos, T. W.: Parasitic disease in humans: the extent in Canada. Can. med. Ass. J. *120:* 310–312 (1979).

39 Csonka, G. W.: Trichomonal vaginitis treated with one dose of metronidazole. Br. J. vener. Dis. *47:* 456–458 (1971).

40 Cuckler, A. C.; Kupferberg, A. B.; Millman, N.: Chemotherapeutic and tolerance studies on amino-nitro-thiazoles. Antibiot. Chemother. *5:* 540–550 (1955).

41 Dainer, M. J.: Untoward reaction of Flagyl (metronidazole). Am. J. Obstet. Gynec. *133:* 939–940 (1979).

42 Danzig, S.; Hatchuel, W. L. F.: Single dose treatment of giardiasis with tinidazole. S. Afr. med. J. *52:* 708 (1977).

43 Darrow, W. W.; Wiesner, P. J.: Personal prophylaxis for venereal diseases. J. Am. med. Ass. *233:* 444–446 (1975).

44 Davie, G.: *Giardia* infestation. S. Afr. med. J. *52:* 260 (1977).

45 Davies, R. B.; Hibler, C. P.: Animal reservoirs and cross-species transmission of *Giardia;* in Jakubowski, Hoff, Water-borne transmission of giardiasis, pp. 104–125. Proc. Symp. 1978 (US Environmental Protection Agency, Cincinnati 1979).

46 Dennerstein, G.: Effective treatment of vaginitis. Drugs *19:* 146–151 (1980).

47 Diamond, L. S.: The establishment of various trichomonads of animals and man in axenic cultures. J. Parasit. *48:* 488–490 (1957).

48 Durel, P.; Roiron, V.; Siboulet, H.; Borel, L. J.: Trial of an antitrichomonal derivative of imidazole (8823 RP). C. r. Soc. fr. Gynéc. *29:* 36–45 (1959).

49 Dykers, J. R., Jr.: Single-dose metronidazole. Am. J. Obstet. Gynec. *132:* 703–704 (1978).

50 Eastham, E. J.; Douglas, A. P.; Watson, A. J.: Diagnosis of *Giardia lamblia* infection as a cause of diarrhoea. Lancet *ii:* 950–951 (1976).

51 Editorial: Drugs for parasitic infections. Med. Lett. *21:* 105–112 (1979).

52 Editorial: Sexually transmitted diseases (extract from the annual report of the Chief Medical Officer of the Department of Health and Social Security for the year 1977). Br. J. vener. Dis. *55:* 225–229 (1979).

53 Editorial: Sexually transmitted disease surveillance 1978. Br. med. J. *ii:* 1375–1376 (1979).

54 Editorial: Giardiasis and water. Lancet *i:* 1176 (1980).

55 Editorial: Physicians' Desk Reference® *34:* 1601–1602 (1980).

56 Edwards, D. I.: Mechanism of antimicrobial action of metronidazole. J. Antimicrob. Chemother. *5:* 499–502 (1979).

57 Edwards, D. I.; Shanson, D.: Metronidazole inactivation by aerobes. J. antimicrob. Chemother. *6:* 402–403 (1980).

58 Edwards, D. I.; Thompson, E. J.; Tomusange, I.: Inactivation of metronidazole by aerobic organisms. J. antimicrob. Chemother. *5:* 315–316 (1979).

59 Evans, B. A.; Catterall, R. D.: Nifuratel compared with metronidazole in the treatment of trichomonal vaginitis. Br. med. J. *ii:* 335–336 (1970).

60 Evans, B. A.; Catterall, R. D.: Nitrimidazine compared with metronidazole in the treatment of vaginal trichomoniasis. Br. med. J. *iv:* 146–147 (1971).

61 Fanta, D.; Gebhart, W.; Gross, W.; Kokoschka, E. M.; Söltz-Szöts, J.; Thurner, J.: Results of routine screening for sexually transmitted diseases in Austria over a six-year period. Br. J. vener. Dis. *55:* 147–148 (1979).

62 Felman, Y. M.; Riccardi, N. B.: Incidence and epidemiology of sexually transmitted diseases. Curr. ther. Res. *26:* 665–674 (1979).

63 Fernex, M.; Jeunet, F.; Richle, R.: Development of a nitroimidazole derivative (Ro 7-0207) for the treatment of amoebiasis, lambliasis and trichomoniasis; in Daikos, Progress in Chemotherapy, vol, I, pp. 978–982. Proc. 8th Int. Congr. Chemother., Athens 1973 (Hellenic Society for Chemotherapy, Athens 1974).

64 Filice, F. P.: Studies on the cytology and life history of a *Giardia* from the laboratory rat. Univ. Calif., Berkeley, Publ. Zool. *57:* 53–146 (1952).

65 Fleury, F. J.; Van Bergen, W. S.; Prentice, R. L.; Russel, J. G.; Singleton, J. A.; Standard, J. V.: Single dose of two grams of metronidazole for *Trichomonas vaginalis* infection. Am. J. Obstet. Gynec. *128:* 320–322 (1977).

66 Forsgren, A.; Forssman, L.: Metronidazole-resistant *Trichomonas vaginalis*. Br. J. vener. Dis. *55:* 351–353 (1979).

67 Fouts, A. C.; Kraus, S. J.: *Trichomonas vaginalis:* reevaluation of its clinical presentation and laboratory diagnosis. J. infect. Dis. *141:* 137–143 (1980).

68 Fowler, W.; Hussain, M.: Nifuratel (Magmilor) in trichomonal vaginitis. Br. J. vener. Dis. *44:* 331–333 (1968).

69 Gardner, H. L.: Urogenital trichomoniasis; in Finegold, Metronidazole, pp. 72–78. Proc. Int. Conf., Montreal 1976 (Excerpta Medica, Amsterdam 1977).

70 Gazder, A. J.; Banerjee, M.: Single dose therapy of giardiasis with tinidazole and metronidazole. Drugs *15:* suppl. 1, pp. 30–32 (1978).

71 Giannini, A. J.: Side effects of metronidazole. Am. J. Psychiat. *134:* 329–330 (1977).

72 Gillin, F. D.; Diamond, L. S.: Clonal growth of *Giardia lamblia* trophozoites in a semisolid agarose medium. J. Parasit. *66:* 350–352 (1980).

73 Goldacre, M. J.; Watt, B.; Loudon, N.; Milne, L. J. R.; Loudon, J. D. O.; Vessey, M. P.: Vaginal microbial flora in normal young women. Br. med. J. *i:* 1450–1453 (1979).

74 Granitzka, S.: Short-term therapy of urogenital trichomoniasis with a new nitroimidazole derivative (Ornidazole/Tiberal, Roche); in Williams, Geddes, Chemotherapy, vol. III, pp. 179–184. Proc. 9th Int. Congr. Chemother., London 1975 (Plenum Press, New York 1976).

75 Green, E.; Lynch, D. M.; McFadzean, J. A.; Pugh, I. M.: Treatment of giardiasis. Br. med. J. *iii:* 411–412 (1974).

76 Hartong, W. A.; Gounley, W. K.; Arvanitakis, C.: Giardiasis: clinical spectrum and functional-structural abnormalities of the small intestinal mucosa. Gastroenterology *77:* 61–69 (1979).

77 Heginbotham, D.: Trichomoniasis: recognition and treatment. Curr. Therap. *18:* 33, 35, 37, 38, 40 (1977).

78 Heiss, H.: Zur Behandlung der *Trichomoniasis vaginalis*. Wien. med. Wschr. *121:* 30–33 (1971).

79 Heiss, H.: Klinische Auswertung aktiver Arzneimittel gegen *Trichomonas vaginalis* im Doppel-Blindversuch. Wien. med. Wschr. *121:* 832–834 (1971).

80 Heyworth, P. G.; Gutteridge, W. E.; Ginger, C. D.: Further studies on the purine and pyrimidine metabolism in *T. vaginalis*. J. Protozool. *25:* 9 B, abstr. 213 (1978).

81 Heyworth, R.; Simpson, D.; McNeillage, G. J. C.; Robertson, D. H. H.; Young, H.: Isolation of *Trichomonas vaginalis* resistant to metronidazole. Lancet *ii:* 476–478 (1980).

82 Hillström, L.; Pettersson, L.; Pálsson, E.; Sandström, S. O.: Comparison of ornidazole and tinidazole in single-dose treatment of trichomoniasis in women. Br. J. vener. Dis. *53:* 193–194 (1977).

83 Hofstetter, A.: Neue Medikamente: Tiberal® Roche. Urologe, A *16:* 308–309 (1977).

84 Hollander, D. H.: Colonial morphology of *Trichomonas vaginalis* in agar. J. Parasit. *62:* 826–828 (1976).

85 Honigberg, B. M.: Trichomonads of importance in human medicine; in Kreier, Parasitic protozoa, vol. II, pp. 275–454 (Academic Press, New York 1978).

86 Honigberg, B. M.; Livingston, M. C.: In vitro sensitivity of *Trichomonas vaginalis* to metronidazole; in Corradetti, Proc. 1st Int. Congr. Parasitology, Rome 1964, vol. I, p. 365 (Pergamon Press, Oxford/Tamburini Editore, Milan 1966).

87 Hotho, H.: *Trichomonas vaginalis* und zytologischer Befund. Arch. Geschwulstforsch. *47:* 455–461 (1977).

88 Howes, H. L., Jr.; Lynch, J. E.; Kivlin, J. L.: Tinidazole, a new protozoal agent: effect on *Trichomonas* and other protozoa. Antimicrob. Agents Chemother. *1969:* 261–266 (1970).

89 Ingham, H. R.; Hall, C. J.; Sisson, P. R.; Tharagonnet, D.; Selkon, J. B.: Inactivation of metronidazole by aerobic organisms. J. antimicrob. Chemother. *5:* 734–735 (1979).

90 Iyngkaran, N.; Lee, E. L.; Robinson, M. J.: Single dose treatment with Tiberal of *Giardia lamblia* infection in children. Scand. J. infect. Dis. *10:* 243–246 (1978).

91 James, D. G.: Traveller's diarrhoea. J. Antimicrob. Chemother. *3:* 5–6 (1977).

92 Jankó, M.: Single dose treatment of giardiasis with tinidazole in children. 4th Int. Congr. Parasitol., Warsaw, 1978, section D, p. 92.

93 Jarrol, E. L., Jr.; Bingham, A. K.; Meyer, E. A.: *Giardia* cyst destruction: effectiveness of six small-quantity water disinfection methods. Am. J. trop. Med. Hyg. *29:* 8–11 (1980).

94 Jirovec, O.; Petru, M.: *Trichomonas vaginalis* and trichomoniasis. Adv. Parasitol. *6:* 117–188 (1968).

95 John, J.; Squires, S.: Abnormal forms of *Trichomonas vaginalis*. Br. J. vener. Dis. *54:* 84–87 (1978).

96 Jokipii, A. M. M.; Jokipii, L.: Comparative evaluation of two dosages of tinidazole in the treatment of giardiasis. Am. J. trop. Med. Hyg. *27:* 758–761 (1978).

97 Jokipii, L.; Jokipii, A. M. M.: Comparison of four dosage schedules in the treatment of giardiasis with metronidazole. Infection *6:* 92–94 (1978).

98 Jokipii, L.; Jokipii, A. M. M.: Single dose metronidazole and tinidazole as therapy for giardiasis: success rates, side effects, and drug absorption and elimination. J. infect. Dis. *140:* 984–988 (1979).

99 Jokipii, L.; Jokipii, A. M. M.: In vitro susceptibility of *Giardia lamblia* trophozoites to metronidazole and tinidazole. J. infect. Dis. *141:* 317–325 (1980).

100 Kane, P. O.; McFadzean, J. A.; Squires, S.: Absorption and excretion of metronidazole. II. Studies on primary failures. Br. J. vener. Dis. *37:* 276–277 (1961).

101 Karapetyan, A. E.: Methods of *Lamblia* cultivation. Tsitologiya, Moskva *2:* 379–384 (1960).

102 Kavousi, S.: Giardiasis in infancy and childhood: a prospective study of 160 cases with comparison of quinacrine (Atabrine) and metronidazole (Flagyl). Am. J. trop. Med. Hyg. *28:* 19–23 (1979).

103 Kawamura, N.: Metronidazole and tinidazole in a single large dose for treating urogenital infections with *Trichomonas vaginalis* in men. Br. J. vener. Dis. *54:* 81–83 (1978).

104 Keighley, E. E.: Trichomoniasis in a closed community. 100 percent follow up. Br. med. J. *ii:* 93–95 (1962).

105 Keighley, E. E.: Trichomoniasis in a closed community: efficacy of metronidazole. Br. med. J. *i:* 207–209 (1971).

106 Keystone, J. S.; Krajden, S.; Warren, M. R.: Person to person transmission of *Giardia lamblia* in day care nurseries. Can. med. Ass. J. *119:* 241–242 (1978).

107 Khambatta, R. B.: Metronidazole in giardiasis. Ann. trop. Med. Parasit. *65:* 487–489 (1971).

108 Knight, R.: Giardiasis, isosporiasis and balantidiasis. Clin. Gastroenterol. *7:* 31–47 (1978).

109 Komaroff, A. L.; Cohen, A. B.; McCue, J.: Alternatives to metronidazole. J. Am. med. Ass. *235:* 2081–2082 (1976).

110 Korner, B.; Jensen, H. K.: Sensitivity of *Trichomonas vaginalis* to metronidazole, tinidazole, and nifuratel in vitro. Br. J. vener. Dis. *52:* 404–408 (1976).

111 Korte, W.: Epidemiologie, Pathologie und Klinik der Infektion mit *Trichomonas vaginalis*. Med. Klin. *68:* 99–106 (1973).

112 Kozlowska, D.; Wichrowska, B.: The effect of chlorine and its compounds used for disinfection of water on *Trichomonas vaginalis*. Wiad. parazyt. *22:* 433–435 (1976).

113 Krishnamurthy, K. A.; Saradhambal, V.: Single dose therapy of giardiasis: a comparative study of tinidazole and metronidazole in pediatric patients. Indian Pediat. *15:* 51–56 (1978).

114 Kuberski, T.: Evaluation of the indirect hemagglutination technique for study of *Trichomonas vaginalis* infections, particularly in men. Sex. transm. Dis. *5:* 97–102 (1978).

115 Kulda, J.; Nohynková, E.: Flagellates of the human intestine and of intestines of other species; in Kreier, Parasitic protozoa, vol. II, pp. 1–138 (Academic Press, New York 1978).

116 Kurnatowska, A.: Comparison of the efficacy of anti-trichomonal drugs in cases of trichomoniasis restricted to the vagina. Wiad. parazyt. *25:* 417–425 (1979).

117 Lawrence, R. M.: Infections of the female genital tract; in Hoeprich, Infectious diseases; 2nd ed., pp. 443–454 (Harper & Row, Hagerstown 1977).

118 Legator, M. S.; Connor, T. H.; Stoeckel, M.: Detection of mutagenic activity of metronidazole and niridazole in body fluids of humans and mice. Science *188:* 1118–1119 (1975).

119 Leite, E. V.; Gonçalves, A. L. C.; Costa, D. G. L. da; Costa Filho, R. L. da; Podkameni, N.: Comparison between ornidazole and metronidazole in intestinal

giardiasis – a double blind clinical trial. Revta Inst. Med. trop. S. Paulo *18:* 28–35 (1976).

120 Levi, G. C.; Avila, C. A de; Neto, V. A.: Efficacy of various drugs for treatment of giardiasis. A comparative study. Am. J. trop. Med. Hyg. *26:* 564–565 (1977).

121 Lindmark, D. G.: Energy metabolism of the anaerobic protozoon *Giardia lamblia.* Molec. biochem. Parasit. *1:* 1–12 (1980).

122 Lindmark, D. G.; Müller, M.: Hydrogenosome, a cytoplasmic organelle of the anaerobic flagellate *Tritrichomonas foetus,* and its role in pyruvate metabolism. J. biol. Chem. *248:* 7724–7728 (1973).

123 Lindmark, D. G.; Müller, M.: Antitrichomonad action, mutagenicity, and reduction of metronidazole and other nitroimidazoles. Antimicrob. Agents Chemother. *10:* 476–482 (1976).

124 Lindner, J. G. E. M.; Plantema, F. H. F.; Vos, N. M. de; Hoogkamp-Korstanje, A. A.: Reaction of the vaginal flora to ornidazole in patients with cervicitis. Chemotherapy *25:* 243–248 (1979).

125 Lloyd, D.; Lindmark, D. G.; Müller, M.: Respiration of *Tritrichomonas foetus.* J. Parasit. *65:* 466–469 (1979).

126 Lövgren, T.; Salmela, I.: In vitro sensitivity of *Trichomonas vaginalis* and *Candida albicans* to chemotherapeutic agents. Acta path. microbiol. scand., B, Microbil. *86:* 155–158 (1978).

127 Lumsden, W. H. R.; Robertson, D. H. H.; McNeillage, G. J. C.: Isolation, cultivation, low temperature preservation, and infectivity titration of *Trichomonas vaginalis.* Br. J. vener. Dis. *42:* 145–154 (1966).

128 MacDonald, T. T.; Ferguson, A.: Small intestinal epithelial cell kinetics and protozoal infection in mice. Gastroenterology *74:* 496–500 (1978).

129 Madanagopalan, N.; Prabhakar Rao, U.; Somasundaram, A.; Lakshmipathi, T.: A correlative study of duodenal aspirate and faeces examination in giardiasis, before and after treatment with metronidazole. Curr. med. Res. Opin. *3:* 99–103 (1975).

130 Maestrone, G.; Semar, R.: Experimental intravaginal infection with *Trichomonas foetus* in guinea pigs. Chemotherapia *12:* 137–145 (1967).

131 Mahony, J. D. H.; Harris, J. R. W.; Farrer, C. J.: Nimorazole and metronidazole in the treatment of trichomonal vaginitis. Br. J. clin. Pract. *29:* 71–72 (1975).

132 Mandoul, R.; Dargelos, R; Millan, J.: Destruction des protozoaires intestinaux de la souris par un dérivé nitré de l'imidazole. Bull. Soc. Path. exot. *54:* 12–16 (1961).

133 Marion-Landais, G.; Heotis, J. P.; Herrett, R. J.; Diaz, J. R.: Nonabsorption of furazolidone from the vagina in women. Curr. ther. Res. *18:* 510–512 (1975).

134 Mason, P. R.: Serodiagnosis of *Trichomonas vaginalis* infection by the indirect fluorescent antibody test. J. clin. Path. *32:* 1211–1215 (1979).

135 Masry, N. A. E.; Farid, Z.; Miner, W. E.: Treatment of giardiasis with tinidazole. Am. J. trop. Med. Hyg. *27:* 201–202 (1978).

136 Matheson, I.; Hernborg Johannessen, K.; Bjørkvoll, B.: Plasma levels after a single oral dose of 1.5 g ornidazole. Br. J. vener. Dis. *53:* 236–239 (1977).

137 McCann, J.; Choi, E.; Yamasaki, E.; Ames, B. N.: Detection of carcinogens as mutagens in the *Salmonella*/microsome test: assay of 300 chemicals. Proc. natn. Acad. Sci. USA *72:* 5135–5139 (1975).

138 McCann, J. S.; Horner, T.; Shepherd, I.; Quin, N.: 2-day treatment of trichomoniasis with nimorazole. Br. J. vener. Dis. *50:* 375–376 (1974).

139 McCann, J. S.; Mahony, D. H.; Harris, J. W. R.: Comparison of nitrimidazine and metronidazole in the treatment of trichomonal vaginitis. Br. J. vener. Dis. *48:* 387–390 (1972).

140 Meerovitch, E.: Cultivation of *Trichomonas vaginalis;* in Taylor, Baker, Methods in cultivating parasites in vitro, pp. 33–37 (Academic Press, London 1978).

141 Mehrotra, S. N.: Treatment of giardiasis with single dose of metronidazole (Flagyl) in children. Pediat. Clins India *10:* 145–147 (1975).

142 Meingassner, J. G.: Comparative studies on the trichomonacidal activity of 5-nitroimidazole-derivatives in mice infected s. c. or intravaginally with *T. vaginalis.* Experientia *33:* 1160–1161 (1977).

143 Meingassner, J. G.; Georgopoulos, A.; Patoschka, M.: Intravaginale Infektionen der Ratte mit *Trichomonas vaginalis* und *Candida albicans.* Z. Tropenmed. Parasit. *26:* 395–398 (1975).

144 Meingassner, J. G.; Havelec, L.; Mieth, H.: Studies on strain sensitivity of *Trichomonas vaginalis* to metronidazole. Br. J. vener. Dis. *54:* 72–76 (1978).

145 Meingassner, J. G.; Mieth, H.: Cross-resistance of trichomonads to 5-nitroimidazole-derivatives. Experientia *32:* 183–184 (1976).

146 Meingassner, J. G.; Mieth, H.: Die Wirksamkeit bekannter systemisch wirksamer Trichomonazide im Infektionsmodell *Trichomonas vaginalis*/Ratte. Arzneimittel-Forsch. *27:* 638–639 (1977).

147 Meingassner, J. G.; Mieth, H.; Czok, R.; Lindmark, D. G.; Müller, M.: Assay conditions and the demonstration of nitroimidazole resistance in *Tritrichomonas foetus.* Antimicrob. Agents Chemother. *13:* 1–3 (1978).

148 Meingassner, J. G.; Stockinger, K.: Untersuchungen zur Identifikation Metronidazol-resistenter *Trichomonas vaginalis*-Stämme in vitro. Z. Hautkr. (in press, 1981).

149 Meingassner, J. G.; Thurner, J.: Strain of *Trichomonas vaginalis* resistant to metronidazole and other 5-nitroimidazoles. Antimicrob. Agents Chemother. *15:* 254–257 (1979).

150 Mettler, L.: Wirkungsvolle Kurzzeitbehandlung der Trichomonaden-Infektion im Bereich des weiblichen Genitale. Therapiewoche *28:* 6095–6098 (1978).

151 Meyer, E. A.: *Giardia lamblia:* isolation and axenic cultivation. Expl Parasit. *39:* 101–105 (1976).

152 Meyer, E. A.; Jaroll, E. L.: Giardiasis. Am. J. Epidem. *111:* 1–12 (1980).

153 Meyer, E. A.; Radulescu, S.: *Giardia* and Giardiasis. Adv. Parasitol. *17:* 1–47 (1979).

154 Meyers, E.; Chang, C. A.: The use of phenolphthalein monophosphate to enhance bioautography with *Trichomonas vaginalis.* J. Antibiot. *32:* 846–848 (1979).

155 Meyers, J. D.; Kuharic, H. A.; Holmes, K. K.: *Giardia lamblia* infection in homosexual men. Br. J. vener. Dis. *53:* 54–55 (1977).

156 Michaels, R. M.: Chemotherapy of trichomoniasis. Adv. Chemother. *3:* 39–108 (1968).

157 Michaels, R. M.; Peterson, L. J.; Stahl, G. L.: Substituted dithiocarbamates and related compounds as trichomonacides. J. Pharm. Pharmac. *15:* 107–113 (1963).

158 Michaels, R. M.; Strube, R. E.: Antitrichomonal agents 5-nitrothiazoles, 5-nitropyridines and 5-nitropyrimidines. J. Pharm. Pharmac. *13:* 601–610 (1961).

159 Mischer, P.; Söltz-Szöts, J.; Thurner, J.: Kurzzeitbehandlung der Trichomoniasis. Z. Hautkr. *51:* 465–468 (1976).

160 Moffett, M.; McGill, M. I.; Schofield, C. B. S.; Masterton, G.: Nitrimidazine in the treatment of trichomoniasis. Br. J. vener. Dis. *47:* 173–176 (1971).

161 Moore, G. W.; Sogandares-Bernal, F.; Dennis, M. V.; Root, D. M.: *Giardia lamblia:* antigenic analyses of somatic extracts and secretory-excretory products. Abstr. 80th Annu. Meet. Am. Soc. Microbiol, Miami Beach 1980, p. 293, C 110.

162 Morgan, B. B.; Lombard, L.; Pierce, A. E.: Chemotherapy of *Trichomonas foetus* infections in rabbits. Proc. Soc. exp. Biol. Med. *70:* 243–246 (1949).

163 Most, H.: Treatment of common parasitic infections of man encountered in the United States (second of two parts). New Engl. J. Med. *287:* 698–702 (1972).

164 Müller, M.: Mode of action of metronidazole on anaerobic micro-organisms; in Phillips, Collier, Metronidazole, pp. 223–228. Proc. 2nd Int. Conf., Geneva 1979 (Royal Society of Medicine and Academic Press, London/Grune & Stratton, New York 1979).

165 Müller, M.: The hydrogenosome; in Gooday, Lloyd, Trinci, The eukaryotic microbial cell, pp. 127–142 (Cambridge University Press, Cambridge 1980).

166 Müller, M.; Lindmark, D. G.: Uptake of metronidazole and its effect on viability in trichomonads and *Entamoeba invadens* under anaerobic and aerobic conditions. Antimicrob. Agents Chemother. *9:* 696–700 (1976).

167 Müller, M.; Meingassner, J. G.; Miller, W. A.; Ledger, W. J.: Three metronidazole-resistant strains of *Trichomonas vaginalis* from the USA. Am. J. Obstet. Gynec. *138:* 808–812 (1980).

168 Nedvedova, H.; Kulda, J.: Pathogenicity of a virulent *Trichomonas vaginalis* strain for the laboratory rat after intravaginal inoculation. J. Protozool. *25:* 39A, abstr. 117 (1978).

169 Notowicz, A.; Stolz, E.; Koning, G. A. J. de: First experiences with single-dose treatment of vaginal trichomoniasis with carnidazole (R 25831). Br. J. vener. Dis. *53:* 129–131 (1977).

170 Nygaard, B.; Kjaersgaard, H.; Korner, B.; Jensen, R. H.: Single dose treatment with ornidazole (Tiberal®) and seven day treatment with metronidazole (Flagyl®) for vaginal trichomoniasis. Ugeskr. Laeg. *139:* 524–526 (1977).

171 O'Connor, B. H.; Adler, M. W.: Current approaches to the diagnosis, treatment, and reporting of trichomoniasis and candidosis. Br. J. vener. Dis. *55:* 52–57 (1979).

172 Owen, R. L.; Nemanic, P. C.; Stevens, D. P.: Ultrastructural observations on giardiasis in a murine model. I. Intestinal distribution, attachment and relationship to the immune system of *Giardia muris.* Gastroenterology *76:* 757–769 (1979).

173 Pai, V. R.; Joshi, V.; Kale, S. S.; Sule, C. R.: A preliminary study of single dose therapy with metronidazole (Flagyl) in giardiasis. Indian Practner *24:* 301–304 (1971).

174 Pai, V. R.; Wadia, F. F.; Dange, M.; Sule, C. R.; Kale, S. S.: Naxogen (Nitrimidazine) in giardiasis. J. Ass. Physns India *22:* 531–533 (1974).

175 Paredes, F. R.; Hawkins, D. F.: Sensitivity of *Trichomonas vaginalis* to chemotherapeutic agents. J. Obstet. Gynaec. Br. Commonw. *80:* 86–88 (1973).
176 Pathak, U. N.; Sur, S. K.; Farrand, R. J.: Comparison of metronidazole/nystatin and nifuratel in the treatment of vaginitis. Br. J. clin. Pract. *29:* 270–272 (1975).
177 Pettersson, T.: The effect of tinidazole (Fasigyn®) in the treatment of giardiasis resistant to metronidazole; in Daikos, Progress in chemotherapy, vol. I, pp. 963–965. Proc. 8th Int. Congr. Chemother., Athens 1973 (Hellenic Society for Chemotherapy, Athens 1974).
178 Pettersson, T.: Single dose tinidazole therapy for giardiasis. Br. med. J. *i:* 395 (1975).
179 Piekarski, G.; Saathoff, M.: Neuere Ergebnisse der *Trichomonas-vaginalis*-Forschung. Z. angew. Bäder- u. Klimaheilk. *23:* 27–43 (1976).
180 Pugh, R. J.; Newton, R. W.: Giardiasis in infancy and childhood. Practitioner *224:* 393–397 (1980).
181 Ralph, E. D.; Clarke, D. A.: Inactivation of metronidazole by anaerobic and aerobic bacteria. Antimicrob. Agents Chemother. *14:* 377–383 (1978).
182 Rao, H. T. M.; Shenoy, D. R.: Single-dose oral treatment of vaginal trichomoniasis with tinidazole and metronidazole. J. Int. med. Res. *6:* 46–49 (1978).
183 Rein, M. F.: Treatment of sexually transmitted diseases. Drug Ther. *7:* 39–41, 45, 47, 48 (1977).
184 Rendtorff, R. C.: The experimental transmission of *Giardia lamblia* among volunteer subjects; in Jacubowski, Hoff, Water-borne transmission of giardiasis, pp. 64–79. Proc. Symp. 1978 (US Environmental Protection Agency, Cincinnati 1979).
185 Richle, R.; Scholer, H. J.; Angehrn, P.; Fernex, M.; Hummler, H.; Jeunet, F.; Schärer, K.; Schüpbach, M.; Schwartz, D. E.: Grundlagen der Chemotherapie von Trichomoniasis und Amoebiasis mit Ornidazol. Arzneimittel-Forsch. *28:* 612–625 (1978).
186 Roberts-Thomson, I. C.; Mitchell, G. F.: Giardiasis in mice. I. Prolonged infections in certain mouse strains and hypothymic (nude) mice. Gastroenterology *75:* 42–46 (1978).
187 Roberts-Thomson, I. C.; Mitchell, G. F.: Protection of mice against *Giardia muris* infection. Infect. Immunity *24:* 971–973 (1979).
188 Roberts-Thomson, I. C.; Stevens, D. P.; Mahmoud, A. A. F.; Warren, K. S.: Acquired resistance to infection in an animal model of giardiasis. J. Immun. *117:* 2036–2037 (1976).
189 Roberts-Thomson, I. C.; Stevens, D. P.; Mahmoud, A. A. F.; Warren, K. S.: Giardiasis in the mouse: an animal model. Gastroenterology *71:* 57–61 (1976).
190 Rodermund, O.-E.; Piekarski, G.: Zur Trichomonadenurethritis des Mannes. Ein Beitrag zur epidemiologischen Situation von *Trichomonas vaginalis* heute sowie zur Ätiopathogenese nicht-gonorrhoischer Urethritiden des Mannes. Z. Hautkr. *54:* 481–486 (1979).
191 Rodin, P.; King, A. J.; Nicol, C. S.; Barrow, J.: Flagyl in the treatment of trichomoniasis. Br. J. vener. Dis. *36:* 147–151 (1960).
192 Roe, F. J. C.: Metronidazole: tumorigenicity studies in mice, rats and hamsters; in Finegold, Metronidazole, pp. 132–137. Proc. Int. Conf., Montreal 1976 (Excerpta Medica, Amsterdam 1977).

193 Roe, F. J. C.: Metronidazole: review of uses and toxicity. J. antimicrob. Chemother. *3:* 205–212 (1977).
194 Roitman, I.; Heyworth, P. G.; Gutteridge, W. E.: Lipid synthesis by *T. vaginalis.* Ann. trop. Med. Parasit. *72:* 583–585 (1978).
195 Rollo, I. M.: Chemotherapy of parasitic diseases; in Goodman, Gilman, The pharmacological basis of therapeutics; 5th ed., pp. 1018–1089 (Macmillan, New York 1975).
196 Root, D. M.; Beckwith, D.; Clough, K.; Van Voorhis, D.: *Giardia lamblia:* detection of antigens by enzyme labelled immunosorbent assay. Abstr. 80th Annu. Meet. Am. Soc. Microbiol., Miami Beach 1980, p. 293, C111.
197 Rosenkranz, H. S.; Speck, W. T.: Studies on the significance of the mutagenicity of metronidazole for *Salmonella typhimurium;* in Finegold, Metronidazole, pp. 119–125. Proc. Int. Conf., Montreal 1976 (Excerpta Medica, Amsterdam 1977).
198 Roy, R. B.; Laird, S. M.; Heasman, L.: Treatment of trichomoniasis in the female: a comparison of metronidazole and nimorazole. Br. J. vener. Dis. *51:* 281–284 (1975).
199 Ruebush, T. K., II.; Juranek, D. D.; Brodsky, R. E.: Diagnosis of intestinal parasites by state and territorial public health laboratories, 1976. J. infect. Dis. *138:* 114–117 (1978).
200 Rust, J. H.: An assessment of metronidazole tumorigenicity: studies in the mouse and rat; in Finegold, Metronidazole, pp. 138–144. Proc. Int. Conf., Montreal 1976 (Excerpta Medica, Amsterdam 1977).
201 Rustia, M.; Shubik, P.: Induction of lung tumors and malignant lymphomas in mice by metronidazole. J. natn. Cancer Inst. *48:* 721–729 (1972).
202 Rustia, M.; Shubik, P.: Experimental induction of hepatomas, mammary tumors, and other tumors with metronidazole in noninbred Sas: MRC (WI) BR rats. J. natn. Cancer Inst. *63:* 863–868 (1979).
203 Saeed, A.; Roy, R. B.; Huq, M. A.: Two-day treatment of trichomoniasis in the female – a comparison of metronidazole and nimorazole. Br. J. clin. Pract. *34:* 41–44 (1980).
204 Salih, S. Y.; Abdalla, R. E.: Symptomatic giardiasis in Sudanese adults and its treatment with tinidazole. J. trop. Med. Hyg. *80:* 11–13 (1977).
205 Salles, J. M. C.; Costa, C. A.; Matos, L. F.: Appraisal of the activity of nitrimidazine in giardiasis and genital trichomoniasis. Hospital *77: 1689–1697 (1970).*
206 Santler, R.; Thurner, J.: Untersuchungen über die Ansteckungsmöglichkeit durch *Trichomonas vaginalis.* Wien. klin. Wschr. *86:* 46–49 (1974).
207 Santler, R.; Thurner, J.; Poitschek, C.: Trichomoniasis. Z. Hautkr. *51:* 757–761 (1976).
208 Sawyer, P. A.; Brodgen, R. N.; Pinder, R. M.; Speight, T. M.; Avery, G. S.: Tinidazole: a review of its antiprotozoal activity and therapeutic efficacy. Drugs *11:* 423–440 (1976).
209 Schneider, J.: Traitement de la giardase (lambliase) par la métronidazole. Bull. Soc. Path. exot. *54:* 84–95 (1961).
210 Schnell, J. D.; Rüther, C.: Therapie kombinierter Vaginalinfektionen von *Trichomonas vaginalis* und Sprosspilzen. Ein kontrollierter Doppelblindvergleich von Metronidazol und Clotrimazol. Geburtsh. Frauenheilk. *34:* 551–557 (1974).
211 Schnitzer, R. J.: Chemotherapy of trichomonad infections; in Schnitzer, Hawk-

ing, Experimental chemotherapy, vol. I, pp. 289–331 (Academic Press, New York 1963).

212 Schubert, E.; Stehr, K.; Harms, S.; Lamina, J.: Determination of protozoans in 998 pediatric fecal samples. Eur. J. Pediat. *133:* 183 (1980).

213 Semgat, A. K.; Grewal, M. S.; Chakravarti, R. N.; Broor, S. L.; Deka, N. C.; Chhuttani, P. N.: Experimental giardiasis in albino rats. Indian J. med. Res. *64:* 1015–1018 (1976).

214 Serup, J.; Jensen, R. H.: Oral treatment of *Trichomoniasis vaginalis* with ornidazole (Tiberal®) and tinidazole (Fasigyn®). A controlled investigation. Ugeskr. Laeg. *140:* 1483–1484 (1978).

215 Siboulet, A.: Current epidemiological aspects of urogenital trichomoniasis; in Finegold, Metronidazole, pp. 83–86. Proc. Int. Conf., Montreal 1976 (Excerpta Medica, Amsterdam 1977).

216 Singh, B.; Cutter, J. C.; Utidjian, H. M. D.: Studies on development of a vaginal preparation providing both prophylaxis against venereal disease, other genital infection and contraception. III. In vitro effect of vaginal contraceptive and selected vaginal preparations of *Candida albicans* and *Trichomonas vaginalis.* Contraception *5:* 401–411 (1972).

217 Singh, R. N.; Gupta, B. D.; Gupta, M.; Kochar, S.: A comparative study of furazolidone and metronidazole in giardiasis. Indian J. Pediat. *44:* 183–188 (1977).

218 Sköld, M.; Gnarpe, H.; Hillström, L.: Ornidazole: a new antiprotozoal compound for treatment of *Trichomonas vaginalis* infection. Br. J. vener. Dis. *53:* 44–48 (1977).

219 Smith, J. W.; Wolfe, M. S.: Giardiasis. A. Rev. Med. *31:* 373–383 (1980).

220 Soyka, E.: The problem of *Trichomonas vaginalis* in children; in Williams, Geddes, Chemotherapy, vol. III, Special problems in chemotherapy, pp. 161–167. Proc. 9th Int. Congr. Chemother., London 1975 (Plenum Press, New York 1976).

221 Spech, H. J.: Lambliasis: Das Profil einer Durchfallserkrankung. Dt. med. Wschr. *103:* 2008–2012 (1978).

222 Sternadel, Z.; Peksa, A.: Comparative study of the effectiveness of antitrichomonal drugs. Wiad. parazyt. *23:* 623–624 (1977).

223 Stevens, D. P.; Frank, D. M.; Mahmoud, A. A. F.: Thymus dependency of host resistance to *Giardia muris* infection: studies in nude mice. J. Immun. *120:* 680–682 (1978).

224 Stevens, D. P.; Roberts-Thomson, I. C.: Giardiasis: animal model: experimentally induced giardiasis. Am. J. Path. *90:* 529–532 (1978).

225 Strickland, G. T.: Chemotherapy of parasitic diseases; in Seligson, CRC handbook series in clinical laboratory science, sect. E, vol. II, pp. 363–391 (CRC Press, Cleveland 1977).

226 Suriyanon, V.; Nelson, K. E.; Ayudhya, V. C. N.: *Trichomonas vaginalis* in a perinephric abscess. A case report. Am. J. trop. Med. Hyg. *24:* 776–780 (1975).

227 Swarz, H.: International experience with a new single 2 gram dose of tinidazole ('Fasigyn'). Curr. med. Res. Opin. *2:* 181–187 (1974).

228 Tapsall, J. W.; Puglisi, J.; Smith, D. D.: *Trichomonas vaginalis* infections in Sydney. Med. J. Aust. *i:* 193–194 (1979).

229 Taylor, A.; Baker, J. R.: The cultivation of parasites in vitro, pp. 92–108 (Blackwell, Oxford 1968).
230 Taylor, M. B.; Berghausen, H.; Heyworth, P. G.; Messenger, N.; Rees, L. J.; Gutteridge, W. E.: Subcellular localization of some glycolytic enzymes in parasitic flagellated protozoa. Int. J. Biochem. *11:* 117–120 (1980).
231 Thin, R. N.; Symonds, M. A. E.; Booker, R.; Cook, S.; Langlet, F.: Double-blind comparison of a single dose and a five-day course of metronidazole in the treatment of trichomoniasis. Br. J. vener. Dis. *55:* 354–356 (1979).
232 Thompson, R. G.; Karandikar, D. S.; Leek, J.: Giardiasis an unusual cause of epidemic diarrhoea. Lancet *i:* 615–616 (1974).
233 Thurner, J.; Meingassner, J. G.: Isolation of *Trichomonas vaginalis* resistant to metronidazole. Lancet *ii:* 738 (1978).
234 Tinkler, A. E.: Nimorazole compared with metronidazole in the treatment of vaginal trichomoniasis. Practitioner *212:* 115–119 (1974).
235 Tsai, Y. H.; Price, K. E.: Experimental models for the evaluation of systemic trichomonacides. Chemotherapy *18:* 348–357 (1973).
236 Underhill, R. A.; Peck, J. E.: Causes of therapeutic failure after treatment of trichomonal vaginitis with metronidazole: comparison of single-dose treatment with a standard regimen. Br. J. clin. Pract. *28:* 134–136 (1974).
237 Valent, M.; Catar, G.; Mikova, L.; Janoska, A.: Study of the resistance of *Trichomonas vaginalis* to Metronidazol Spofa. J. Protozool. *24:* 16A, abstr. 113 (1977).
238 Videau, D.; Niel, G.; Siboulet, A.; Catalan, F.: Secnidazole. Br. J. vener. Dis. *54:* 77–80 (1978).
239 Visvesvara, G. S.: Axenic growth of *Giardia lamblia* in Diamond's TPS-1 medium. Trans. R. Soc. trop. Med. Hyg. *74:* 213–215 (1980).
240 Visvesvara, G. S.; Healy, G. R.: The possible use of an indirect immunofluorescent test using axenically grown *Giardia lamblia* antigens in diagnosing giardiasis; in Jakubowski, Hoff, Water-borne transmission of giardiasis, pp. 53–62. Proc. Symp. 1978 (US Environmental Protection Agency, Cincinnati 1979).
241 Voogd, C. E.; Van der Stel, J. J.; Jacobs, J. J. J. A. A.: The mutagenic action of nitroimidazoles. I. Metronidazole, nimorazole, dimetridazole and ronidazole. Mutat. Res. *26:* 483–490 (1974).
242 Wagner, J. D.; Josey, W. E.: Treatment-resistant trichomoniasis. J. Am. med. Ass. *239:* 2035 (1978).
243 Wallin, J.: Sexuell übertragbare Erkrankungen: Die gegenwärtige Situation in Schweden. Hautarzt *31:* 233–236 (1980).
244 Warhurst, D. C.; Wright, S. G.: Cryopreservation of *Giardia intestinalis.* Trans. R. Soc. trop. Med. Hyg. *73:* 601 (1979).
245 Weinbach, E. C.; Clagett, C. E.; Keister, D. B.; Diamond, L. S.; Kon, H.: Respiratory metabolism of *Giardia lamblia.* J. Parasit. *66:* 347–350 (1980).
246 Weitgasser, H.: Die Behandlung der *Trichomoniasis vaginalis* mit Tiberal® Roche. Wien. med. Wschr. *126:* 162–165 (1976).
247 Weltman, R.: New metronidazole study: some reassuring findings for now. J. Am. med. Ass. *239:* 1371 (1978).
248 Werkman, H. P. T.; Meuwissen, J. H. E. T.: Single-dose treatment of giardiasis with ornidazole in children. Lancet *ii:* 1373 (1979).

249 Wildfeuer, A.: Die Chemotherapie der vaginalen Trichomoniasis und Candidosis der Maus. Arzneimittel-Forsch. *24:* 937–943 (1974).

250 Wilson, A.; Ackers, J. P.: Urine culture for the detection of *Trichomonas vaginalis* in men. Br. J. vener. Dis. *56:* 46–48 (1980).

251 Wolfe, M. S.: Giardiasis. J. Am. med. Ass. *233:* 1362–1365 (1975).

252 Wolfe, M. S.: Giardiasis. New Engl. J. Med. *298:* 319–321 (1978).

253 Woodcock, K. R.: Treatment of trichomonal vaginitis with a single oral dose of metronidazole. Br. J. vener. Dis. *48:* 65–68 (1972).

254 Woodcock, K. R.: Two-day treatment with metronidazole in vaginal trichomoniasis. Br. J. vener. Dis. *48:* 383–386 (1972).

255 Wright, R. A.; Judson, F. N.: Relative and seasonal incidences of the sexually transmitted diseases. Br. J. vener. Dis. *54:* 433–440 (1978).

256 Wright, S. G.; Tomkins, A. M.: Quantitative histology in giardiasis. J. clin. Path. *31:* 712–716 (1978).

257 Wright, S. G.; Tomkins, A. M.; Bryceson, A. D. M.: Metronidazole in giardiasis; in Finegold, Metronidazole, pp. 98–104. Proc. Int. Conf., Montreal 1976 (Excerpta Medica, Amsterdam 1977).

258 Wright, S. G.; Tomkins, A. M.; Ridley, D. S.: Giardiasis: clinical and therapeutic aspects. Gut *18:* 343–350 (1977).

Dr. J. G. Meingassner, Sandoz Forschungsinstitut,
Brunnerstrasse 59, A-1235 Vienna (Austria)

Antibiotics Chemother., vol. 30, pp. 203–223 (Karger, Basel 1981)

Leishmaniasis

P. Kern[1]

Department of Medicine, Bernhard-Nocht-Institut für Schiffs- und Tropenkrankheiten, Hamburg, FRG

Introduction

Human leishmaniasis comprises a heterogeneous spectrum of diseases [1]. Three major forms are generally distinguished: cutaneous leishmaniasis, mucocutaneous leishmaniasis, and visceral leishmaniasis of which the latter is potentially lethal [2, 3]. They are caused by various species of the protozoan parasite Leishmania and transmitted by female sandflies (Phlebotomus, Sergentomyia, and Lutzomyia). Therefore, the occurrence of leishmaniasis is generally restricted to those areas where vectors are present. Military personnel, travellers, and people working in endemic areas may acquire the disease and import it into nonendemic areas [4]. The incubation period varies from months to several years. Figures on the incidence and prevalence of human leishmaniasis are not available [2]. Other forms of transmission, i. e., via blood transfusion or contagion should also be considered [5, 6]. Endemic foci with sporadic diseases are seen in the Mediterranean countries, in the Middle East, in India and in Africa, the so-called Old World leishmaniasis, and in Central and South America, the so-called New World leishmaniasis.

[1] The excellent secretarial assistance of Mrs. *T. Thiede* is gratefully acknowledged.

Biology of Infection and Taxonomy

Leishmanias appear in two distinct morphological forms: the flagellated promastigote in the insect vector and the unflagellated amastigote in the mammalian host (Leishman-Donovan bodies). The amastigote is an obligate intracellular parasite of macrophages. The parasite multiplies rapidly by binary fission finally leading to the rupture of the macrophage. The parasites are released and infect further macrophages or are ingested during blood meal by female sandflies. In that case the leishmania transform into flagellated promastigotes within the sandfly's gut, undergo a series of morphological variations and again multiply rapidly. The flagellated parasites migrate into the proboscis and are eventually inoculated into the skin of a further vertebrate host when the sandfly takes another blood meal. The promastigotes are rapidly cleared by mononuclear phagocytes and lose their flagellum, thus resembling an amastigote form, whereby the parasite's life cycle is now completed, having passed through a vertebra and an insect host. The different species and possible strains of leishmanias are adapted to specific hosts including man (obligatory or accidental), mammalian animals, lizzards, and sandflies of different genera and species [7, 8]. With few exceptions, the different species and strains of leishmanias cannot be distinguished by light microscopy. Present taxonomy of leishmanias includes the epidemiology, the clinical pictures in man, the ultrastructural morphology of he parasites, their characteristics in in vivo and in vitro cultures, the analysis of enzyme patterns, and the buoyant density of kinetoplastic deoxyribonucleic acid, host-vector specificity, and immunological tests. New classifications of leishmanias have been published with special reference to those species occurring in Central and South America [1, 7, 8]. At the present time, four groups can clearly be distinguished: *Leishmania donovani* complex, *Leishmania tropica* complex, *Leishmania mexicana* complex, and *Leishmania brasiliensis* complex (see 'Glossary').

Clinical Disease, Diagnosis and Pathology

The mounting scientific knowledge on the biological differences of Leishmania species in the last years should not prevent clinicians from looking at the principal pathophysiological events involved. Infection in man ranges from mild, self-curing to severe fatal disease. The inoculated leishmanias multiply in macrophages and lead to a varying granuloma formation. It may be restricted to the initial site of infection. However, local or systemic metastases may follow immediately, later, after spontaneous cure, or even after chemotherapy [9]. The metastases may also be restricted to the skin, but can spread into the nasopharyngeal mucosa. Furthermore, the leishmanias may immediately colonize from the initial site of inoculation into the visceral organs, i. e. spleen, liver, lymph nodes, bone marrow, leading to a life-threatening disease. However, even after treatment a respread into the skin is possible and suggested to be of importance in maintaining the transmission in the Indian type of Kala Azar [8].

Cutaneous Leishmaniasis [8, 10–13]

This includes a rather complex spectrum of diseases caused by different species and strains of leishmania [*L. tropica* complex, *L. mexicana* complex]. Its manifestation depends largely upon the cell-mediated immunity of the host, ranging from anergic diffuse cutaneous forms to the ultrasensitive recidiva forms. The self-healing form, i. e., Oriental sore, falls between the two extremes. Several weeks after bite by a sandfly and the inoculation of leishmania, a small lesion in the skin appears, ulcerates and becomes crusted (fig. 1, 3). The ulcer heals spontaneously after several months and leaves behind a typical scar. Secondary bacterial infection may change the clinical picture. The lesions may vary widely in number and in localization. Sometimes several ulcers occur at the same time by either multiple infected sandfly bites or metastatic spread [2, 4, 14]. A spreading along the lymph vessels has also been observed [4, 8] (fig. 2). In cases of recidiva or lupoid form, the ulcer never heals, or it heals and relapses by spreading around the original lesion possibly several years after apparent healing [15]. A diffuse cutaneous form appears at first merely as a small nodule, but metastasizes later to other parts of the skin, forming plaque-like ulcers [16, 17]. However, it does never involve visceral organs.

The diagnosis is based on the clinical picture and the demonstration of leishmania parasites in smears prepared from material from the edges of a nodule. Contaminations of blood or pus should be prevented. An in vitro culture in NNN (Novy, Nicolle, McNeal) media (possible in specialized laboratories) may be helpful and can be used to demonstrate the promastigote form of leishmanias. An ambient temperature of 22–26 °C will reveal an optimal growth. The differentiation of the strain may additionally be accomplished. The intradermal leishmania test (Montenegro test) is of minor value, if at all. Due to the shortage of defined, standardized antigen, a general application will never be justified [10, 18].

1 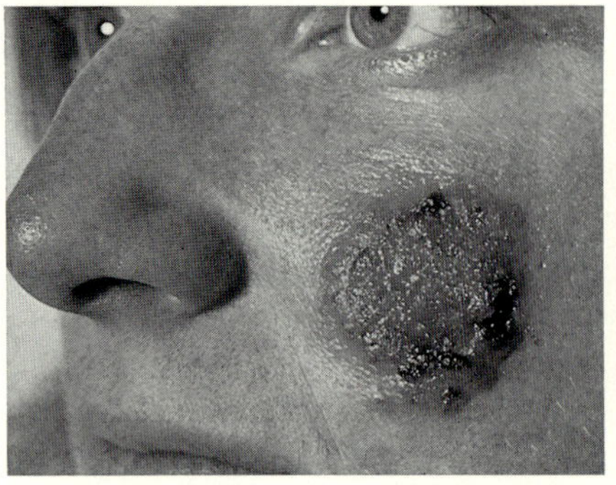 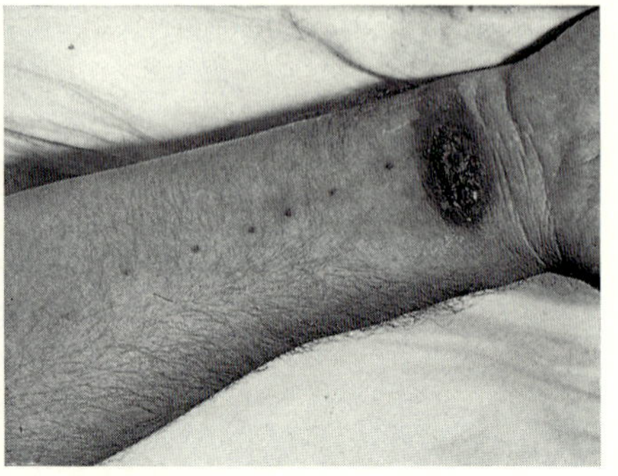 2

Fig. 1. Oriental sore acquired in Saudia Arabia.
Fig. 2. Oriental sore with spread along lymph vessels.

Mucocutaneous Leishmaniasis [8, 11, 19]

Its occurrence is restricted to Brazil and caused by a subspecies of *L. brasiliensis*.

After inoculation of leishmanias, a long-lasting initial lesion may occur which results in a disfiguring scar (fig. 4). Metastases into the nasopharyngeal tissue regularly occur while the initial skin lesion is still active or even many years after the primary ulcer has healed. Chronic rhinitis is the leading clinical symptom, later on the cartilage of the nasopharynx can be destructed to such an extent that a common cavity of mouth and nose results. Mucocutaneous lesions never heal spontaneously [19]. Additional damage may result from secondary bacterial infection and even pneumonia may occur. The diagnosis is based on the clinical picture, the history and scars of cutaneous leishmaniasis (more than 90 % had had a cutaneous lesion before). Except for the very early mucocutaneous granuloma, the parasites are scarce in smears and even culture techniques fail to demonstrate the parasites.

The histological picture is not characteristic and shows chronic granuloma formation. Inoculation of the tissue suspension into hamsters' nose and feet may lead to a diagnostic granuloma formation, but it takes 6 to 12 months until amastigotes can be recovered. The leishmanian test is also of limited value because specific antigen is not generally available. Antibody tests may be of diagnostic help when performed in laboratories specialized for this investigation.

3
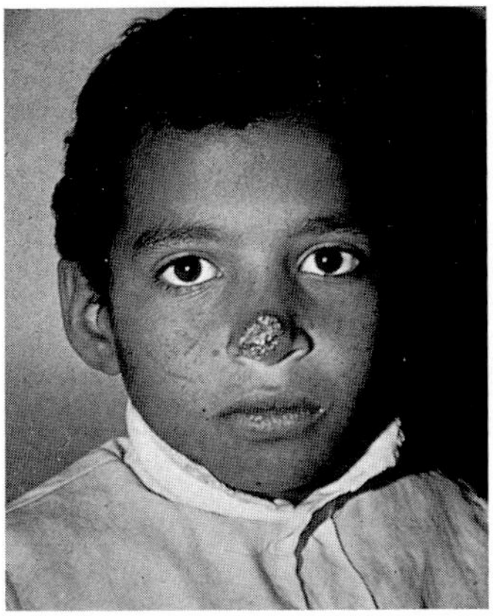

Fig. 3. Oriental sore of the nose, acquired in Saudi Arabia.

4
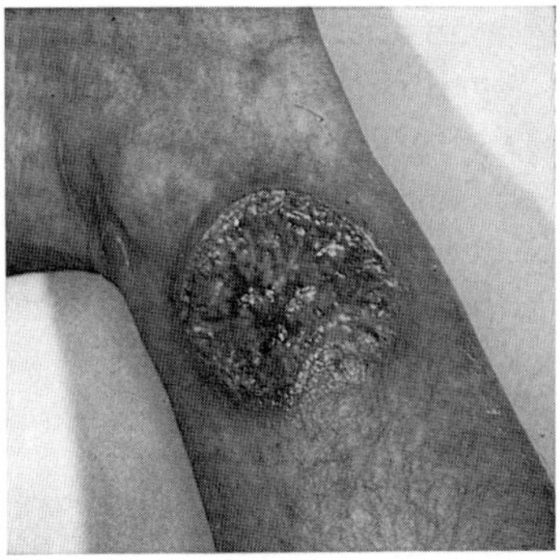
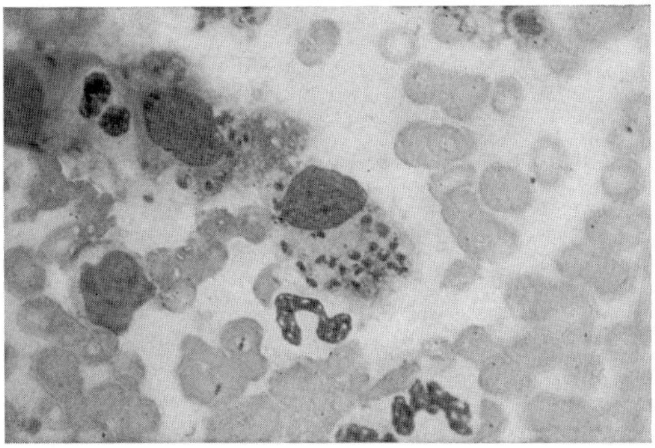
5

Fig. 4. Cutaneous Leishmaniasis, acquired in the Amazonas region, Brazil.

Fig. 5. Bone marrow smear: amastigote *Leishmania donovani* within macrophages.

Visceral Leishmaniasis [11, 20–23]

Kala Azar has a widespread geographical distribution and leads to severe illness which often ends fatally [2, 3]. Differences in the clinical picture are observed, depending on the geographical occurrence, but also visceral organs, i. e., liver, spleen, lymph nodes, tonsils, etc., as well as into the bone marrow (fig. 5). Enlargement and dysfunction of these organs leads to severe sequelae.

The diagnosis is based on the clinical findings: weight loss, night sweats, intermittent fever, hepatosplenomegaly, lymphadenopathy, pancytopenia, bleeding disorder and imbalance of serum proteins due to an excessive increase in gammaglobulins. Specimens of the bone marrow or liver are necessary to establish diagnosis. Amastigotes within macrophages can be identified on smears from Pappenheim-stained bone marrow specimens or can be grown in in vitro cultures up to 6 weeks.
Leishmanin Skin Test (Montenegro Test) with specific standardized antigen becomes positive only after treatment [25]. Its use is therefore restricted to epidemiological surveys. Antibody levels measured by different test systems are of great help, but cross-reactivity between leishmanias and trypanosomes and group-specific cross-reactivity among various leishmanias seriously limit the reliability of many test systems [8].

Haematology [26, 27]

The occurring pancytopenia has stimulated a number of investigations. There is a marked bone-marrow hyperplasia together with megaloblastic or dimorphic changes in erythropoiesis, increase in plasma cells, mononuclear phagocytes and eosinophilic myelocytes. Red cell survival is shortened. Autoimmune mechanisms have been considered for the rapid destruction of red cells. Shifts of the circulating pools as well as an enhanced abnormal sequestration are probably also involved, commonly referred to as hypersplenism. Numerous aspects of anemia, granulocytopenia, and thrombocytopenia are not fully elucidated.

Pathology [24, 28–31]

Biopsy specimens reveal many organisms in histiocytes of the skin. This histiocytic reaction is followed by a granulomatous reaction later on, characterized by increasing numbers of lymphocytes, plasma cells, epitheloid cells and giant cells. In visceral leishmaniasis, phagocytic cells of the reticulo-endothelial system multiply to an enormous extent. They also harbour large numbers of amastigotes. Thus, the organs become greatly enlarged.

The polar appearance of cutaneous leishmaniasis was compared with the spectrum of diseases in leprosy [7, 13]: diffuse cutaneous leishmaniasis, as an anergic state, and the lupoid or mucocutaneous leishmaniasis, as hypersensitive forms. However, in a careful histopathological study, *Ridley* [13] stated that there are fundamental differences between the two diseases despite the many points in common. In the anergic state of diffuse cutaneous leishmaniasis, the T lymphocyte action is completely abolished [17]. This can be due to suppressor factors released by macrophages while on the particular strain of leishmania involved. A dermal form, the so-called post-Kala-Azar cutaneous leishmaniasis, is observed in India. The natural reservoir differs from one area to the other. Domestic or wild animals usually harbor the parasite; however, in the Indian form of Kala Azar man is the natural reservoir. In general, it affects children more often than adults and shows a male to female preponderance of 4:1 [20, 24]. The leishmanias spread from the initial site of inoculation into the harboring parasites or to the individual's failure to react. Cure requires T/B cell cooperation whereby an adequate T/B balance is essential [28]. The strong antibody response without concomitant T-cell response seen in visceral leishmaniasis is of no help in curing the leishmaniasis.

In cases with hypersensitivity reaction there is an overshoot of cellular immune reaction, thus the inflammatory lesions persist together with an inadequate elimination of parasites. Lymphocytes and plasma cells are present in large quantities, but the type of the histological lesion is unpredictable. Uncontrolled T cell aggression leads to an ongoing inflammation. The self-healing form of cutaneous leishmaniasis is characterized by an adequate T cell response and also a moderate antibody response. As a result, there will be an intensive inflammatory reaction at the site of infection, as well as the specific elimination of Leishmania-bearing phagocytic mononuclear cells [28].

In vivo and in vitro Infection Models

Essential information on immunopathology of leishmaniasis has been accumulated in laboratory animals [8, 28]. Guinea pigs and hamsters infected with *Leishmania enrietti* developed a self-curing cutaneous manifestation, analogous to human infection with *L. tropica* [32]. Mice infected with *L. tropica* have a different susceptibility and disease pattern depending on the strain involved: highly resistant (C57 Black/6, NZB), transiently infected (CBA/H, C3H/He and A/J), chronically infected (BALB/c, DBA/2) and highly susceptible (nude mice) [33–35]. Hamsters and mice were suitable models of visceral leishmaniasis when infected with *L. donovani*. On the other hand, the guinea pig is resistant to human pathogenic leishmanias. From studies in mice it became evident that the susceptibility and the resistance to a protozoan parasite is governed by a single gene or tight linkage group mapped on chromosome 1 [36, 37]. It is of particular interest that the immune response locus (Ir) closely related to the H2 locus in mice is not concerned with the leishmania infection.

Leishmania transform readily into the promastigote form in vitro [38]. Cultures of amastigotes are only possible when leishmanias are grown together with macrophages. The phagocytosed parasites multiply in vitro within the macrophage host [39]. Several studies on mechanisms of macrophage activation have been performed using this model [40, 41]. Besides this, drug sensitivity studies using that in vitro model have been reported recently [42]. Pentavalent antimony, pentamidine, and amphothericin B were examined and were found to eliminate 90–100 % of amastigotes within the macrophage cultures. In contrast, the promastigotes in cell-free media were much less sensitive to the major antileishmanial drugs [43]. Thus, the in vitro macrophage amastigote culture seems to offer a model for drug testing which resembles the in vivo situation [42].

The immunopathological network in healing, protecting or exaggerating murine leishmaniasis has been studied extensively for *L. tropica* and *L. donovani* [28, 41, 44–50]. Macrophages are the key cells in the immunopathological process. But T cell responses are of primary importance, as has been shown in the nude mice model. In which way specific T lymphocytes eliminate leishmania parasites is not quite clear. Other infection disease models, such as infections with *Listeria monocytogenes* or *Mycobacteria leprae,* or tumor immunology have not yielded a clear-cut answer up to now.

Leishmania antigens can be discovered on infected macrophages, whereby one can conclude that antigenic material is presented to the immune system. Sensitized T lymphocytes may release specific factors (lymphokines) which transform macrophages via surface receptors into an activated state and finally lead to an intracellular kill of parasites. In that case, the parasitophorus vacuole undergoes fusion with lysosomes which apparently destroy the parasite. However, Leishmanias survive if they can prevent the phagolysosome formation, or escape from the vacuolar apparatus, or withstand the toxic milieu of the phagolysosome environment. They also escape the specific immune attack if parasites' antigens are not expressed on the macrophages' membrane. On the other hand, the infected macrophages might be targets of cytotoxic lymphocytes, thus eliminating the parasite-bearing host cell. B cell activation might be necessary as well, because otherwise T cell immunity appears to be inefficient.

One can summarize that leishmanias possibly cause disturbances within the immunocompetent cells as well as macrophages. This leads to a number of immunopathological events resembling clinical disease.

Current Therapy

Cutaneous Leishmaniasis

No single chemotherapeutic regimen has been proved to be satisfactory in treating cutaneous leishmaniasis [10]. Since the lesions heal spontaneously, it is difficult to evaluate the effectiveness of drugs by the methods at hand. Several trials using compounds effective in other protozoan diseases showed negative results. As the scar formation is typical for the Oriental sore, it is necessary to avoid secondary bacterial infections and to keep the lesions clean. Various efforts are being made to enhance healing of the ulcer, including local radiation, cauterization, kryotherapy, or local infiltration with antileishmanial drugs [10, 51]. In areas where the lesions heal spontaneously, specific treatment is unnecessary. In the case of long-lasting (over 6 months) or disfiguring lesions, drug treatment with pentavalent antimonials is advisable despite the side effects (see below). Treatment is mandatory in those areas known to be endemic for *L. brasiliensis* infections to prevent skin relapses as well as involvement of the nasopharyngeal tissue. Regular follow-up examinations should be advised. For plastic surgery of disfiguring facial lesions, at least 1 year should have passed after effective medical treatment [2].

Mucocutaneous and Visceral Leishmaniasis

Curative chemotherapy cannot be guaranteed by the limited range of available drugs. The full participation of the host's immune system is as important as drug treatment for the cure of leishmanial infection whether a viscero- or dermatotropic manifestation.

Antimony Compounds [43, 52]

The use of antimonials to treat leishmaniasis is nearly historical, and they are still in use today. Despite its toxicity, tartar emetic (antimony III potassium tartrate) was found to achieve an effective leishmanicidal effect. Other trivalent antimonials, i. e., stibophen, anthiomaline, were tested and found to be as effective and less toxic. They have been widely used until pentavalent antimonials were discovered and introduced into the treatment of leishmaniasis. The exact parasiticidal action of the pentavalent

Table I. Pentavalent antimony compounds

Pentostam	sodium stibogluconate (sodium antimony (V) gluconate) stable solution of 100 mg/ml application i. m. or i. v. by slow infusion, hospitalization required sensitivity test of 200 mg initially necessary treatment: 600 mg/day for 10–14 days
Glucantime	meglumin antimoniate (antimony (V) N-methyl-glutamin) stable aqueous solution, 300 mg/ml application: i. m. or i. v. by slow infusion, hospitalization required treatment: 3,000 mg/day for 10–20 days
Diamidine	
Pentamidine	lomidine stable solution, 200 mg/ml application i. m., hospitalization required treatment: 3–4 mg/kg body weight/day for 14 days side effects: reversible renal dysfunction, possibly late neuropathies, blood sugar imbalance by i. v. application hypersensitivity reactions
Antibiotics	
Amphothericin B	fungizone stable solution, 50 mg/ampoule application i. v. per slow infusion in 5 % dextrose, hospitalization required treatment: 1st day 1 mg, 2nd day 5 mg, 3rd day 10 mg, then increasing every day to a total amount of 1 mg/kg body weight or 1.5 mg/kg body weight per day total dose: 2 g side effects: hypersensitivity reactions, diminished by adding 25–50 mg hydrocortison per infusion, hepatic and renal failure, pancytopenia

antimonial (Sb V) is not defined. The compound was also considered to play a role in the host's defense to eradicate the infection. Due to toxicity, similar to that of arsenicals, it is of limited use, particularly regarding large or prolonged dosage or use in malnourished individuals. Pentostam and glucantime (table I) are now in common use. There appears to be only little difference in the efficacy of both drugs. Only occasional side effects and ECG changes have been reported. Other pentavalent antimonials are less commonly used, i. e., neostibosan (ethylstibamine) and ureastibamin (carbostibanin, carbantin and stiburea).

Several years ago, in vivo drug sensitivity tests were conducted in hamsters and mice using *L. donovani, L. tropica* and *L. brasiliensis*. It was found that the curative effect is dose related. However, recent data using genetically defined animal species as well as defined leishmanial isolates are scarce.

Recent pharmacological studies revealed that the Sb V plasma level peaks immediately after intravenous infusion, whereas after intramuscular application the drug diffusion from the site of injection takes some time [53]. Lower plasma levels for prolonged periods of time are achieved. By measuring plasma and urine levels in normal individuals or patients with visceral leishmaniasis, an accumulation of Sb V was not observed. This is in contrast to trivalent antimonials which are bound to the erythrocytes and thus have completely different pharmacological properties. Whether extra- to intracellular shift of pentavalent antimonials occurs and causes toxic symptoms is unknown. The observation of effective (Sb V) treatment and the observation of toxic side effects in a Kenyan boy with renal failure suggests that renal function may be an important limiting factor.

Acute drug-related symptoms may occur in visceral leishmaniasis. They resemble the symptoms of serum sickness and are thought to be due to the massive destruction of parasites. These symptoms can be overcome by administering corticosteroids together with the pentavalent antimonial [54].

Single treatment courses are sufficient in cases with Indian, Chinese or South American Kala-Azar. At least three courses should be given in cases of Mediterranean or East African Kala-Azar as well as in the case of South American (Brazil) cutaneous and mucocutaneous leishmaniasis [2].

Diamidines

Beside its trypanocidal activity, the effect in the treatment of leishmaniasis is still debatable. Two compounds have gained some attention [8, 43]: pentamidine and stilbamidine. Despite their toxicity, they may be considered for treatment in obstinate antimony-resistant cases.

Antibiotics

Amphothericin B is a potent antileishmanial drug. Due to severe toxicity, its use is restricted to the treatment of advanced cases of mucocutaneous leishmaniasis not responding to antimonials. The drug must be given by slow intravenous infusion, and hospitalization is mandatory.

Rifampicin trials for treatment of cutaneous leishmaniasis have been conducted in Kuwait, however, the results were not conclusive [8, 10].

Other Antileishmanial Drugs

Biguanide (Cycloguanilpaomate, Cycloguanilemboate, Camolar). Repository action is achieved by the intramuscular 'single shot' application. Good results have been obtained against the American cutaneous leishmaniasis; however, conflicting results have been reported from Ethiopia [8, 10]. As the results cannot be adequately assessed in cases of cutaneous leishmaniasis because of spontaneous regression, the drug has not received further consideration.

In South America, human drug trials have been conducted using nifurtimox (Lampit) or rochagan in treating mucocutaneous leishmaniasis [55]. The results do not favor either drug. Antimonials still are the most effective drugs.

Supportive Therapy

Kala-Azar is a wasting disorder and needs intensive supportive care. Besides adequate diet, bedrest, etc., attention should be paid to concurrent bacterial infections which often cause death due to pancytopenia. Individual support of malfunctions must be given. Transfusions are indicated in case of severe anemia.

New Advances

Drug Carriers

Screening of antiprotozoal or new drugs has been disappointing. Even treatment with the available drugs cannot guarantee a cure of the infection. Therefore, the elaboration of the immunopathological events was of essential importance for new developments.

Similar to leishmanias or other intracellular parasites, liposomes were found to be phagocytosed by mononuclear cells only. They are rapidly cleared from the bloodstream. The bilayer vesicles serve as capsules for a variety of substances entrapped within the aqueous interspaces. Thus, particles loaded with antimonials seem to offer the ideal vehicle to achieve a high drug concentration in close proximity to intracellular parasites. The phagolysosome formation within the leishmania-infected macrophage and the lysomotrophic properties of liposomes support the close connection. A number of recent reports deal with drug carriers [56–62]. In C57 B1 mice infected with *L. donovani* (LV9 line), the entrapped stibogluconate was 200 times more effective than the free drug [57], and even more effective in NMMI mice [58]. The master/*L. donovani* infection model was investigated by others [59, 60]. A 700-times more effective therapy was achieved with meglumine antimoniate entrapped liposomes as compared to the free drug.

8-aminoquinolines showed a marked action on *L. donovani* in mice and hamsters [64]. The most active compound out of the 274 tested was WR 6026 which was discovered for its antimalarial activity. Recent investigations in the hamster/*L. donovani* model revealed a greater efficacy than that of meglumin antimoniate in the treatment of a 17-day infection. Liposome encapsulated WR 6026 was found to be the most potent antileishmanial principle, even 2.5–6.6 times more effective than encapsulated meglumine antimoniate, or more than 1,000 times more effective than the free meglumine antimoniate [60]. Hemolytic crisis induced by 8-aminoquinolines may be a major drawback, but a 50% suppression of leishmanias was achieved with a dosage below the level causing clinical hemolysis in humans.

Liposome encapsulated drugs undoubtedly enhance their efficacy against visceral leishmaniasis in small animals. However, several problems must be solved before liposomes can be used for human leishmaniasis, i. e., an optimum liposome composition must be formulated, an optimum route of administration must be found, an optimal leishmanicidal drug must be identified as well as immunological factors have to be considered. It appears that the antileishmanial drug is not effective on its own, but requires the support of the host's immune response. Furthermore, both host differences in metabolizing the drug and differences in sensitivity of different parasite isolates have to be taken into consideration. Toxicological aspects may be strongly influenced by the factors mentioned. Whether liposomes per se without drug act as immunostimulants is still unknown [61]. Unspecific immunostimulants might also enhance the efficacy of drugs, even in the encapsulated form. A chain of questions related to the immunological defense and intracellular killing of amastigotes has to be answered.

While most experiments have been performed in models resembling visceral leishmaniasis, the situation in cutaneous leishmaniasis is much less clear. However, it was found that liposomes entrapped with pentostam can suppress cutaneous lesions to a far greater extent than the free drug [63]. Whether circulating macrophages take up drug-loaded liposomes and infiltrate the skin lesions or act as an unspecific stimulus has not been tested.

Experimental results from *L. donovani*-infected hamsters indicated that orally administered tetracycline, either given alone or in combination with leishmanicidal drugs or liposomes reduced mortality due to leishmaniasis considerably [60].

Immunotherapy and Vaccination

Dialyzable extracts of human leukocytes (transfer factor) have been shown to exert immune modulating capacities [65]. Their effect was tested in various conditions of deficient cell-mediated immunity. A small clinical trial of transfer factor therapy in human cutaneous leishmaniasis revealed a beneficial effect in 10 out of 12 patients treated [66]. However, many critical points have to be solved, and much work has to be done [67].

Since cutaneous leishmaniasis is a self-healing lesion, it is a medical problem only when disfiguring facial scars develop. According to an old custom in the Middle East, children were vaccinated with material taken from lesions to prevent nasty scars. Scientific attempts to immunize against cutaneous leishmaniasis are numerous [for review see 8, 68]. Living cultures of *L. tropica* promastigotes have been used with varying success [51], but bacterial, mycoplasmal or viral contamination of the vaccine made it a dangerous procedure. A standardized procedure for *L. tropica* vaccine was therefore proposed [69]. There are no recent reports about its use and effectiveness.

Killed parasites as vaccines in man have been used recently in a trial in South America [70]. A link between vaccine inoculation and protection was suggested, but it is unproven.

Future Prospects

With regard to the immunopathological events, the Leishmania model provides a remarkable tool for studying various mechanisms, i. e., macrophage-parasite interaction, macrophage activation, T-B cell cooperation, T cell-mediated lysis of phagocytes, T cell cytotoxicity, etc. However, numerous problems, i. e., intracellular survival of certain host-parasite combinations, specific action of drugs, etc., are not yet solved.

Liposomes seem to offer an ideal vehicle for transporting effective drugs into the phagocytic cells. However, several problems have to be solved until carrier liposomes can be utilized in human leishmaniasis.

Vaccination and transfer factor therapy seem to offer another prospect, but no substantial progress has been achieved. Considering 12 million human leishmaniasis cases throughout the world [71, 72], further efforts are mandatory to understand and control the disease.

Glossary

Aleppo boil	see cutaneous leishmaniasis
Acute cutaneous leishmaniasis	wet, rural, zoonotic form caused by *L. tropica* major transmitted by *Phlebotomus* sp. recorded mammalian host: Gerbils, sand rat
Amastigote	nonflagellated leishmania, only observed in the mammalian host's macrophages
Baghdad boil	see cutaneous leishmaniasis
Chiclero's ulcer	cutaneous, rarely diffuse cutaneous, leishmaniasis (Central America), caused by *L. mexicana mexicana* transmitted by *Lutzomyia* sp. recorded mammalian host: forest rodents, man only accidental host
Chronic cutaneous leishmaniasis	cutaneous leishmaniasis (Venezuela) caused by *L. mexicana pifanoi* transmitted by *Lutzomyia* sp. recorded mammalian host: forest rodents, man accidental host

Glossary (continued)

Cutaneous leishmaniasis	dry, urban, anthroponotic form caused by *L. tropica* minor transmitted by *Phlebotomus* sp. recorded mammalian host: man, dog
Delhi boil	see cutaneous leishmaniasis
Diffuse cutaneous leishmaniasis	caused by *L. tropica* (aethiopica) or *L. mexicana pifanoi* transmitted by *Phlebotomus* sp. recorded mammalian host: rock hyraxes, man rarely accidental host
Espundia	see cutaneous and mucocutaneous leishmaniasis (Brazil)
Kala Azar	see visceral leishmaniasis
Leishmania donovani complex includes	*L. donovani* *L. infantum* *L. chagasi*
Leishmania tropica complex includes	*L. tropica* minor *L. tropica* major *L. tropica* aethiopica
Leishmania mexicana complex includes	*L. mexicana mexicana* *L. mexicana amazonensis* *L. mexicana pifanoi* *L. enrietti* (not infecting man)
Leishmania brasiliensis complex includes	*L. brasiliensis brasiliensis* *L. brasiliensis guyanensis* *L. brasiliensis panamensis* *L. brasiliensis peruviana* *L. hertigi* (not infecting man)
Leptomonad	flagellated leishmaniasis, only observed in sandflies or mimicked in in vitro cultures

Glossary (continued)

Mucocutaneous leishmaniasis	caused by *L. brasiliensis brasiliensis* transmitted by *Lutzomyia* sp. recorded mammalian host: forest rodents, man only accidental host
Oriental sore	see cutaneous leishmaniasis
Pian-bois	cutaneous leishmaniasis caused by *L. brasiliensis guyanensis* transmitted by *Lutzomyia* sp. man accidental host
Post-Kala-Azar disease	cutaneous manifestation after visceral manifestations of Kala-Azar have subsided
Promastigote	flagellated leishmania, only observed in sandflies or mimicked in in vitro cultures
Sandfly	only vector for *Leishmania* sp. *Phlebotomus, Lutzomyia, Sergentomyia*
Uta	cutaneous leishmaniasis (parts of Peru and Argentina) caused by *L. peruviana* transmitted by *Lutzomyia* sp. recorded mammalian host: dog
Visceral leishmaniasis	(1) caused by *L. donovani* transmitted mainly by *Phlebotomus* sp. recorded mammalian host: man (2) caused by *L. infantum* transmitted by *Phlebotomus* sp. recorded mammalian host: dog, fox, etc., man only accidental host (3) caused by *L. chagasi* (South America) transmitted by *Lutzomyia* sp. recorded mammalian host: fox, dog, man only accidental host

References

1 Lainson, R.; Shaw, J. J.: Epidemiology and ecology of leishmaniasis in Latin America. Nature, Lond. *273:* 595 (1978).

2 Marsden, P. D.: Leishmaniasis. New Engl. J. Med. *300:* 350 (1979).

3 Anon: Problems with leishmaniasis. Br. med. J. *ii:* 1179 (1978).

4 Bienzle, U.; Ebert, F.; Dietrich, M.: Cutaneous leishmaniasis in eastern Saudi Arabia. Epidemiological and clinical features in a nonimmune population living in an endemic area. Tropenmed. Parasit. *29:* 188 (1978).

5 Symners, W.: Leishmaniasis acquired by contagion. Lancet *i:* 127 (1960).

6 Shaw, P. K.; Quigg, L. T.; Allain, D. S.; et al.: Autochthonous dermal leishmaniasis. Am. J. trop. Med. Hyg. *25:* 788 (1976)

7 Bray, R. S.: Leishmania. A. Rev. Microbiol. *28:* 189 (1974).

8 Zuckermann, A.; Lainson, R.: Leishmania; in Kreyer, Parasitic protozoa, vol. 1, p. 58 (Academic Press, New York 1977).

9 Dostrovsky, A.: Relapses in cutaneous leishmaniasis. Ann. trop. Med. Parasit. *30:* 267 (1936).

10 Dowlati, Y.: Cutaneous leishmaniasis. Int. J. Dermatol. *18:* 362 (1979).

11 Ward, R. D.: New World leishmaniasis. A review of the epidemiological changes in the last three decades. Proc. 15th. Int. Congr. Ent., Washington 1977, p. 505.

12 Bryceson, A. D. M.: A diffuse cutaneous leishmaniasis in Ethiopia. Immunological studies. Trans. R. Soc. trop. Med. Hyg. *64:* 380 (1970).

13 Ridley, D. S.: The pathogenesis of cutaneous leishmaniasis. Trans. R. Soc. trop. Med. Hyg. *73:* 150 (1979).

14 Nadim, A.; Seyedi-Rashti, M. A.; Ashi, J.: Cutaneous leishmaniasis in Saudi Arabia. Bull. Soc. Path. Exot. *72:* 237 (1979).

15 Petit, J. H. S.: Chronic (lupoid) leishmaniasis. Br. J. Derm. *74:* 27 (1962).

16 Bryceson, A. D. M.: Diffuse cutaneous leishmaniasis in Ethiopia. I. The clinical and histological feature of the disease. Trans. R. Soc. trop. Med. Hyg. *63:* 708 (1969).

17 Convit, J.; Pinardi, M. E.; Rondoss, J.: Diffuse cutaneous leishmaniasis. A disease due to immunological defect of the host. Trans. R. Soc. trop. Med. Hyg. *66:* 603 (1972).

18 Pampiglione, J.; Manson-Bahr, P. E. C.; La Placa, M.; et al.: Studies on Mediterranean leishmaniasis. IV. The leishmania skin test in cutaneous leishmaniasis. Trans. R. Soc. trop. Med. Hyg. *70:* 62 (1976).

19 Marsden, P. D.; Monata, R. R.: Mucocutaneous leishmaniasis: a review of clinical aspects. Revta Soc. bras. Méd. trop. *9:* 309 (1975).

20 Nadim, A.; Navid-Hamidid, A.; Javadian, E.; et al.: Present status of kala-azar in Iran. Am. J. trop. Med. Hyg. *27:* 25 (1978).

21 Krampitz, H. E.: Neuere Erkenntnisse über die geographische Verbreitung der Leishmaniasen in der alten Welt; in Jusatz, Geomedizin in Forschung und Lehre (Steiner, Wiesbaden 1979).

22 Pampiglione, S.; La Placa, M.; Schlick, G.: Studies on Mediterranean leishmaniasis. I. An outbreak of visceral leishmaniasis in northern Italy. Trans. R. Soc. trop. Med. Hyg. *68:* 349 (1974).

23 Aikat, B. K.; Sahaya, S.; Pathania, A. G. S.; et al.: Clinical profile of cases of Kala-azar in Bihar. Indian J. med. Res. *70:* 563 (1979).

24 Neafie, R. C.; Connor, D. H.: Visceral leishmaniasis; in Binford, Connor, Pathology of tropical and extraordinary diseases. An atlas, vol. I (Armed Forces Institute of Pathology, Washington 1976).

25 Pampiglione, S.; Manson-Bahr, P. E. C.; La Placa, M.; et al.: Studies on Mediterranean leishmaniasis. III. The leishmanian skin test in Kala-Azar. Trans. R. Soc. trop. Med. Hyg. *69:* 60 (1975).

26 Aikat, B. K.; Mohanty, D.; Pathania, A. G. S.; et al.: Haematological investigations in kala-azar patients in Bihar. Indian J. med. Res. *70:* 571 (1979).

27 Woodruff, A. W.; Topley, E.; Knight, R.; et al.: The anaemia of kala azar. Br. J. Haematol. *22:* 319 (1972).

28 Belehu, A.; Louis, J. A.; Pugin, P.; et al.: Immunopathological aspects of leishmaniasis. Springer Semin. Immunopathol. *2:* 399 (1980).

29 Bryceson, A. D. M.; Bray, R. S.; Wolstencroft, R. A.; et al.: Immunity in experimental leishmaniasis of the guinea pig. Clin. exp. Immunol. *7:* 301 (1970).

30 Aikat, B. K.; Pathania, A. G. S.; Sehgal, Shobha; et al.: Immunological responses in Indian kala-azar. Indian J. med. Res. *70:* 583 (1979).

31 Turk, J. L.; Bryceson, A. D. M.: Immunological phenomena in leprosy and related diseases. Adv. Immunol. *13:* 209 (1971).

32 Kretschmar, W.: Immunität bei der *Leishmania enrietti* Infektion des Meerschweinchens. Tropenmed. Parasitol. *16:* 277 (1965).

33 Mitchell, G. F.: Responses to infection with metazoan and protozoan parasites in mice. Adv. Immunol. *28:* 451 (1980).

34 Howard, J. G.; Hale, C.; Ling Chan-Liew, W.: Immunological regulation of experimental cutaneous leishmaniasis. I. Immunogenetic aspects of susceptibility to *Leishmania tropica* in mice. Parasit. Immunol. *2:* 303 (1980).

35 Rezai, H. R.; Farrell, J,; Soulsby, E. L.: Immunological responses of *L. donovani* infection in mice and significance of T. cell in resistance to experimental leishmaniasis. Clin. exp. Immunol. *40:* 508 (1980).

36 Bradley, D. J.: Regulation of Leishmania populations within the host. II. Genetic control of acute susceptibility of mice to *Leishmania donovani* infection. Clin. exp. Immunol. *30:* 130 (1977).

37 Bradley, D. J.; Taylor, B. A.; Blackwell, J.; et al.: Regulation of Leishmania populations within the host. III. Mapping of the locus controlling susceptibility to visceral leishmaniasis in the mouse. Clin. exp. Immunol. *37:* 7 (1979).

38 Evans, D. A.: Kinetoplastida; in Taylor, Baker, Methods of cultivating parasites in vitro, p. 63 (Academic Press, London 1978).

39 Berman, J. D.; Dwyer, D. M.; Wyler, D. J.: Multiplication of Leishmania in human macrophages in vitro. Infect. Immunity *26:* 375 (1979).

40 Handman, E.; Burgess, A. W.: Stimulation by granulocytemacrophage colony-stimulating factor of *Leishmania tropica* killing by macrophages. J. Immun. *122:* 1134 (1979).

41 Mauel, J.: The biology of the macrophage-leishmania interaction; in van den Bossche, The host-invader interplay, p. 165 (Elsevier/North Holland Biomedical Press, Amsterdam 1980).

42 Berman, J. D.; Wyler, D. J.: An in vitro model for investigation of chemotherapeutic agents in leishmaniasis. J. infect. Dis. *142:* 83 (1980).
43 Berman, E.: Chemotherapy of leishmaniasis; in Schnitzer, Hawking, Experimental chemotherapy, vol. 1, p. 257 (Academic Press, New York 1963).
44 Handman, E.; Ceredig, R.; Mitchell, G. F.: Murine cutaneous leishmaniasis. Disease patterns in intact and nude mice of various genotypes and examination of some difference between normal and infected macrophages. Aust. J. exp. Biol. med. Sci. *57:* 9 (1979).
45 Howard, J. G.; Hale, C.; Liew, F. Y.: Immunological regulations of experimental cutaneous leishmaniasis. III. The nature and significance of specific suppression of cell-mediated immunity in mice highly susceptible to Leishmania tropica. J. exp. Med. *152:* 594 (1980).
46 Behin, R.; Mauel, J.; Sordat, B.: *Leishmania tropica.* Pathogenicity and in vitro macrophage function in strains of inbred mice. Expl Parasit. *48:* 81 (1979).
47 Poulter, L. W.: Mechanisms of Immunity to leishmaniasis. I. Evidence for a changing basis of protection in self-limiting disease. Clin. exp. Immunol. *39:* 14 (1980).
48 Poulter, L. W.: Mechanisms of immunity to leishmaniasis. II. Significance of the intra-macrophage localization of the parasite. Clin. exp. Immunol. *40:* 25 (1980).
49 Arredondo, B.; Perez, H.: Alteration of the immune response associated with chronic experimental leishmaniasis. Infect. Immunity *25:* 16 (1979).
50 Bjorvatin, B.; Neva, F. A.: Experimental therapy of mice infected with *Leishmania tropica.* Am. J. trop. Med. Hyg. *28:* 480 (1979).
51 Egoz, N.; Michaeli, D.: Epidemiological, immunological and clinical problems of cutaneous leishmaniasis in Israel. A review. Rev. int. Serv. Santé Armées *51:* 151 (1978).
52 Harvey, S. C.: Heavy metals; in Goodman, Gilman, The pharmacological basis of therapeutics (MacMillan, New York 1975).
53 Rees, P. H.; Keating, M. J.; Kager, P. A.; et al.: Renal clearance of pentavalent antimony (sodium stibogluconate). Lancet *ii:* 226 (1980).
54 Pugin, P.; Miescher, P. A.: Le Kala-azar. Etude clinique et physiopathologique à propos d'un nouveau cas observé en Suisse. Schweiz. med. Wschr. *109:* 265 (1979).
55 Marsden, P. D.; Cuba, C. C.; Barreto, A. C.; et al.: Nifurtinox in the treatment of South American leishmaniasis. Trans. R. Soc. trop. Med. Hyg. *73:* 391 (1979).
56 Gregoriadis, G.: The carrier potential of liposomes in biology and medicine. New Engl. J. Med. *195:* 704–765 (1976).
57 Black, C. D. V.; Watson, G. L.; Ward, R. J.: The use of Pentostam liposomes in the chemotherapy of experimental leishmaniasis. Trans. R. Soc. trop. Med. Hyg. *71:* 550 (1977).
58 New, R. R. C.; Chance, M. L.; Thomas, S. C.; et al.: Antileishmanial activity of antimonials entrapped in liposomes. Nature, Lond. *272:* 55 (1978).
59 Alving, C. R.; Steck, E. A.; Chapman, W. L.; et al.: Therapy of leishmaniasis. Superior efficacies of liposome encapsulated drugs. Proc. natn. Acad. Sci. USA *75:* 2959 (1978).

60 Alving, C. R.; Steck, E. A.; Chapman, W. L.; et al.: Liposomes in Leishmaniasis. Therapeutic effects of antimonial drugs, 8-aminoquinolines and tetracycline. Life Sci. *26:* 2231 (1980).
61 Peters, W.: Therapy of intracellular parasitic infections with lysomotropic drugs; in van den Bossche, The host-invader interplay, p. 567 (Elsevier/North Holland Biomedical Press, Amsterdam 1980).
62 Steck, E. A.: Host-protozoa-drug interactions in targeted chemotherapy; in van den Bossche, The host-invader interplay, p. 575 (Elsevier/North Holland Biomedical Press, Amsterdam 1980).
63 Chance, M. L.; New, R. R. C.: The use of liposomes in the treatment of experimental cutaneous and visceral leishmaniasis; in van den Bossche, The host-invader interplay, p. 659 (Elsevier/North Holland Biomedical Press, Amsterdam 1980).
64 Kinnamon, K. E.; Steck, E. A.; Loizeaux, P. S.: The antileishmanial activity of lepidines. Am. J. trop. Med. Hyg. *27:* 751 (1978).
65 Khan, A.; Kirkpatrick, C. H.; Hill, N. O.: Immune regulators in transfer factor (Academic Press, New York 1979).
66 Sharma, M.; Firouz, R.; Ala, F.; et al.: Transfer factor therapy in human cutaneous leishmania infection (CLI). A double-blind clinical trial; in Khan, Kirkpatrick, Hill, Immune regulators in transfer factor, p. 563 (Academic Press, New York 1979).
67 Grob, P. J.; Arrenbrecht, S.: Indications and limitations for transfer factor therapy; in Steffen, Ludwig, Clinical immunology and allergy, developmental immunology, vol. 14 (Elsevier/North Holland Biomedical Press, Amsterdam 1981).
68 Cox, F. E. G.: Immunisation against parasitic infection; in van den Bossche, The host-invader interplay, p. 525 (Elsevier/North Holland Biomedical Press, Amsterdam 1980).
69 Handman, E.; Spira, D. T.; Zuckermann, A.; et al.: Standardization and quality control of *Leishmania tropica* vaccine. J. biol. Stand. *2:* 11 (1974).
70 Mayriuk, W.; Da Costa, C. A.; Magalhaes, P. A., et al.: A field trial of a vaccine against American dermal leishmaniasis. Trans. R. Soc. trop. Med. Hyg. *73:* 385 (1979).
71 Mahmoud, A. A. F.; Warren, K. S.: Algorithms in the diagnosis and management of exotic diseases XXIV. Leishmaniases. J. infect. Dis. *136:* 160 (1977).
72 Marinkelle, C. J.: The control of leishmaniasis. Bull. Wld Hlth Org. *58:* 807 (1980).

Dr. P. Kern, Department of Medicine, Bernhard-Nocht-Institut für Schiffs- und Tropenkrankheiten, Bernhard-Nocht-Strasse 74, D-2000 Hamburg 4 (FRG)

Antibiotics Chemother., vol. 30, pp. 224–256 (Karger, Basel 1981)

Malaria

M. Dietrich, P. Kern[1]

Department of Medicine, Bernhard-Nocht-Institut für Schiffs- und Tropenkrankheiten, Hamburg, FRG

Introduction

In human malaria 1 of 2 species generally prevails, *Plasmodium vivax* (tertian malaria) or *Plasmodium falciparum* (malignant tertian malaria). Two other species, *Plasmodium ovale* (tertian malaria) and *Plasmodium malariae* (quartan malaria) are of regional importance only. Plasmodia are transmitted by Anopheles species as vectors. Occasionally, vertical transmission during pregnancy, during delivery or maternal-fetal transfusion, transmission by blood transfusion, organ transplantation, or possibly by repeated use of contaminated syringes among drug addicts may occur [1–5].

Malaria is endemic in many tropical and subtropical countries, for its generation is dependent on the warmer climates. The disease is still an enormous threat to many millions of people in those countries. According to the World Health Organization, moderate to high risk is present in 92 countries [6, 7]. It has attracted further importance in the last 10 years because of an increasing morbidity throughout the world, and the occurrence of parasite strains which are less susceptible or resistant to previously effective antimalarial agents [8].

Recent figures from more moderate climates in Europe report hypoendemic foci in Turkey [6, 9], a few autochthonous cases [10, 11], but increasing numbers of imported cases [9, 12, 13].

The development of drug-resistant plasmodial strains and contradictory recommendations have complicated the treatment and chemoprophylaxis of

[1] The excellent secretarial assistance of Mrs. *T. Thiede* is gratefully appreciated.

malaria. New drugs and drug combinations are under trial at present. Therefore, current concepts of treatment and chemoprophylaxis of drug-resistant malaria have to be adapted to the recent advances in drug development.

Parasite Cycle and Biology of Infection

Infected mosquitos inject sporozoites into human blood by bite. These infective stages of the parasite are cleared readily from the circulation, but mature to schizonts within the parenchymal cells of the liver. During this pre-erythrocytic stage of infection, the subject remains free of symptoms. After variable intervals, the liver cells liberate the matured merozoites into the bloodstream. The trophozoites mature within the red blood cell, and erythrocytic schizogony occurs. The erythrocyte bursts and merozoites are liberated again. Other red blood cells are infected, and a synchronous maturation and liberation leads to fever attacks every 2 or 3 days, depending on the species involved. In the case of severe *P. falciparum* infection, overlapping cycles lead subsequently to constant fever without characteristic spikes as in tertian or in quartan malaria. Some of the trophozoites develop into sexually differentiated forms (gametocytes). The gametocytes do not cause clinical disease, but are infective for female mosquitos. Under certain environmental conditions (night temperature above 15–16 °C), fertilization of gametocytes results in the development of sporozoites. They, again, are infective for man, thus closing the cycle.

While infection with *P. falciparum* or *P. malariae* follows this cycle, tertian malaria sporozoites or exoerythrocytic stages (i. e., *P. vivax, P. ovale*) can transform into dormant stages (cryptocyte, hypnocyte) which do not cause clinical symptoms, but may lead to malarial disease months or years after infection [14]. This phenomenon – defined as 'relapse' – can be observed both after treated malaria as well as after prophylactic suppression by certain antimalarial agents after leaving the endemic area.

Clinical Disease and Pathology

Spiking chills and fever attacks at regular intervals are the leading symptoms. Other findings such as malaise, abdominal discomfort, diarrhoea, vomiting, fluid balance disturbances, aching muscles, headache, etc., are frequent.

Haemopoietic System

Erythrocytes are the target cells during the blood stage of infection. Due to the synchronous growth of plasmodia within the red blood cells, the cells rupture simultaneously and are captured by the reticulo-endothelial system [15]. Haemolysis may continue for several weeks after the clearance of malarial parasites [16, 17]. The degree of anaemia does not correspond to the degree of malarial infection. Other factors, such as immunologically mediated mechanisms, could possibly be involved [17]. Transient depression of haematopoiesis, i. e., erythropoiesis, has been postulated [18–20]. Current knowledge, based on in vitro bone marrow investigations, demonstrates ineffective erythropoiesis and reduced rate of erythropoietic proliferation to be the most important factors [19, 21, 22].

Thrombocytopenia is associated with malaria and is related to the degree of parasitaemia [23]. The life span of platelets is shortened. Enhanced turnover and pooling of platelets within the spleen plays a role in the mechanisms of thrombocytopenia. Moderate granulocytopenia can be observed occasionally.

Kinetic studies indicate that this is a result of shifted pools, but also lacking possibility to mobilize bone marrow reserves [24].

Haemostaseology

In severe cases, moderate fibrinolysis can be observed. Disseminated intravascular coagulation, however, is not a usual complication. Consumption coagulopathy is rarely seen [25–27].

Lung

Pulmonary oedema is one of the complications of severe falciparum malaria resulting from renal failure which can hardly be overcome by diuretic treatment. However, pulmonary oedema may develop in the absence of fluid overload. The vascular damage may play an important role in the interstitial lung disease [28–30].

Liver and Spleen

Transient enlargement of these organs is commonly observed, due to the expansion of the reticulo-endothelial system. Malaria pigment is stored in vast quantities which leads macro- and microscopically to findings of a brown-coloured organ. A moderate fatty degeneration of hepatocytes is seen. Conjugated bilirubinaemia and elevated transaminases stress the hepatocellular disturbances [22, 31, 32].

Kidney

Hypoxia and obstruction of the microvascular system leads to a transitory renal failure. Malarial immune complexes are localized in the glomerular membrane [17]. These deposits are also transient and can only be detected by kidney biopsy which, however, is not a routine procedure in malaria. Combination of vascular and lower nephron nephropathy coincides with glomerular lesions [17, 33].

Chronic malarial nephropathy is characterized by the following findings: nephrotic syndrome, lack of response to antimalarial therapy, poor response to corticosteroids. Immune complex deposits leading to the nephrotic syndrome play a dominant role [34, 35]. Autoimmune mechanisms are possibly involved at later stages of the chronic nephropathy, leading ultimately to renal failure [17].

Brain

Cerebral malaria is the most deleterious form of *P. falciparum* infection. Prodromal symptoms, such as headache, fatigue, and fever are followed by psychomotorial unrest, agitations, transitory focal signs, delirium, and end in a deep coma or death [28, 36, 37]. The pathogenesis is still unknown, immune pathological mechanisms are likely to be involved [17].

Immune System

Innates of malaria endemic areas acquire a state of resistance to the infection by immunologically mediated mechanisms. Multiplication of plasmodia is kept under control [38, 39]. Natural immunity to malaria is a feature of the host in which case the infection is inhibited further on. This may be exemplified by the innate resistance of man to avian or rodent plasmodia. Genetic factors, such as haemoglobin anomalies or enzyme deficiencies play an other important role [40, 41]. The nonspecific perturbations of the immune responsiveness include polyclonal B cell activation and immunosuppression [17]. Several factors may account for this diverse immune response. It was speculated that modulations of macrophage function are related to the amount of phagocytosed parasitic material thus generating helper as well as suppressor activity [38]. Some observations in immunosuppressed individuals seem to support those observations [42, 43].

Acquired immunity describes the situation in which the host has raised defense mechanisms which lead to protection from renewed infection. In endemic areas, where reinfections are quite numerous, the individuals have protective antibodies against the endemic species of human malaria parasites. Low parasitaemia is often present, but does not lead to clinical symptoms. Such a state of immunity is acquired slowly, so that infants and young children do not have that protection. 'Sterile' immunity is never achieved. Therefore, immunologically protected subjects are called semi-immune. The prenatal or postnatal transfer of antibodies leads to a passive immunity and weakens subsequent reinfection of the homologous strain of the relevant species of malaria parasite during the first few months of newborn life [39].

Other Clinical Entities

Blackwater Fever. This is an extremely rare complication of severe falciparum malaria. It is characterized by an acute intravascular haemolysis with massive haemoglobinuria, acute renal failure, cerebral symptoms, and disseminated intravascular coagulation [44]. The findings are similar to the haemolytic uraemic syndrome [45, 46]. It was said that repeated infections with *P. falciparum* are predisposing factors [47]. The process resembles that of autoimmune haemolytic anaemia or can also be induced by a drug-dependent type of hypersensitivity reaction, Thus, quinine may cause 'black water fever', as it can apply to indications other than malaria [48, 49]. It is of interest that in previous decades during the quinine era blackwater fever was observed more frequently than today.

Tropical Splenomegaly Syndrome. This syndrome is characterized by an enormous enlargement of the spleen and liver, 'big spleen disease'. Anaemia, elevated malarial antibodies, and high IgM levels are typical features. The IgM is of polyclonal origin, and large amounts of IgM are stored in mononuclear cells. It is postulated that this leads to an expansion of the phagocytic cell system and subsequently to an enlargement of the corresponding organs [17, 50].

Laboratory in vivo and in vitro Infection Models

In vivo Infection Models

Avian Model. Several decades ago experimental drug screening was restricted to avian plasmodia, i. e., *P. relictum, P. cathemerium,* or *P. gal-*

linaceum. The effects of drugs in the avian model and the actual results then obtained in man did not correlate sufficiently [51].

Rodent Models. A new era was started after the discovery of a rodent infection model in the late 1940s [52]. Infections with *P. berghei* in the laboratory mouse were extremely valuable, and the experimentally possible cyclical transmission of *P. berghei* through the mosquito has further increased its value [51, 53]. The characteristics of *P. berghei-P. yoelii* complex are mainly the predilection for reticulocytes in the circulation. It can be adapted to rat and hamster species. *P. vinckey* and subspecies as well as *P. chabaudi* and subspecies have a predilection for mature erythrocytes. Differences of the morphology and the enzyme composition are the distinguishing features [54].

For drug screening, strains have been developed that are more or less resistant to particular drugs. This could be achieved with *P. berghei* and others, both in cyclical transmission and blood infection models [51, 55, 56].

Simian Models. The first reports of *P. cynomolgi* in rhesus monkeys date back to 1941 [57]. The model was greatly improved and was found to be quite similar to the *P. vivax* infection in man. The drug effects could be related to the schizontocidal action as well as to the causal prophylactic and anti-relapse property [58]. *P. cynomolgi* was utilized for systematic evaluation of the prophylactic and curative properties of 8-aminoquinolines which led to the discovery and identification of primaquine [59]. *P. cynomolgi* counterparts *P. vivax* infections, whereas *P. knowlesii* resembles the pattern of *P. falciparum* infection. It is believed that secondary exoerythrocytic stages do not occur [51, 60]. Drug-resistant strains of *P. knowlesii* served as a valuable tool in experimental drug screening [60–62]. Numerous attempts have been made to apply human plasmodia to apes. However, only splenectomized animals were suitable [63]. Later, it was found that *Aotus trivirgatus* (owl monkey) could be infected with strains of *P. vivax* and *P. falciparum* [64, 65]. This was the animal model for antimalarial chemotherapy which had long been looked for. Human drug-resistant vivax and falciparum strains can both be adapted to the owl monkey model.

Drug testing has been improved enormously and conclusions can be drawn concerning the infection in man [66]. Established drug-resistant strains are available, i. e., chloroquine-resistant strain (Smith's strain), as well as 8-aminoquinoline-resistant strains of *P. vivax* (Chesson strain) [56, Annex 4]. The animal models have also been used for other investigations [51, 53]. This led to the discovery of the blood cycles of plasmodia, the basis for relapses, origin of gametocytes, as well as to the unterstanding of various pathophysiological mechanisms, etc. [67, 68]. It has been postulated that *P. chabaudi* is a suitable model for cerebral malaria. However, despite initial efforts the strain could not be maintained and was lost [69]. Immunization protocols have been started and applied to simian or human strains in the simian models [70].

In vitro Infection Models

In vitro models are helpful for many purposes, i. e., in order to gather information on the biology and biochemistry of the parasite, to measure the activity of certain drugs, to obtain parasitic material for vaccines, etc. [8, 70–72]. In principle, there are two major in vitro methods available: the short-term culture technique (macro- or micro-method) [73] and the continuous cultivation technique [74]. The short-term cultures are well suited for studies of drug sensitivity, i. e., for 4-aminoquinolines or mefloquine, but not for those drugs which act through metabolites. In principle, defibrinated blood is cultured in a defined medium and under defined conditions. After 24 h, the inhibition of schizont maturation in the presence of drug is measured on a thick film. When cultivating a drug-resistant strain, the schizont growth is not inhibited up to defined dose levels. However, the in vitro test system does not allow conclusions about the degree of resistance concerned. While for the macrotechnique large quantities of blood are required, the microtechnique is much more practical for everybody and also has a higher success rate, and it will soon replace the macromethods [8]. Commercially available tissue culture plates containing defined drug concentrations will allow worldwide screening to detect falciparum strains that are resistant to chloroquine, mefloquine or quinine. It should be mentioned that the test can be read after 24 h, so that treatment can then be adapted according to the laboratory result.

Under defined conditions, several stages of human plasmodia in animal species can be maintained in vitro using the continuous cultivation technique [74]. It has not been possible to culture a single isolation through a complete cycle. Presumably, this is related to the different environmental conditions in which the parasite grows. It is applied to several areas of research, i. e., membrane antigen, development of immunoserological and serological tests, strain differences, as well as experimental immunization programmms [70, 71]. Furthermore, the mode of action of drugs and drug resistance can also be studied more easily in an in vitro test system than in the in vivo models. Biochemical studies, such as differences in metabolic pathways and enzyme characteristics, are facilitated [70, 71].

Current Treatment and Chemoprophylaxis of Malaria

Terms and Definitions

As described above, the life cycle of human pathogenic plasmodia has important characteristics as to whether drug susceptibility is concerned. The target of causal prophylaxis is to achieve a lethal effect on the developmental stages prior to blood schizonts. Certain drugs, as quinine and 4-aminoquinoline affect only blood schizonts. Thus, exoerythrocytic stages of the parasite in the case of *P. vivax* and *P. ovale* infections are not influenced. On the other hand, pre-erythrocytic stages can be destroyed by folic acid antagonists (dihydrofolate reductase inhibitors; DHF) often referred to as antifols. Unfortunately, no drug is available to destroy sporozoites. The action during the life cycle of each drug is, therefore, of considerable interest when giving treatment or prophylactic recommendations to patients [7, 47, 56, 75].

Clinical prophylaxis indicates the prevention of symptoms by suppressive agents without necessarily preventing the establishment of exoerythrocytic stages. However, the infected individual is kept free from clinical symptoms while taking the suppressive drug. Clinical attacks may occur at varying intervals after suppressive medication is stopped.

Clinical curative recommendations are given in order to relieve the symptoms without causing complete destruction of malaria parasites in the body. This regimen is often followed in endemic regions where the chance of reinfection is high in the individual immunity set up.

The term *'radical cure'* describes the action of the drug or drug combinations which destroy blood schizonts leading to clinical symptoms, as well as tissue stages of *P. vivax* and *P. ovale,* as well as elimation of gametocytes. It is only advisable to those living in susceptible, previously freed malaria regions or to those who are not entering endemic areas any more. 8-Aminoquinolines subsequent to or simultaneously with 4-aminoquinolines are regularly prescribed.

While relapses derive from dormant exoerythrocytic stages in the case of *P. vivax* or *P. ovale* infection [14], *recrudescence* describes the situation of renewed parasitaemia at a microscopically detectable level, usually within weeks from the first day of treatment. *Sensitivity* to drugs is defined as clearance from asexual parasites within 7 days of initiation of treatment (drug dose, application and time are defined). *Resistance* grade I describes the situation where parasites have disappeared at day 7, but do reoccur within 21 days. In grade II resistance, parasitaemia is substantially diminished at day 7, and grade III resistance indicates the unresponsiveness of plasmodia to the drug given [77].

Current Used Drugs (see also table V)

Quinine

Quinine is the chief alkaloid of cinchona, the bark of the Cinchona tree, originally indigenous to certain regions of South America. Until early 1930, this alkaloid was the only chemotherapeutic agent for the specific treatment of malaria. Synthetic drugs relegated its use as the drug of choice.

The mode of action is not completely understood. Similar to chloroquine, quinine intercalates with desoxyribonucleic acid (DNA), but it binds to probably more than one side [8, 75]. Quinine is effective both as a suppressive drug and able to control or avoid clinical attacks. Its action is primarily schizontocidal for vivax as well as for falciparum infections. There is some gametocidal activity against *P. vivax, P. ovale,* and *P. malariae*. Quinine lacks a causal prophylactic and curative property (table I). 'Resistance' has been described very early in this century [78] and decreased drug sensitivity can be seen in vivo and in vitro models nowadays.

Quinine can be described as a general protoplasmic poison and affects various organ systems. Therefore, side effects are pronounced, but are as a rule dose-related. Overdosage or hypersensitivity leads to marked neurological and gastrointestinal disturbances and can cause death due to central nervous system involvement [75]. It is also believed that quinine plays an important role in blackwater fever [17, 48].

At the present time, quinine is a valuable drug for treating acute attacks of chloroquine-resistant falciparum malaria, especially in combination with sulfonamides, antifols, tetracyclines or other compounds (table III).

Table I

	Blood schizontocidal		Primary tissue schizontocidal		Secondary tissue		
	falciparum	vivax	falciparum	vivax	schizontocidal vivax	gametocital falciparum	gametocital vivax
Acridines	+	+	–	–	–	–	+
Quinine	+	+	–	–	–	–	±
4-Aminoquinolines	+	+	–	–	–	–	–
8-Aminoquinolines	–	±	+	+	+	+	+
Diaminopyrimidines	+	+	+	–	?	–	–
Biguanides	+	+	+	–	–	–	–
Sulfonamides	+	±	–	–	–	–	–
Sulfones	+	±	–	–	–	–	–
Tetracyclines	±	?	+	?	?	?	?
Quinoline methanols	+	+	–	–	–	–	–

4-Aminoquinolines (Chloroquine, Hydroxychloroquine, Amodiaquine)

Chloroquine was synthesized as early as 1934, but consequent studies on its antimalarial activity had only been performed after a time delay of 10 years [75, 79, 80].

The molecular mechanisms of drug action on Plasmodia are not fully understood. Intercalation with DNA is thought to induce the lethal effect on asexual blood schizonts. Chloroquine blocks acid proteases and peptidases in the phagosomes of intraerythrocytic parasites. This leads to an amino acid deprivation. Pigment clumping will be the result of disturbed metabolism [81]. Chloroquine is selectively taken up by the parasite, and the concentration of the drug found in infected erythrocytes is more than 100 times higher than in noninfected erythrocytes.

Despite its antimalarial activity, the substance has anti-inflammatory properties and is also used against rheumatic diseases as well as in the treatment of photoallergic reactions [75]. The antimalarial activity is primarily directed against blood schizonts (table I). In the acute malaria attack it rapidly controls parasitaemia and clinical symptoms. The drug is

Table II. Treatment of acute malaria attack

Generic name	Day 1	Day 2	Day 3	Day 4	Day 5	Total dose
Chloroquine (base)	900 mg	300 mg	300 mg	(300 mg)	–	1.5(–1.8) g
Amodiaquine (base)	600 mg given at once	400 mg	400 mg	(400 mg)	–	1.4(–1.8) g
Quinine (dihydrochlorate or sulphate)	3×500 mg	3×500 mg	2×500 mg	2×500 mg	2×500 mg/day days 5–10	8.0–11.0 g 7–10 days
Pyrimethamine and Sulfadoxine	75 mg + 1,500 mg	single dose				

not a causal but a suppressive prophylactic agent. Therefore, it does not prevent the establishment of infection (exoerythrocytic stages of all four human malaria species).

Reports of drug resistance of *P. falciparum* strains were published as early as in the 1960s [82–84]. Due to the large scale application of chloroquine's prophylactic measure in different parts of the world, resistant strains developed in South America and Southeast Asia [85]. At the present time, chloroquine resistance reaches up to 80% in some parts of Southeast Asia as well as in South America [86]. There are also reports from East Africa concerning chloroquine resistance of falciparum malaria [87].

Side effects with doses recommended for malaria suppression or therapy are usually slight. They include gastrointestinal symptoms, dizziness, headache, and pruritus [47]. They are short in duration and without adverse consequences. Pruritus was especially reported from West Africa, and it was independent of the presence or absence of malaria parasites in the blood [88].

Large overdoses of chloroquine (taken with the intention to commit suicide) lead to neurological, respiratory and cardiovascular disturbances. Neurological manifestations include drowsiness, visual disturbances, and convulsive seizures. Death is often preceded by hyperexcitability. Cardiovascular manifestations include vasodilatation and hypotension. Furthermore, decreased myocardial contractility and finally cardiac arrest is seen [89]. The effects are similar to those observed with quinine or quinidine.

Table III. Other drug combinations for treatment of 4-aminoquinoline resistant and multi-resistant *P. falciparum* infections

Generic name	Day 1	Day 2	Day 3	Day 4	Day 5	Total dose
Quinine +	2 g	2 g	2 g	–	–	6 g
Sulfadoxine +	2 g	2 g	2 g	2 g	2 g	10 g
Pyrimethamine	50 mg	50 mg	50 mg	50 mg	50 mg	250 mg
Quinine +	2 g	2 g	2 g	–	–	6 g
Sulfadoxine +	2 g	2 g	2 g	2 g	2 g days 5–10	20 g
Tetracycline	1 g	1 g	1 g	1 g	1 g days 5–10	10 g
Mefloquine	1.0–1.5 g single dose					1.5 g

The chronic toxic effects are of much greater importance. Medium doses of chloroquine taken continuously over a long period of time may cause effects due to the selective accumulation of chloroquine in melanin-containing cells, i. e., retina. Furthermore, disturbances of the vestibular and acoustical organ, as well as myopathy, mostly referred to as neuropathy or neuromyopathy, have been found following treatment of certain chronic diseases like rheumatoid arthritis. The side effects have only been observed if a certain dose level of at least 100 g was exceeded within a few months [47, 90]. Aplastic anaemia was observed in a case after use of chloroquine-sulphate [90a].

For amodiaquine drug-induced agranulocytosis has been reported [91]. The observation of teratogenic effects of chloroquine is restricted to few observations despite worldwide use of chloroquine since over 30 years in malaria treatment and suppression [89]. Respective communications have to be taken with caution. Therefore, chloroquine must be assumed to be safer during pregnancy for the mother as well as for the fetus than malaria infection (table II, IV).

8-Aminoquinolines (Primaquine, Quinocide, Pamaquine)

Pamaquine was the first of the 8-aminoquinoline antimalarials to be introduced into medicine [92]. During a large-scale antimalarial programme, several hundreds of derivatives of 8-aminoquinoline were explored, and primaquine was chosen as the most effective drug [59, 93].

The mechanisms of antimalarial action are not understood.

Table IV. Chemoprophylaxis af malaria (currently used)

Drug	Dosage, mg (adults)	Frequency	Acquires resistance	Remarks
Quinine	500 mg	daily	possible	suppressive drug
Chloroquine	300 mg (base)	weekly	regionally for *P. falciparum* not for *P. vivax*	suppressive
Amodiaquine	300–400 mg (base)	weekly	regionally for *P. falciparum* not for *P. vivax*	suppressive
Proguanil	100–200 mg	daily	regionally frequent for *P. falciparum* and *P. vivax*	suppressive and causal prophylactic (*P. falciparum*)
Chlorproguanil	20–40 mg	weekly	regionally frequent for *P. falciparum* and *P. vivax*	suppressive and causal prophylactic (*P. falciparum*)
Pyrimethamine	25 mg	weekly	regionally frequent for *P. falciparum* and *P. vivax*	suppressive and causal prophylactic (*P. falciparum*)
Mefloquine	500 mg	weekly	not observed	suppressive drug
Pyrimethamine + chloroquine	25 mg + 150 mg (base)	weekly	regionally	suppressive for *P. falciparum* and *P. vivax* causal prophylactic for *P. falciparum*
Pyrimethamine + sulfadoxine	25 mg + 500 mg	weekly	known for *P. vivax* regionally for *P. falciparum*	suppressive and causal prophylactic
Pyrimethamine + dapsone	12.5 mg + 100 mg	weekly	?	suppressive and causal prophylactic
Primaquine (disphosphate)	15 mg (base)	fortnightly	5–30 %	toxicity in higher doses, haemolysis, methaemoglobinemia, 'kernikterus' in newborn

Table V

Generic name	Some brand names
Quinacrine	Atebrin (no longer in use)
Quinine	Quinine (-sulfate, -dihydrochloride) Quinimax
Chloroquine (-diphosphate)	Resochin, Aralen, Avlochlor
Chloroquine (-sulphate)	Nivaquine
Amodiaquine (-dihydrochloride)	Camoquine, Flavoquine
Amodiaquine (base)	Basoquine
Primaquine (diphosphate)	Primaquine
Quinocide (dihydrochloride)	Quinocid
Pyrimethamine	Daraprim, Erbaprelina, Malocide, Pyrimethamine Heyl
Proguanil (hydrochloride)	Paludrine, Chlorguanide, Bigumal
Chlorproguanil (hydrochloride)	Lapudrine
Cycloguanil (-emboate)	Camolar
Sulfadiazine	Sulfazine, Diazine
Sulfadoxine	Fanasil, Fanasulf, Fanzil
Sulfalene	Kelfizine
Sulfadimethoxine	Madribon
Dapsone (DDS)	Daphone, Avlosulfone
Acedapsone	Camilan, Hansolar
Mefloquine	(not yet available for clinical use)

One of the early recognized features of 8-aminoquinolines was their ability to destroy gametocytes of *P. falciparum* [51, 80]. This holds true even today for those strains of *P. falciparum* which are multi-drug resistant [94]. As shown in table I, 8-aminoquinolines are also highly active against the primary exoerythrocytic forms of *P. vivax* and *P. falciparum.* This causal prophylactic effect is obtained with well-tolerated doses, too. This activity is of little practical value. The drug is ineffective against the asexual blood forms of *P. falciparum,* whereas the activity against *P. vivax* can be obtained with higher doses. The great clinical value of primaquine is radical curative treatment of vivax and ovale malaria. Southeast Asian strains of *P. vivax* can relapse more frequently in a given period of time than can other strains endemic elsewhere. Those strains have exoerythrocytic stages that are more resistant to primaquine than strains from other geographical regions. Higher doses of drug are therefore necessary [95–97]. With 15 mg/day over 14 days, a 5% failure rate can be assumed, rising regionally up to 30% [98].

The drug is well tolerated in the usual therapeutic dosis (15–45 mg/day). Mild to moderate abdominal cramps and epigastric distress have occurred in individuals given larger doses [75]. Granulocytopenia was a rare complication of therapy and is usually associated with overdosage [91].

Haemolytic anaemia is the most serious and life-threatening side effect. A concomitant deficiency of glucose-6-phosphate dehydrogenase in those patients was already observed as early as in 1950 [99]. Furthermore, using a daily dose of 15 mg for 14 days, it might induce haemolytic crisis and a shortened red cell survival in certain ethnic groups. Thus, 20 mg daily might be the upper limit [100]. The drug causes oxidative haemolysis in patients with G-6-PD deficient erythrocytes [101].

Primaquine is the only available and generally very effective anti-relapse compound. It can be used in those areas where reinfection is less likely and a concomitant glucose-6-phosphate dehydrogenase deficiency can be ruled out (table IV). Reports on decreasing sensitivity (Chesson's strain) have to be taken into account.

Dihydrofolate Reductase Inhibitors ('Antifolic Compounds')

Biguanides (Proguanil, Chloroproguanil, Cycloguanil Emboat)

The first reports on the antimalarial activity of biguanides go back to 1945 [102]. The compound is converted in the body into a triacine derivative, that is, an active inhibitor of the enzyme dihydrofolate reductase. This enzyme catalyzing the reduction of dihydrofolate to tetrahydrofolate is of vital importance to cells and the biosynthesis of purines, pyrimidine and certain amino acids. Protozoa have, in general, either lost or never had the ability to use preformed folate [103] and they need a supply of PABA (para-aminobenzoic acid) to produce their own. Quantitative differences in the binding to parasite and host dihydrofolate reductase is of main importance for its action. As shown in table I, chloroproguanil acts on blood schizonts of *P. falciparum* and *P. vivax*. While the schizontocidal effect is achieved slowly, the main importance is its action on the exoerythrocytic tissue stages of *P. falciparum*. This turns the drug into a causal prophylactic antimalarial agent. It also has some effect on gametocytes which renders them noninfectious for mosquitos [51]. Due to the widespread use, resistance has been developed quite rapidly and to a point where tolerated doses would not be efficient.

A combination with other drugs will be discussed later. There are only minor side effects.

Diaminopyrimidines (Pyrimethamine, Trimethoprim)

Since 1951, pyrimethamine has been used widely for prophylaxis and suppression of malaria [104, 105]. The pharmacological action resembles that described for biguanides, but its potential is greatly enhanced [75]. Pyrimethamine is ineffective as an antibacterial agent although extremly effective as an antimalarial. Trimethoprim, on the other hand, is effective as an antibacterial, but less as an antimalarial agent. Pharmacokinetic properties render pyrimethamine more effective than the active metabolite of proguanil. Its causal prophylactic activity and suppressive activity are identical to those of the biguanides (table I). Unfortunately, plasmodial resistance to this compound developed early throughout the world [105]. Side effects have been reported, but only excessive doses may cause haematological abnormalities, in particular megaloblastic anaemia [107]. The dose of pyrimethamine should, therefore, not be increased over that recommended for prophylactic use.

Compounds with inhibitory activity of the dihydrofolate reductase are mainly of prophylactic importance (table IV). The effective combinations with antifols and other drugs (table II) will be discussed later.

Sulfonamides (Sulfalene, Sulfadoxine, Sulfadiazine, Sulfadimethoxine)

After the introduction of sulfonamides as antimalarial compounds during the 1940s, large numbers of studies were reported not earlier than in the 1960s [108, 112]. Especially long-acting sulfonamides have attracted the interest for treatment or prophylaxis of malaria. The pharmacological basis of their antimalarial properties is again the inhibition of biosynthesis of desoxynucleotides. While pyrimethamine and proguanil inhibit dihydrofolate reductase, sulfonamides and sulfones compete with the 4-aminobenzoic acid (PABA) and inhibit dihydropteroat synthetase. Thus, the reduction of dihydrofolate to tetrahydrofolate cannot take place. While different pharmacokinetic properties are inherent to the mentioned compounds, the antimalarial effect is only directed against blood schizonts of *P. falciparum* and to a lesser degree of *P. vivax* (table I).

It is fortunate that little use has been made of these compounds alone in the treatment of malaria. Thus, only drug combinations are presently used (table II, IV). Side effects, i. e., allergic reactions and haematological complications, are seen quite often [109].

Sulfones (Dapsone, Acedapsone)

The antimalarial properties of sulfones were recognized several decades ago [110]. The pharmacological mechanisms resemble those of sulfonamides. Their activity is therefore similar and mainly directed against asexual blood forms of *P. falciparum,* whereas *P. vivax* schizonts do not respond (table I). Their suppressive activity is only used in combination with other drugs (table IV).

Side effects were, unfortunately, frequent. The most common untoward effect is haemolysis of varying degrees. This develops in almost every individual treated with 200–300 mg Dapsone per day. The strongly oxidant drug can produce methaemoglobinaemia, sulphhaemoglobinaemia, and Heinz body formation in normal subjects at therapeutic doses. Glucose-6-phosphate dehydrogenase-deficient individuals will respond with a varying degree of haemolysis [101]. Dapsone may occasionally produce agranulocytosis as well [91].

As an antimalarial drug it is used only in combination with other drugs (table IV).

Drug Combinations [56, 111]

The report on drug resistance to all major antimalarial compounds in the early 1960s prompted many researchers to use combinations of antiparasitic agents for treatment or prophylaxis (table II–IV). Two effects can be distinguished: (1) the additive effect, i. e., a suppressive drug combined with a causal prophylactic drug or anti-relapse drug, and (2) the potentiating effect – a combination of compounds which act synergistically, i. e., inhibitors of dihydrofolate reductase, and sulfonamides or sulfones.

4-Aminoquinolines and 8-Aminoquinolines

A combination of those drugs for causal prophylaxis has been used widely to protect US Army personnel in the Vietnam War, but did not protect them against chloroquine-resistant *P. falciparum* infection. Amodiaquine and primaquine are in use for causal prophylaxis (table IV) [76].

4-Aminoquinolines or Quinine and Dihydrofolate Reductase Inhibitors

Those combinations are widely in use. Current recommendations include chloroquine and pyrimethamine. The antimalarial effect of both drugs is additive, that means chloroquine exerts its suppressive effect, whereas pyrimethamine acts as a causal prophylactic agent, especially for *P. falciparum*. However, this combination is not suitable to prevent relapses from *P. vivax* and *P. ovale* or to protect from infection by strains resistant to either drug.

Dihydrofolate Inhibitors and Sulfonamides or Sulfones

These combinations have extensively been studied and proved to be useful in individuals with multiresistant strains of *P. falciparum* [112, 113]. Parasitaemia is suppressed by sulfonamides, and pyrimethamine acts on the pre-erythrocytic stages [112, 113, 117]. The two drugs used in combination were more active than either one alone [114–116]. Sulfadoxine potentiates pyrimethamine to about 100-fold activity.

Several combinations have been studied and effective doses elaborated. At the present time, combinations of pyrimethamine (12.5 mg) and Dapsone (100 mg), i. e. Maloprim®, pyrimethamine (25 mg) and sulfadoxine (500 mg), i. e. Fansidar®, are in use (table II, IV). Despite its recommendation for Southeast Asia and South America (areas with chloroquine-resistance), its superiority is limited. Several reports indicate increasing resistance of *P. falciparum* strains to the drugs in question [86, 118–121].

Other drug associations against chloroquine-resistant falciparum malaria are presently in use (table III). Quinine has turned out to be of essential importance for acute malaria attack (table II) [122].

Other Antimalarial Drugs of Less Importance

Tetracyclines

Some antimalarial effect has been attributed to tetracyclines several years ago [123]. The clearance of fever and parasitaemia was generally slower than with the classical antimalarials (table I). Their value vas recently been reappraised in order to cope with multi-drug-resistant *P. falciparum* infections [124].

Tetracyclines show a marked blood schizontocidal activity and have some effect against primary tissue schizonts [51]. However, their use for treatment or prophylaxis of malaria is limited because other drugs are available. The compound can only be used in combination with quinine, dihydrofolate reductase inhibitors or 4-aminoquinolines in cases of multi-drug-resistant falciparum infection (table III) [125].

Quinacrines

Quinacrine is an acridine derivative introduced for antimalarial therapy in the 1930s [75]. Due to its toxicity, it is no longer in use at the present time [56]. It is also of minor value in those individuals with chloroquine-resistant falciparum strains because resistance will also be directed to quinacrine [126].

Supportive Therapy

Despite chemotherapy of malaria attack, supportive measures are necessary in severe falciparum malaria [28, 126–129]. Non-immune patients should be hospitalized. At the time of admission, most patients will have a marked hypotension. A marked haemoconcentration might also be present. Fluid balancing is therefore very important.

Blood transfusions need not to be given, but may be necessary in cases of acute haemolysis or other forms of severe anaemia. Iron, vitamin B_{12}, or folinic acid are possibly unnecessary. Treatment with heparin is only effective if disseminated intravascular coagulation is proven by laboratory test.

Cerebral malaria may be treated with corticosteroids. The anti-oedema therapy will include the administration of mannite and/or furosemide, or other diuretics.

In case of renal failure, dialysis is necessary. Pulmonary oedema, due to fluid imbalance, may be treated with dialysis. In cases with toxic oedema, only assisted or controlled ventilation with high oxygen supply will be effective. Treatment of severe liver failure includes complete blood exchange [130].

Convulsions, more often seen in children than in adults, are treated with parenteral or oral diazepam or paraldehyde.

New Advances

Quinolinemethanols [66]

WR 142 490, Generic Name: Mefloquine. This new antimalarial drug is one of the most promising compounds. The mode of action and its biochemical pathways are not fully understood. Ii the rodent and simian models, Mefloquine has been shown to be a highly effective blood schizontocide [72, 131]. The pharmacological data obtained so far are promising. The mean blood half-time is about 14 days, with a range of 6–23 days. Because of that wide range, occasional treatment failure may occur when the drug is used as a single dose in the treatment of acute attacks.

Several clinical studies have been performed. A dosage of 1.0–1.5 g was found to be effective in treating acute attacks. The suppressive prophylactic activity is also established. 0.25–0.5 g per week is an efficient dosis [132].

Resistance to Mefloquine has been accomplished in the rodent model. It was found that little or no cross-resistance to chloroquine will occur in either the highly chloroquine-resistant or in the moderately resistant lines of *P. berghei* [72].

The suppressive prophylactic activity of the drug against *P. falciparum* and *P. vivax,* administered either weekly or bi-weekly, is dramatic (table I). However, treatment of acute attacks in areas with chloroquine-resistant strains has been found to be inadequate [133]. Combinations with dihydrofolate reductase inhibitors are presently under investigation.

WR 30 090. Despite its early discovery, the antimalarial activity in man was not tested until 1970 [59]. In avian, simian and rodent models the drug appeared to be superior to quinine. Cross-resistance to chloroquine was not found in *P. falciparum* infected owl monkeys [66]. The pharmacological action is not yet understood. It exerts a good suppressive activity against *P. vivax* and *P. falciparum,* but no tissue schizontocidal activity. Cross-resistance was examined in the rodent model and found to be present only with the highly chloroquine-resistant strain of *P. berghei.* In humans, radical cure was achieved in approximately 90 % of the cases with multiresistant *P. falciparum* infection (Phillipine Per strain, Malayan Tailor strain, and Vietnamese Smith's strain) [66, 134]. No drug-related side effects were seen.

Phenanthrenemethanols [66]

WR 33 063. In the avian model, the drug was found to have an enhanced efficacy against *P. gallinaceum* as compared to quinine. However, it was ineffective orally against blood-induced *P. cynomolgi* infections in rhesus monkeys, or infections with the Malayan Camp or Vietnamese Smith's strains of *P. falciparum* in owl monkeys. Clinical studies revealed that treatment with 400 mg 4 × daily for 3 days led to a cure of infection by chloroquine-resistant Camp strain. Higher dosage regimen was necessary to cure from the severely chloroquine-resistant Smith's strain. Several clinical trials were performed, i. e., comparison of quinine, WR 33 063 and other compounds. The cure rate was 92 %. Few observations of RI resistance are noted [134–136]. Suppressive prophylactic activity was evaluated. It demonstrated no tissue schizontocidal activity. Only minor side effects were reported.

WR 122 455. In the rodent model, it was found that the drug resembled a rapid blood schizontocide against P. *berghei,* highly resistant to primaquine, pyrimethamine, and cycloguanil. It was also moderately effective against a chloroquine-resistant line, but inactive against highly chloroquine-resistant lines. The resistance was stable, even in the absence of drug reselection pressure. The mode of action is assumed to be like that of chloroquine.

Few clinical studies have been performed. No conclusion can yet be drawn. The drug is very well tolerated, but seemed to produce mild gastrointestinal symptoms.

WR 171 669. Despite its potent antimalarial effect, only few studies have been performed. In the rodent model, it cured all mice of blood-induced *P. berghei* infection. In the Aotus *P. falciparum* test model the drug was less potent than WR 122 455. In the few phase II studies with *P. falciparum* infection, a radical cure was obtained in all of 9 patients. In those cases no side effects were observed.

Quinazolines [66]

WR 158 122. The synthesis of this compound was reported in 1974. Quinazolines resemble agents with folate antagonistic properties. In the animal models, rapid antimalarial activity was observed. The compound has been tested in the owl monkey model alone or in combination with sulfonamides, the combination of WR 158 122 with sulfonamides produced a marked potentiation [137]. Rapid development of resistance was observed when subcurative doses were used. Furthermore, cross-resistance to pyrimethamine-resistant strains was found.

Only few clinical studies have been carried out with inconsistent results. Toxicity studies revealed haematological disturbances due to its folate antagonism.

Dihydrotriazine [56]

WR 38 839 (Clociguanil) and WR 99 210. These drugs are closely related to cycloguanil and act as dihydrofolate reductase inhibitors. Clinical studies have been performed in combination with sulfonamides.

Quinghaosu [138, 139]

This drug has been studied in China. It is an old chemical entity known as Quinghao, the active principle of the plant *Artemisia annua.* As an antimalarial, it was studied in several animal models as well as in humans infected with *P. vivax* and *P. falciparum.* It appears to be at least as effective as quinine and to better tolerated. The main disadvantage are the necessity of giving it parenterally and the relatively high recrudescence rate.

Floxacrine [140]

Hoe 991. This compound was synthesized in 1972 and underwent extensive studies for its antimalarial activity in various test systems. It was found to be highly effective against drug-sensitive and drug-resistant *P. berghei* strains and affected asexual intraerythrocytic stages of *P. berghei.* The action was found to be comparable to that of mepacrine and amodiaquine. Toxicity studies were promising; however, the drug had to be withdrawn from further clinical studies [141].

Malaria Vaccine [69, 70]

Evidence has been accumulated in the last years showing that animal hosts can be effectively immunized by plasmodial antigens. Great progress has been made in obtaining pure antigen preparations as a prerequisite of vaccine production. The effect was shown to be species-specific and also stage-specific, i. e., vaccination with sporozoites protected against newly inoculated sporozoites, etc. Vaccination against blood-schizont-antigen preparations using irradiated asexual parasites (attenuated parasites) have shown partial protection to a subsequent challenge with viable plasmodia. The immunization against gametocytes was designed to block fertilization in the mosquito gut. However, the results were poor.

Immunization against sporozoites would be the optimal technique leading to complete protection against plasmodial infection. In the animal model, this was found to be effective. Studies of malaria vaccination in man have posed complex problems in relation to their procedure and the evaluation of results. Only few observations have been reported. Infected irradiated mosquitos were fed on human volunteers who were later challenged with infected nonirradiated sporozoites. Immunization resulted in complete protection. However, in all instances, the protection was species-specific.

Interestingly, nonspecific protection was seen in rodent models when animals were concurrently infected with immunostimulatory bacterial, such as *Corynebacterium parvum*. Thus, much emphasis of future research work has to be laid on the specific role of the immune system.

Future Prospects

During the past decades, numerous efforts have been made in several countries to eradicate malaria. A satisfactory success was achieved initially. Unfortunately, many of these activities were not pursued properly or were discontinued completely. Rapidly developing resistance of mosquitos to insecticides and the ban on effective insecticides due to their toxic and teratogenic properties added to the problems of eradicating malaria. The reappearance of malaria in countries formerly very successful in its eradication and the vast epidemic areas, for instance in the Indian subcontinent, indicate that malaria is now again threatening increasing numbers of people. It is estimated that worldwide more than a million children die of malaria every year. Furthermore, the rapid development of resistance rate I to III in Southeast Asia, even to new drug combinations that have been in use for only a few years and were effective in a very high percentage, demonstrates a vast and growing problem which is not only limited to some parts of Southeast Asia. A regional resistance to pyrimethamine up to 80% in East Africa and single cases of chloroquine resistance in East Africa are a warning. Furthermore, a spread of these resistances has to be expected due to the increasing traffic, both of tourists and businessmen, from continent to continent and from country to country. Other strains will be imported not only into countries with moderate climates, such as the United States or Europe, where imported cases have been tenfold in the last few years, but also into tropical countries with endemic malaria.

Although malaria will attack a greater part of the world population in the next years than in the past two decades, new drugs developed, but not yet in the market, together with various combinations of antimalarial agents may be sufficient to cure those who are infected with malaria. However, to prevent infection using prophylactic agents with suppressive activity only must be regarded with great caution when applied to populations on a large scale. Efforts should be made to perform regional eradication programs using all means available, e. g. destroying breeding sites for mosquitos, use of insecticides, and at the same time radical cure of the people living in this region.

The complex problems in malarial vaccination, i. e. production of antigen in large quantities and the species-specific action of the vaccines which allow only a short-lived partial protection will remain and amount to serious handicaps in the vaccination against malaria at the present time. There is considerable hope that these problems of vaccination will be overcome, but only in several years from now.

In conclusion, one may state that the threat of malaria is increasing. Future aspects in the control of malaria will be located in the field of chemotherapy for the next few years and in immunization programs, possibly in the next decade.

Glossary

Cure, clinical	Drugs which terminate the clinical attack, but do not necessarily eradicate the infection
Cure, radical	Drugs which terminate the clinical attack and destroy erythrocytic as well as exoerythrocytic stages of the parasite, especially *P. vivax/P. ovale* infection
Drug resistance	Drugs which lead to a clearance only shortly or not at all defined by the Standard or Extended Test:
Grade I (RI)	Clearance of asexual parasitaemia, followed by recrudescence
Grade II (RII)	Marked reduction of asexual parasites, but no clearance
Grade III (RIII)	No marked reduction of asexual parasites
Gametocidal	Drugs which destroy the sexual stages and eliminate the reservoir for the mosquitos

Glossary (continued)

Immunes	
Non-immune	Man not raised in endemic areas
Semi-immune	Individuals born in endemic areas
Incubation time	Interval between infection and first occurrence of clinical symptoms
Malaria	
Connatal	Vertical transmission or maternal transfusion after birth
Induced	Transmission by transfusion
Introduced	Transmission by mosquito bite
Prepatent period	Maturation time of exoerythrocytic stages until erythrocytic parasitaemia can be demonstrated
Prophylaxis	
Causal	Erythrocytic infection is prevented by a drug or a drug combination which destroys primary liver schizonts or sporozoites
Suppressive	Erythrocytic infection cannot establish because drugs destroy early erythrocytic forms
Recrudescence	Renewed parasitaemia at a microscopically detectable level after treatment
Relapse	Reoccurrence of infection from 'secondary' tissue stages after a variable symptom-free period
Relapse, anti-relapse drugs	Compounds which act mainly on the secondary exoerythrocytic (cryptocytic) stages of *P. vivax, P. ovale*
Rieckmann Test	In vitro sensitivity test of *P. falciparum* to all directly acting blood schizontocidal drugs
Schizontocidal	
Blood	Drugs which destroy erythrocytic stages
Tissue	Compounds acting on exoerythrocytic stages

Glossary (continued)

Sporontocidal	Compounds given to the vertebra host to prevent the development of sporogenic stages in the mosquito
Transmission	
Cyclical	Experimental infections induced by sporozoites deriving from colonized mosquitos *(Anopheles stephani)* via bite or preparations from crushed mosquitos
Vertical	Fetal infections during pregnancy
WHO Standard Field Test	Drug sensitivity test for 7 days: its value is limited because resistance of grade I will be missed
WHO Extended Field Test	Drug sensitivity test for 28 days

References

1 Wenzel-Simon, A.; Bienzle, U.; Bauer, K.; et al.: Konnatale Malaria. Klin. Paediat. *189:* 404 (1977).

2 Exter, J. L.; Renaud, H.; Monnet, P.: Paludisme congénital à *Plasmodium vivax.* Nouv. Presse méd. *9:* 455 (1980).

3 Dover, A. S.; Schultz, M. G.: Transfusion-induced malaria. Transfusion *11:* 353 (1971).

4 Singal, M.; Shaw, P. K.; Lindsay, R. C.; et al.: An outbreak of introduced malaria in California possibly involving secondary transmission. Am. J. trop. Med. Hyg. *26:* 1 (1977).

5 Lefavour, G. S.; Pierce, J. C.; Frame, J. D.: Renal transplant-associated malaria. J. Am. med. Ass. *244:* 1820 (1980).

6 Anon: Synopsis of the world malaria situation, 1978. Wkl. Epidem. Rec. Relevé épidém. hebd. *55:* 193 (1980).

7 Anon: WHO Expert Committee on Malaria. 7th Rep. WHO Tech. Rep. Ser. No. 640 (1979).

8 Wernsdorfer, W. H.; Kouznetsov, R. L.: Drug-resistant malaria – occurrence, control, and surveillance. Bull. Wld Hlth Org. *58:* 341 (1980).

9 Weise, H. J.: Malariaeinschleppungen in die Bundesrepublik Deutschland einschliesslich Berlin (West) unter besonderer Berücksichtigung der letzten 5 Jahre (1973–1977). Bundesgesundhbl. *22:* (1979).

10 Guillausseau, P. J.; Drouet, L.; Garin, Y.; et al.: Paludisme autochtone à *Plasmodium falciparum.* Une nouvelle observation parisienne. Nouv. Presse méd. *9:* 456 (1980).

11 Larcan, A.; Laprevote-Heully, M. C.; Voydeville, G.; et al.: Une nouvelle observation de paludisme autochtone avec contamination probable dans un aéroport international de la région parisienne. Ann. intern. Méd. *129:* 411 (1978).
12 Anon: Epidemiology malaria in Britain 1979. Br. med. J. *ii:* 281 (1980).
13 Weise, H.-J.: Malariaepidemiologie in Europa; in Dietrich, Schönfeld, Hahnenklee-Symposium 1979 (Editiones Roche, Basel 1980).
14 Krotowski, W. A.; Krotowski, D. M.; Garnham, P. C. C.; et al.: Relapses in primate malaria. Discovery of two populations of exoerythrocytic stages. Preliminary note. Br. med. J. *i:* 153 (1980).
15 Omanaga, U.: Possible pathogenic mechanism of hemolysis in malaria. J. trop. Pediat. envir. Child Hlth *24:* 230 (1978).
16 Folayan Esan, G. J.: Haematological aspects of malaria. Clin. Haematol. *4:* 247 (1975).
17 Houba, V.; Lambert, P. H.; Mackey, L. J.; et al.: Immunopathology of malaria. Springers Semin. Immunopathol. *2:* 359 (1980).
18 Srichaikul, T.; Panikbutr, N.; Jeumtrakul, P.: Bone marrow changes in human malaria. Ann. trop. Med. Parasit. *61:* 40 (1967).
19 Srichaikul, T.; Siriawawakul, T.: Ferrokinetics in patients with malaria. Haemoglobin synthesis and normoblast in vitro. Trans. R. Soc. trop. Med. Hyg. *70:* 244 (1976).
20 Abdalla, S.; Weatherall, D. J.; Wickramasinghe, S. N.; et al.: The anaemia of *P. falciparum* malaria. Br. J. Haemat. *46:* 171 (1980).
21 Woodruff, A. W.; Ausdell, V. E.; Pettit, L. E.: Cause of anaemia in malaria. Lancet *i:* 1055 (1979).
22 Dietrich, M.; Dörmer, P.; Kern, P.; et al.: Evidence for ineffective erythropoiesis in human malaria. Blut (submitted, 1980).
23 Horstmann, R. D.; Dietrich, M.; Bienzle, U.; et al.: Malaria-induced thrombocytopenia. Blut *42:* 160 (1981).
24 Dale, D. C.; Wolff, S. M.: Studies of the neutropenia of acute malaria. Blood *41:* 197 (1973).
25 Fletcher, J. R.; Butler, T.; Kopriva, C. J.; et al.: Acute *Plasmodium falciparum* malaria. Vital capacity blood gases and coagulation. Archs intern. Med. *129:* 617 (1972).
26 Srichaikul, T.; Puwasatien, P.; Puwasatien, P.; et al.: Complement changes and disseminated intravascular coagulation in *Plasmodium falciparum* malaria. Lancet *i:* 770 (1975).
27 Rasche, H.: Blutgerinnungsstörungen bei Malaria: in Dietrich, Schönfeld, Hahnenklee-Symposium. Malaria – Diagnose – Klinik – Therapie, pp. 77 (Editiones Roche, Basel 1980).
28 Hall, A. P.: The treatment of severe falciparum malaria. Trans. R. Soc. trop. Med. Hyg. *71:* 367 (1977).
29 Martell, R. W.; Kallenbach, J.: Zwi, S.: Pulmonary edema in falciparum malaria. Br. med. J. *i:* 1763 (1979).
30 Blanlœil, Y.; Bason, D.; Lajartre, A. Y. de: et al.: Oedème du poumon non hémodynamique au cours d'un accès pernicieux palustre. Nouv. Presse méd. *9:* 2024 (1980).

31 Deller, J. J., Jr.; Cifarelli, P. S.; Berque, S.; et al.: Malaria hepatitis. Milit. Med. *132:* 614 (1967).

32 Ramachandran, S.; Perera, M. V. F.: Jaundice and hepatomegaly in primary malaria. J. trop. Med. Hyg. *79:* 207 (1976).

33 Ehrich, J. H. H.: Pathogenese der Malaria-Nephropathien; in Dietrich, Schönfeld, Hahnenklee-Symposium. Malaria – Diagnose – Klinik – Therapie, pp. 53–73 (Editiones Roche, Basel 1980).

34 Allison, A. C.; Houba, V.; Hendrickse, R. G.; et al.: Immune complexes in the nephrotic syndrome of African children. Lancet *i:* 1232 (1969).

35 Weise, M.; Ehrich, J. H. H.; Votter, A.: Nierenbeteiligung bei Malaria. Klin. Wschr. *54:* 651 (1976).

36 Toro, G.; Roman, G.: Cerebral malaria. A disseminated vasculomyelinopathy. Archs Neurol. *35:* 271 (1978).

37 Vietze, G.: Malaria and other protozoal diseases affecting the nervous system. Trends Neurosci. *3:* 152 (1980).

38 Luzzatto, L.: Genetics of red cells and susceptibility to malaria. Blood *54:* 961 (1979).

39 Cohen, S.: Mechanisms of malaria immunity. Trans. R. Soc. trop. Med. Hyg. *71:* 283 (1977).

40 Wyler, D. J.: Cellular aspects of immunoregulations in malaria. Bull. Wld Hlth Org. *57:* suppl. 1, p. 239 (1979).

41 Bienzle, U.; Guggenmoos-Holzmann, J.; Luzzatto, M.: Malaria and erythrocyte G6PD variants in West Africa. Am. J. trop. Med. Hyg. *28:* 619 (1979).

42 Tapper, M. L.; Armstrong, D.: Malaria complicating neoplastic disease. Archs intern. Med. *136:* 807 (1976).

43 Duperval, R.; Longpré, B.; Madarnas, P.: Unexplained falciparum malaria in a patient with chronic lymphocytic leukemia. Can. med. Ass. J. *121:* 1585 (1979).

44 Maegraith, B.: Blackwater fever anuria. Trans. R. Soc. trop. Med. Hyg. *38:* 1 (1944).

45 Gasser, V. C.; Gautier, R.; Steck, A.; et al.: Hämolytisch-urämische Syndrome: Bilaterale Nierenrindennekrosen bei akuten erworbenen hämolytischen Anämien. Schweiz. med. Wschr. *38:* 905 (1955).

46 Kaplan, B. S.; Thomson, P. D.; De Chadarevian, T. P.: The hemolytic-uraemic syndrome. Pediat. Clins N. Am. *23:* 761 (1976).

47 Bruce-Chwatt, L. J.: Essential malariology, p. 69 (Heinemann, London 1980).

48 Foy, H.; Kondi, A.: The correlation between blackwater fever, malaria, quinine and atebrin. Ann. trop. Med. Parasit. *44:* 309 (1950).

49 Webb, R. F.; Ramirez, A. M.; Hocken, A. G.; et al.: Acute intravascular haemolysis due to quinine. N. Z. med. J. *91:* 14 (1980).

50 Greenwood, B. M.; Fakunle, Y. M.: The tropical splenomegaly syndrome. The role of the spleen in the immunology of parasitic diseases, p. 229 (Schwabe, Basel 1979).

51 Peters, W.: Chemotherapy and drug resistance in malaria (Academic Press, London 1970).

52 Vincke, J. H.; Lips, M.: Un nouveau Plasmodium d'un rongeur sauvage du Congo. *Plasmodium berghei* n. sp. Annls Soc. belge Méd. trop. *28:* 97 (1948).

53 Killick-Kendrick, R.; Peters, W.: Rodent malaria (Academic Press, London 1978).
54 Landau, J.; Boulard, Y.: Life cycles and morphology; in Killick-Kendrick, Peters, Rodent malaria (Academic Press, London 1978).
55 Peters, W.; Howells, R. E.: Chemotherapy; in Killick-Kendrick, Peters, Rodent malaria (Academic Press, London 1978).
56 Anon: Chemotherapy of malaria and resistance to antimalarials. Report of a WHO scientific group. Tech. Rep. Ser. No. 529 (World Health Organization, Geneva 1973).
57 Coggeshall, L. T.: The selective action of sulfanilamid on the parasites of experimental malaria in monkeys in vivo and in vitro. J. exp. Med. *71:* 13 (1940).
58 Schmidt, L. H.; Genther, C. S.: The antimalarial properties of 2.4 diamino-5-p-chlorophenyl-6-ethylpyrimidine (Daraprim). J. Pharmac. exp. Ther. *107:* 61 (1953).
59 Wiselogle, F. Y.: A survey of antimalarial drugs 1941–1945, vol. 1 (Edwards, Ann Arbor 1946).
60 Coggeshall, L. T.; Maier, J.: Determination of the activity of various drugs against the malaria parasite. J. infect. Dis. *69:* 108 (1941).
61 Ramakrishnan, S. P.: Experimental selection of drug-resistant Plasmodia. A review of results up to 1962. Proc. 7th Int. Congr. Trop. Med. Malar., Rio de Janeiro 1963, vol. 5, p. 474.
62 Schmidt, L. H.; Rossan, R. N.; Fradkin, R.; et al.: Studies on the antimalarial activity of 1,2-dimethoxy-4-(bis-diethylaminoethyl)-amine-5-bromobenzene. Bull. Wld Hlth Or. *34:* 783 (1966).
63 Bray, R. S.: Studies on malaria in chimpanzees. VI. *Laverania falcipara.* Am. J. trop. Med. Hyg. *7:* 20 (1958).
64 Geiman, Q. M.; Meagher, M. J.: Susceptibility of a New World monkey to *Plasmodium falciparum* from man. Nature, Lond. *215:* 437 (1967).
65 Schmidt, L. H.: Infections with *Plasmodium falciparum* and *Plasmodium vivax* in the owl monkey-model systems for basic biological and chemotherapeutic studies. Trans. R. Soc. trop. Med. Hyg. *67:* 446 (1973).
66 Rozman, R. S.; Caufield, C. J.: New experimental antimalarial drugs. Adv. Pharmacol. Chemother. *16:* 1 (1979).
67 Nussenzweig, R. S.; Cochrane, A. H.; Lustig, H. J.: Immunologic responses; in Killick-Kendrich, Peters, Rodent malaria (Academic Press, London 1978).
68 Pasvol, G.; Weatherall, D. J.: The red cell and the malaria parasite. Br. J. Haemat. *46:* 165 (1980).
69 Cox, H. W.: Personal commun. (1977).
70 NMRI/US AID/WHO Workshop on the Immunity of Malaria. Bull. Wld Hlth Org. *57:* suppl. 1 (1979).
71 US AID/WHO Workshop on the Biology and in vitro Cultivation of Malaria Parasites. Bull. Wld Hlth Org. *55:* 121 (1977).
72 Peters, W.; Howells, R.; Portus, J.; et al.: The chemotherapy of rodent malaria. XXVII. Studies on mefloquine WR 142,490. Ann. trop. Med. Parasit. *71:* 407 (1977).
73 Rieckmann, K. H.; Campbell, G. H.; Sax, L. J.; et al.: Drug sensitivity of *Plasmodium falciparum.* An in vitro microtechnique. Lancet *i:* 22 (1978).

74 Trager, W.; Jensen, S. B.: Cultivation of malaria parasites. Nature, Lond. *273:* 621 (1978).

75 Rollo, J. M.: Drugs used in the chemotherapy of malaria; in Goodman, Gilman, The pharmacological basis of therapeutics; 5th ed. (McMillan, New York 1975).

76 Lopez-Antuniano, F. J.: Guide to the chemotherapy of human malaria. Pan. Am. Hlth Org. Scient. Publ. No. 373 (1979).

77 Anon: Chemotherapy of malaria. Report of a WHO scientific group. WHO Tech. Rep. Ser. No. 375 (1967).

78 Nocht, B.; Werner, H.: Beobachtungen über die relative Chininresistenz bei Malaria aus Brasilien. Dt. med. Wschr. *36:* 1557 (1910).

79 Butts, D. C. A.: Results on 449 cases of naturally acquired malaria treated with chloroquine. J. natn. Malaria Soc. *9:* 44 (1950).

80 Jeffrey, G. M.; Young, M. D.; Eyles, D. E.: The treatment of *Plasmodium falciparum* infection with chloroquine, with a note on infectivity to mosquitos of primaquine- and pyrimethamine-treated cases. Am. J. Hyg. *64:* 1 (1956)

81 Warhurst, D. C.; Thomas, S. C.: The chemotherapy of rodent malaria. XXXI. The effect of some metabolic inhibitors upon chloroquine-induced pigment-clumping (CIPC) in *Plasmodium berghei.* Ann. Trop. Med. Parasitol. *72: 203* (1978).

82 Maberti, S.: Desarrollo de resistencia a la pirimetamina. Presentación de 15 casos estudiados en Trujillo, Venezuela. Archos venez. Méd. trop. Parasit. méd. *3:* 239 (1960).

83 Moore, D. V.; Lanier, J. E.: Observations on two *Plasmodium falciparum* infections with an abnormal response to chloroquine. Am. J. trop. Med. Hyg. *10:* 5–9 (1961).

84 Harinasuta, T.; Suntharasmai, P.; Viravan, C.: Chloroquine-resistant falciparum malaria in Thailand. Lancet *ii:* 657 (1965).

85 Clyde, D. F.: Treatment of drug-resistant malaria in man. Bull. Wld Hlth Org. *50:* 243 (1974).

86 Bunnag, D.; Harinasuta, T.; Suntharasamai, P.; et al.: Monitoring of antimalarial drugs in the treatment of acute falciparum malaria. Abstr. 453, 10th Int. Congr. Trop. Med. Malaria, Manila 1980.

87 Campbell, C. C.; Chin, W.; Collins, W. E.; et al.: Chloroquine-resistant *Plasmodium falciparum* from East Africa. Lancet *ii:* 1151 (1979).

88 Olatunde, J. A.: Chloroquine-induced pruritus in Lagos, Nigeria. J. Niger. med. Ass. *6:* 28 (1959).

89 Weniger, H.: Review of side effects and toxicity of chloroquine. WHO/Mal/79.906 (1979).

90 Bruce-Chwatt, L. J.: Prolonged malaria prophylaxis. Br. med. J. *i:* 650 (1978).

90a Sleijfer, D. T.; Mulder, N. H.; Nieweg, H. O.: The value of prognostic indices in aplastic anaemia. Blut *42:* 69 (1981).

91 Young, G. A. R.; Vincent, P. C.: Drug-induced agranulocytosis. Clin. Haematol. *9:* 483 (1980).

92 Mühlens, P.: Die Behandlung der natürlichen menschlichen Malaria-Infektion mit Plasmodien. Naturwissenschaft *14:* 1162 (1926).

93 Schmidt, L. H.; Coatney, G. R.: Review of investigations in malaria chemotherapy (USA) 1946 to 1956. Am. J. trop. Med. Hyg. *4:* 208 (1955).

94 Rieckmann, K. H.; McNamara, J. V.; Frischer, H.; et al.: Gametocidal and sporontocidal effects of primaquine and of sulfadiazine with pyrimethamine in a chloroquine-resistant strain of *P. falciparum.* Am. J. trop. Med. Hyg. *17:* 661 (1968).

95 Clyde, D. F.; McCarthy, V. D.: Radical cure of Chesson strain vivax malaria in man by 7, not 14 days of treatment with primaquine. Am. J. trop. Med. Hyg. *26:* 562 (1977).

96 Coatney, G. R.; Cooper, W. C.; Young, M. D.: Studies in human malaria. XXX. A summary of 204 sporozoite-induced infections with the Chesson strain of *Plasmodium vivax.* J. natn. Malaria Soc. *9:* 381 (1950).

97 Fischer, G. U.; Gordon, M. P.; Lobel, H. O.; et al.: Malaria in soldiers returning from Vietnam. Epidemiology, therapeutic and clinical studies. Am. J. trop. Med. Hyg. *19:* 3 (1970).

98 Krotoski, W. A.: Frequency of relapse and primaquine resistance in Southeast Asian vivax malaria. New Engl. J. Med. *303:* 587 (1980).

99 Beutler, E.: The hemolytic effect of primaquine and related compounds. A review. Blood *14:* 103 (1959).

100 Alving, A. S.; Johnson, C. F.; Tarlov, A. R.; et al.: Mitigation of hemolytic effect of primaquine and enhancement of its action against exoerythrocytic forms of Chesson-strain of *Plasmodium vivax* by intermittant regimens of drug administration. Bull. Wld Hlth Org. *22:* 621 (1960).

101 Gordon-Smith, E. C.: Drug induced oxidative hemolysis. Clin. Haematol. *9:* 557 (1980).

102 Adams, AR. D.; Maegraith, B. E.; King, J. D.; et al.: Studies on synthetic antimalarial drugs. XIII. Results of a preliminary investigation on the therapeutic action of 4888 (Paludrine) on acute attacks of benigne tertian malaria. Ann. trop. Med. Parasit. *39:* 225 (1945).

103 Ferrone, R.: Folate metabolism in malaria. Bull. Wld Hlth Org. *55:* 292 (1977).

104 Archibald, H. M.: Preliminary field trials on a new schizontocide. Br. med. J. *ii:* 821 (1951).

105 Clyde, D. F.: Observations on monthly pyrimethamine ('Daraprim') prophylaxis in an East African village. E. Afr. med. J. *31:* 41 (1954).

106 Avery-Jones, S.: Resistance of *P. falciparum* and *P. malariae* to pyrimethamine (Daraprim) following man treatment with this drug. A preliminary note. E. Afr. med. J. *31:* 47 (1954).

107 Scott, J. M.; Weir, D. G.: Drug-induced megaloblastic change. Clin. Haematol. *9:* 587 (1980).

108 Rozman, A.: Chemotherapy of malaria. A. Rev. Pharmacol. *13:* 127 (1973).

109 Weinstein, L.: Sulfonamide and trimethoprim-sulfamethoxazole; in Goodman, Gilman, The pharmacological basis of therapeutics; 5th ed. (McMillan, New York 1975).

110 Leiker, D. L.: Note on sulphone activity in malaria infection. Lepr. Rev. *27:* 66 (1956).

111 Tigertt, W. D.; Clyde, D. F.: Drug resistance in the human malarias. Antibiotics Chemother. *20:* 246 (1976).

112 Richards, W. H. G.: The combined action of pyrimidines and sulfonamides or

sulfones in the chemotherapy of malaria and other protozoal infections. Adv. Pharmacol. Chemother. *8:* 121 (1970).
113 Chin, W.; Contacos, P. G.; Coatney, G. R.; et al.: The evaluation of sulfonamides, alone or in combination with pyrimethamine, in the treatment of multiresistant falciparum malaria. Am. J. trop. Med. Hyg. *15:* 823 (1966).
114 Havas, L.; Hamza, B.; Fernex, M.; et al.: Combinations of folic acid and folinic acid antagonists in human and veterinary medicine. Chemotherapy *19:* 179 (1973).
115 Ebisawa, J.; Komoriya, T.; Kimura, M.; et al.: Morphologic and clinical effect of pyrimethamine-sulfonamide combinations (sulformethoxine-pyrimethamine or sulfamonomethoxine-pyrimethamine on *P. vivax* and its infections). Jap. J. exp. Med. *44:* 151 (1974).
116 Tawil, A. A.: Clearance of falciparum parasitaemia with a single dose sulfadoxine-pyrimethamine in Vientiane, Laos. Southeast Asian J. trop. Med. Publ. Hlth *9:* 409 (1978).
117 Schmidt, L. H.; Harrison, J.; Rossan, R. N.; et al.: Quantitative aspects of pyrimethamine sulphonamide synergism. Am. J. trop. Med. Hyg. *26:* 837 (1977).
118 Tin, F.; Hlaing, N.: Resistance to antimalarials by *Plasmodium falciparum* in Burma. Southeast Asian J. trop. Med. Hyg. Publ. Hlth *8:* 104 (1977).
119 Pearlman, E. J.; Lampe, R. M.; Thiemann, W.; et al.: Chemosuppressive field trials in Thailand. III. The suppression of *Plasmodium falciparum* and *Plasmodium vivax* parasitaemias by a sulfadoxine-pyrimethamine combination. Am. J. trop. Med. Hyg. *26:* 1108 (1977).
120 Rumens, L. W.; Dennis, D. T.; Atmosoedjono, S.: Fansidar resistant falciparum malaria in Indonesia. Lancet *ii:* 580 (1979).
121 Holzer, B.; Keller, H.; Frossard, E., and Stürchler, D.: Ist Plasmodium falciparum, der Erreger der Malaria tropica, jetzt auch gegen Fansidar resistent? Schweiz. Med. Wschr. *110,* 324 (1980).
122 Clyde, D. F.: Treatment of drug-resistant malaria in man. Bull. Wld Hlth Org. *50:* 243 (1974).
123 Colwell, F. J.; Hickmann, R. L.; Intraprasert, R.; et al.: Minocycline and tetracycline treatment of acute falciparum malaria in Thailand. Am. J. trop. Med. Hyg. *21:* 144 (1972).
124 Miller, L. H.; Glew, R. H.; Wyler, D. J.; et al.: Evaluation of clindamycin in combination with Quinine against multidrug resistant strains of *Plasm. falciparum.* Am. J. trop. Med. Hyg. *23:* 565 (1974).
125 Anon: *Plasmodium falciparum* malaria contracted in Thailand resistant to chloroquine and sulfonamide-pyrimethamine. Illinois MMWR *29:* 493 (1980).
126 Wery, M.; Coosemans, M.: La résistance médicamenteuse dans le paladisme. Ann. Soc. belg. Méd. trop. *60:* 137 (1980).
127 Hall, A. P.: The treatment of malaria. Br. med. J. *i:* 323 (1976).
128 Gilles, H. M.: The management and treatment of malaria. A personal view. Ann. Soc. belg. Méd. trop. *60:* 129 (1980).
129 Dietrich, M.; Schönfeld, H.: Hahnenklee-Symposium 1979. Malaria – Diagnose – Klinik – Therapie (Editions Roche, Basel 1980).
130 Nielsen, R. L.; Kower, R. B.; Chin, W.; et al.: The use of exchange transfusion. A potentially useful adjunct in the treatment of fulminant falciparum malaria. Am. J. med. Sci. *277:* 325 (1979).

131 Schmidt, L. H.; Crosby, R.; Rasco, J.; et al.: Antimalarial activities of various 4-quinolinemethanols with special attention to WR 142490 (Mefloquine). Antimicrob. Agents Chemother. *13:* 1011 (1978).

132 Clyde, D. F.; McCarthy, V. C.; Miller, R. M.: Suppressive activity of mefloquine in sporozoite-induced human malaria. Antimicrob. Agents Chemother. *9:* 334 (1976).

133 Hall, A. P.; Doberstyn, E. B.; Karnchanachetanee, C.; et al.: Sequential treatment with quinine and mefloquine or quinine and pyrimethamine-sulfadoxine for falciparum malaria. Br. med. J. *i:* 1626 (1977).

134 Hall, A. P.; Segal, H. E.; Pearlman, E. J.; et al.: Comparison of a 9-phenanthrene methanol (WR 33063), 4-quinoline methanol (WR 30090), and quinine for falciparum malaria in Thailand. Trans. R. Soc. trop. Med. Hyg. *69:* 342 (1975).

135 Segal, H. F.; Chinvanthananond, P.; Laixuthai, B.; et al.: Preliminary study of WR 33 063 in the treatment of falciparum malaria in Northeast Thailand. Am. J. trop. Med. Hyg. *23:* 560 (1974).

136 Arnold, J. D.; Martin, D. C.; Carson, P. E.; et al.: A phenanthrene methanol (WR 33 063) for treatment of acute malaria. Antimicrob. Agents Chemother. *3:* 207 (1973).

137 Schmidt, L.: Studies on the 2,4-diamino-6 substituted quinazolines. III. The capacity of sulfadiazine to enhance the activities of WR 158 122 and WR 159 412 against infections with various drug-susceptible and drug-resistant strains of *Plasmodium falciparum* and *Plasmodium vivax* in owl monkeys. Am. J. trop. Med. Hyg. *28:* 808 (1979).

138 Qinghoasu Antimalaria Coordinating Research Group: Antimalaria studies on qinghoasu. Chin. med. J. *92:* 811 (1979).

139 Peters: Abstract 1722. Trop. Dis. Bull. *77:* 555 (1980).

140 Raether, W.; Finch, I.: Antimalarial activity of floxacrine (HOE 991). I. Studies on blood schizontocidal action of floxacrine against *Plasmodium berghei, P. vinckei,* and *P. cynomolgi.* Ann. trop. Med. Parasit. *73:* 505 (1979).

141 Raether, W.: Personal commun. (1980).

Prof. Dr. M. Dietrich, Department of Medicine, Bernhard-Nocht-Institut für Schiffs- und Tropenkrankheiten, Bernhard-Nocht-Strasse 74, D-2000 Hamburg 4 (FRG)

Antibiotics Chemother., vol. 30, pp. 257–271 (Karger, Basel 1981)

Pneumocystis Carinii Pneumonitis[1]

Walter T. Hughes

Division of Pediatric Infectious Diseases,
Johns Hopkins University School of Medicine, Baltimore, Md., USA

Historical Account

Chagas [2] is believed to have been the first to describe *Pneumocystis carinii.* He reported cyst forms in the lungs of guinea pigs infected with *Trypanosoma cruzi.* However, he mistakenly considered the cysts to be a stage in the life cycle of the trypanosome. *Carini* [1] described similar cysts which he also considered to be schizogomy in the course of *Trypanosoma lewisi.* It was *Delanoe and Delanoe* [4, 5] in Paris who identified the cysts in the lungs of rats without trypanosomiasis and proposed the agent as a separate and new organism. They also suggested the name *Pneumocystis,* since cysts were found only in the lungs, and *carinii* because *Carini* provided them with specimens for comparison. Later, *Chagas, Carini* and others concluded the organism was not a trypanosome.

Interstitial plasma cell pneumonitis had been recognized as a significant problem in European infants. The etiology was discovered to be *P. carinii* by *Van der Meer and Brug* [33] in the Netherlands in 1942. The pneumonitis occurred in endemics and epidemics in nursling homes in Europe following World War II but these have subsided in recent years.

Since 1955, *P. carinii* has been encountered in North America, not in infants, but in children and adults with malignancies, congenital immune deficiency disorders and organ transplant recipients. In these individuals

[1] Acknowledgement: partial support from grant 5 RO1 AI 14769, National Institute of Allergy and Infectious Diseases, National Institutes of Health and the Board for the Hospital for the Consumptives of Maryland (Eudowood).

the infection causes an acute diffuse alveolar pneumonitis rather than interstitial plasma cell pneumonitis of infants. Currently, the infection is encountered primarily in the immunocompromised child and adult.

Epidemiology

P. carinii has been found in the lungs of animals, humans, or both in all parts of the world. The organisms may exist in latent form unassociated with clinical manifestations. In a compromised host a severe pneumonitis may be provoked. It is generally believed, but not proven, that most cases of overt pneumonitis represent activation of latent organisms. The population at risk for the disease is limited almost exclusively to debilitated and marasmic infants, children with congenital immune deficiency disorders, organ transplant recipients, individuals with severe protein-calorie malnutrition, patients with malignancies, those receiving immunosuppressive drugs over prolonged periods of time and certain cases with chronic diseases. Endemics and small epidemics have occurred only in nursling homes with infants. Clusters of cases have been reported from a few cancer centers [3]. However, the contagious nature of the infection has never been ascertained and the mode of transmission is unknown.

Prevalence

The prevalence of *P. carinii* pneumonitis appears to vary with the extent of immunocompromise of the host. In a prospective study of leukemic children, *P. carinii* pneumonitis occurred in 5.0% of those maintained on only one immunosuppressive anticancer drug, in 2.3% receiving 2 drugs, 2.2% receiving 3 drugs, 22.4% receiving 4 drugs and 35.7% of those receiving 3 drugs plus mediastinal irradiation [12]. Serological surveys of normal children show that about three-fourths of this population acquires antibody to *P. carinii* by age 4 years [27, 28].

Pathology

The histopathology of the infantile form of *P. carinii* pneumonitis differs from the childhood and adult form. With the infantile type an extensive plasma cell infiltration of the alveolar septae occurs occupying up to two-thirds of the total lung space. The septae may be 5–20 times the normal thickness [6]. The childhood and adult form occurs in immunocompromised patients and is characterized by an extensive alveolopathy with masses of organisms filling the alveoli. The septae may be thickened with mononuclear inflammatory cells. The total weight of affected lungs may be over twice that of normal. With rare exception the organisms and the disease remain localized to the lungs.

Laboratory in vitro and in vivo Models

An excellent animal model for *P. carinii* has been developed. Findings in the animals have been representative of human disease in all comparative studies to date. Sprague-Dawley rats have been used in most studies. The rats are given prednisone or cortisone acetate, along with an antibiotic such as tetracycline. Within 2–4 months close to 100% of the animals acquire *P. carinii* pneumonitis. Inoculation of *P. carinii* is not required. Apparently the immunosuppression permits replication of latent organisms to establish infection. Other mammals, such as mice and rabbits, have also been used with similar results.

Chemotherapy

Three drug regimens have each been shown to be effective in the treatment of *P. carinii* pneumonitis. These are pentamidine isethionate, pyrimethamine plus sulfadiazine and trimethoprim plus sulfamethoxazole (TMP-SMZ).

Pentamidine Isethionate

Pentamidine is 4:4′-diamidinodiphenoxypentane di-(β-hydroxyethanesulfonate). The drug is available through the manufacturer May & Baker, Ltd. in England and the Parasitic Disease Drug Service at the Center for Disease Control in the United States. The exact mechanism of action against *P. carinii* is unknown; however, some evidence suggests that the drug binds dihydrofolate reductase [36].

Pentamidine was first used by *Ivady and Paldy* [19] in 1958 for the treatment of *P. carinii* interstitial plasma cell pneumonitis in infants. By

1963 these investigators had treated 212 infants [20]. In untreated patients the mortality rate was 50%. With pentamidine therapy the mortality was reduced to 20% by 1959 and when the drug was used early in the course of the disease the mortality rate was 5.0%. Another study showed that marked degeneration of *P. carinii* cysts occurred after the 6th day of treatment and after the 10th day all organisms had been clear from the lungs [32]. Eventually, a mortality rate of 3.0% in infants with the pneumonitis was achieved [20].

When *P. carinii* pneumonitis began to appear in the United States, pentamidine was distributed in this country only through the Center for Disease Control. Through this system, data were collected on essentially all cases of the pneumonitis. Analysis of these reports included cases from November 1967 through December 1970 [37, 38]. Of the first 163 confirmed cases treated with pentamidine, 43% recovered. A total of 404 patients, confirmed plus suspect cases, received pentamidine directed by a standard protocol. These cases experienced several adverse reactions. 189 (47%) had one or more of the following adverse effects: impaired renal function (24%), liver dysfunction (10%), hematologic abnormalities (4%), injection-site reactions (18%), hypoglycemia (6%), hypotension (10%), rashes (2%) and hypocalcemia (1%). However, these reactions are usually reversible with proper management. The best results from pentamidine therapy have been reported in studies from single institutions where complete clinical recovery occurred in 68–75% of those treated with pentamidine [13, 18].

Overall the drug can be considered quite effective since *P. carinii* pneumonitis in the immunocompromised host has a mortality rate of 90–100%. In a study of 107 cases in the United States from 1955 through 1967, 102 (95%) died [25]. In the Center for Disease Control study, 6 patients with *P. carinii* pneumonitis were not treated because pentamidine was not available and all died [37]. Additional information became available through an early study to evaluate amphotericin B in this infection. Of 7 cases treated with this antifungal agent, or no drug, 6 died [9].

Pentamidine is administered intramuscularly in the dosage of 4.0 mg/kg/day for a period of 14 days. The drug is given as a single daily injection. The total dosage should not exceed 56 mg/kg. The drug can be administered intravenously in 5–10 ml of sterile distilled water and infused slowly over a period of 5–10 min. This route is not recommended since the adverse reactions are more severe from intravenous than intramuscular administration.

Table I. Summary of *P. carinii* pneumonitis treated with trimethoprim-sulfamethoxazole [modified from ref. 40]

Reference	Patients	Dose and route mg/kg/day			Clinical response		
		TMP	SMZ	route	TMP-SMZ only	pentamidine after TMP-SMZ	failure
14	20	4–7	20–35	oral	14/20	2/20	4/20
24	8	20	100	oral	5/8	0/8	3/8
26	3	20	100	oral	3/3	0/3	0/3
13	26	20	100	oral	17/26	4/26	5/26
23	5	20	100	oral	4/5	0/5	1/5
3	7	20	100	oral	4/7	2/7	1/7
40	11	10–15	50–75	i. v.	7/11	1/11	3/11
42	22	20	100	oral	17/22	5*/22	8/22

* TMP-SMZ plus pentamidine.

Pyrimethamine-Sulfadiazine

The drug combination pyrimethamine and sulfadiazine was found to be as effective as pentamidine in animals treated for *P. carinii* pneumonitis [8]. This therapy has only been evaluated in a small number of patients. Of the total of 9 patients reported from four studies [7, 21, 30, 31] 5 died, 2 recovered and 2 improved. In a small controlled study, 7 patients with proven *P. carinii* pneumonitis were randomized to receive either pentamidine or pyrimethamine-sulfadiazine [44]. Of the 3 cases treated with pentamidine, 2 recovered and 1 died. 3 of the 4 patients treated with pyrimethamine-sulfadiazine died and 1 recovered.

Trimethoprim-Sulfamethoxazole (table I)

Trimethoprim combined with a sulfonamide was developed for the treatment of bacterial infections and was used extensively before it was considered for the treatment of *P. carinii* infection. Sulfonamides competitively inhibit the incorporation of *p*-aminobenzoic acid into dihydrofolate. Trimethoprim inhibits the progression of microbial dihydrofolic acid to tetrahydrofolic acid; inhibition of this earlier step of purine synthesis eventually inhibits the production of deoxyribonucleic acid. The rationale for the potential efficacy of TMP-SMZ included the following.

Pyrimethamine, a pyrimidine similar to trimethoprim, had been effective in combination with sulfonamides in animal studies and limited studies in humans also indicated these drugs were effective in the treatment and prevention of *P. carinii* pneumonitis. The kinetics of TMP-SMZ permit concentrations of trimethoprim 1.5–3.5 times greater in human lung tissue than in serum. Also, pentamidine isethionate, known to be effective for the treatment of *P. carinii* pneumonitis, inhibits dihydrofolate reductase, as does trimethoprim.

The initial study in animals reported in 1974 [17] showed TMP-SMZ to be effective in both the treatment and prevention of *P. carinii* pneumonia. The cortisone-antibiotic-treated rat served as an excellent animal model to study the effects of these drugs on *P. carinii* pneumonitis. When pneumonitis had developed, TMP-SMZ reduced the mortality rate to 36 % while none of the animals receiving the drug prophylactically acquired the infection. In comparison all of the control animals died with *P. carinii* pneumonitis. The therapeutic effects were more favorable than with pentamidine. Since the drug had been used extensively and safely for the treatment of bacterial infections, clinical evaluation in humans seemed justified.

The first study of TMP-SMZ for the treatment of *P. carinii* pneumonitis in humans was reported in 1975 [14]. This pilot study included patients with mild and moderately severe cases of *P. carinii* pneumonitis who were treated orally with one of two dosage levels of TMP-SMZ. Of 14 children treated with 20 mg TMP and 100 mg SMP/kg/day, 12 recovered and 2 died. Supplemental pentamidine was required in 3 of these patients, 2 who subsequently died and 1 progressively severe case that recovered. 6 other patients were treated with a lower dosage of 4–7 mg of TMP and 20–35 mg SMZ/kg/day. 4 of these patients recovered and 2 died. Both fatal cases and 1 that recovered were also treated with pentamidine. There were no significant adverse effects from pentamidine. This study demonstrated the efficacy and safety of TMP-SMZ in the treatment of *P. carinii* pneumonitis and suggested that the higher dosage level was more effective than the lower one.

When TMP-SMZ was compared to pentamidine isethionate children with cancer and *P. carinii* pneumonitis were randomly assigned to treatment either with TMP-SMZ orally or pentamidine intramuscularly for a course of 14 days [13]. 50 patients were entered sequentially into the study regardless of the severity of the pneumonitis. The dosage was TMP, 20 mg/kg and SMZ, 100 mg/kg/day in four equally divided doses. Pentamidine was given in the single daily dosage of 4.0 mg/kg. All patients were treated with the initial drug regimen for at least 3 days. After this the drug was discontinued and the alternate drug begun if the following criteria were met indicating nonresponse: inability to maintain an arterial oxygen tension (PaO_2) of at least 70 mm Hg without increasing the fraction of inspired oxygen (FiO_2), life-threatening side effects from the drug, or, inability to take the drug. Of the 26 patients initially treated with TMP-SMZ, 20 recovered (77%) – 17 after TMP-SMZ alone and 3 of 9 who were crossed over to pentamidine. Of the 24 patients initially treated with pentamidine isethionate, 18 recovered (75%) 14 of 15 who received only pentamidine and 4 of 9 who were crossed over to TMP-SMZ. Injection site reactions, abnormal values for blood urea nitrogen, creatinine or glucose, or combinations of these occurred in 14 of the 15 patients who were treated with pentamidine alone. Only 1 of the 17 patients treated with TMP-SMZ alone developed any of these abnormalities. The serum levels of TMP and SMZ are summarized in figure 1. Since the serum values for both TMP and SMZ were relatively lower in the 1st day of treatment than those achieved later in course, it seems advisable to start therapy with a 'loading dose' equal to one-half, rather than one-fourth, of the calculated dose. This seems especially important in that the serum values for both TMP and SMZ were lower in the patients who failed to respond than in those who responded favorably.

When available it is desirable to measure serum levels of the drugs, especially in the early course of the infection. 2-hour postdosage serum levels of 3–5 μg/ml of TMP and 100–150 μg of SMZ appear to be appropriate ranges. The 2-week course with either drug seems adequate for most cases. Although both pentamidine and TMP-SMZ are equally effective, TMP-SMZ is preferred because of the lower prevalence of adverse effects.

The intravenous preparation of TMP-SMZ has been evaluated primarily in adults [40]. The drug was administered initially based on the dosage of 10–15 mg TMP and 50–75 mg of SMZ/kg/day intravenously in four equally divided doses. Subsequently the dose was modified to maintain 1½ h postdose serum levels of greater than 5 μg/ml. The intravenous preparation was made by adding a 5.0-ml ampule of 80 mg TMP and 400 mg SMZ to 75 ml of 5% dextrose and administered over a 60-min period. 11 consecutive patients were treated and 7 (64%) recovered. Adverse effects were minor with a skin rash in 1 patient and nausea and vomiting in another.

Although the adverse effects from TMP-SMZ have been few and insignificant in patients treated for *P. varinii* pneumonitis, one can expect at

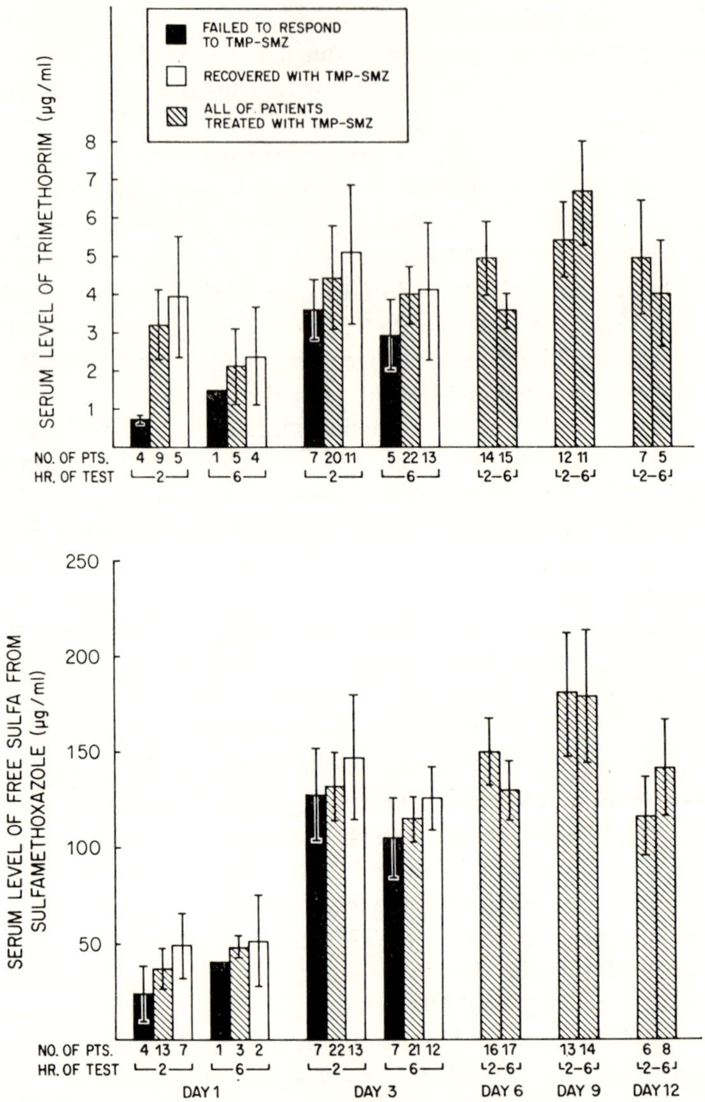

Fig. 1. Serum levels of trimethoprim (TMP) are shown in the top graph and sulfamethoxazole (SMZ) as free sulfa in the bottom graph. All values are reported as the mean ± 1 SE. Levels of drugs on days 1 and 3 are given for the patients who responded (open bars) and those who failed to respond (solid bars) to TMP-SMZ therapy. The shaded bars represent the values for all patients who had determinations of serum drug levels. Specimens of serum were not available for all patients in the study (courtesy *Hughes* et al. [13]).

least the known adverse effects for this drug combination from general use in other infections. The adverse and toxic effects are essentially those of sulfonamides and include: transient skin rashes, nausea, vomiting, diarrhea, allergic reactions, drug fever, toxic nephrosis, agranulocytosis, aplastic anemia, megaloblastic anemia, hemolytic anemia, methemoglobinemia, folic acid deficiency and the Stevens-Johnson syndrome. Except for rashes and gastrointestinal disturbances the other effects are rare.

Comparison of TMP-SMZ and pyrimethamine and sulfamonomethoxine has been done in animal studies. The mortality rate of rats with *P. carinii* pneumonitis treated with pyrimethamine and the sulfonamide was 57 % and with TMP-SMZ, 25 % [43]. Another animal study evaluated pentamidine, TMP-SMZ, trimethoprim, and the combination of pentamidine plus TMP-SMZ [22]. The mortality rates from *P. carinii* pneumonitis were 45 % for pentamidine, 28 % for TMP-SMZ, 93 % for trimethoprim, and 37 % with both pentamidine plus TMP-SMZ.

Supportive Management

P. carinii causes a severe pneumonitis with marked impairment of pulmonary function. Hypoxia with low arterial oxygen tension always occurs, carbon dioxide retention is rarely found and the arterial pH is usually increased. Oxygen should be administered as needed to maintain the PaO_2 above 70 mm Hg. Attempts must be made to keep the fraction of inspired oxygen (FiO_2) below 50 vol% to avoid oxygen toxicity. Assisted or controlled ventilation may be required when the PaO_2 cannot be maintained above 60 mm Hg at FiO_2 of 50 %. Secondary or concomitant bacterial infections should be sought out and treated with appropriate antibiotics. Immunosuppressive drugs should be withheld if the primary disease persists.

Chemoprophylaxis

In animal studies pentamidine has been proven to be ineffective when administered prophylactically in the prevention of *P. carinii* pneumonitis [15]. Furthermore, immunization with *P. carinii* cyst preparations, the administration of rifampin, clindamycin, or pyrimethamine-sulfadiazine were not effective in preventing the pneumonitis in the cortisone-treated rat model [15].

The drug combination sulfadoxine-pyrimethamine was evaluated in the Shiraz Orphanage where *P. carinii* interstitial plasma cell pneumonitis was endemic [29]. Beginning at 1 month of age all infants admitted to the orphanage received either a placebo or sulfadoxine-pyrimethamine in a double-blind investigation. 75 infants were enrolled in the study. 3 of the 42 infants on the placebo died with *P. carinii* organisms in the lungs and 4 developed complement-fixating antibodies suggestive of infection. None of the 33 infants on the drug combination died or had a complement-fixation response.

When TMP-SMZ was tested in the animal model the drug combination administered orally was totally effective in preventing the infection. All of the untreated control animals acquired *P. carinii* pneumonitis while none of those given TMP-SMZ had any evidence of the infection [17]. Since the drug had been used extensively with safety on a long-term basis for the prevention of urinary tract infections and chronic bronchitis, the feasibility of similar prophylaxis for immunocompromised patients at high risk for *P. carinii* pneumonitis seemed warranted.

Children with malignancies receiving intensive immunosuppressive therapy and at unusually high risk for *P. carinii* pneumonitis were selected for a randomized, double-blind, placebo-controlled study [16]. 160 children were randomized to receive either a placebo or TMP-SMZ (150–750 mg/m^2 day) for as long as 2 years. Of the 80 patients receiving the placebo, 17 acquired *P. carinii* pneumonitis, while none of the 80 children receiving TMP-SMZ had the infection ($p = < 0.01$).

When the placebo group was compared to the TMP-SMZ group no significant differences were observed for the findings by physical examination, symptoms, blood counts, mean corpuscular values, platelet estimates done weekly and bone marrow examinations, serum folic acid values, urinalysis, blood urea nitrogen, SGOT, alkaline phosphatase, total protein, albumin, globulin and immunoglobulin G, A and M levels determined at 3-month intervals. Oral candidiasis was the only adverse effect noted from TMP-SMZ prophylaxis.

In 1980 another study of TMP-SMZ prophylaxis was reported [10]. This study also demonstrated efficacy of the prophylaxis in pediatric cancer patients. Skin rashes, neutropenia and gastrointestinal complaints were encountered in some patients but the incidence and magnitude of these side effects were considered to be less than the benefits.

It seems clear that TMP-SMZ prophylaxis is effective only while the patient receives the drug. In animal studies rats pretreated with TMP-SMZ for 6 weeks then placed in germ-free isolators and then immunosuppressed with cortisone subsequently died with *P. carinii* pneumonitis proving that TMP-SMZ did not eradicate the organism [11]. Furthermore, when cancer patients were given TMP-SMZ prophylaxis for only 2 weeks during the early course of anticancer therapy, *P. carinii* pneumonitis was not prevented but only the onset was delayed in comparison to those who did not receive the prophylaxis [41].

Thus, TPM, 5 mg and SMZ, 25 mg/kg/day in two divided doses given orally 12 h apart is effective in the prevention of *P. carinii* pneumonitis. Oral nystatin is suggested as an adjuvant to prevent oral candidiasis.

While TMP-SMZ has been demonstrated to be effective when administered prophylactically the group of patients requiring such management usually are receiving regimens of other drugs, irradiation, of both. Furthermore, physicians, patients and their parents may be preoccupied with the life-threatening primary disease. Under these circumstances, will the antibiotic prophylaxis be utilized when only a relatively small portion of the population at risk will actually acquire the pneumonitis? The studies proving successful prophylaxis for *P. carinii* pneumonitis were carried out under controlled conditions with close monitoring for compliance. Can similar compliance be expected under general management conditions over the necessarily long periods of time? A 3-year study designed to answer this question was recently completed at St. Jude Children's Research Hospital [39]. Annual institutional attack rates for *P. carinii* pneumonitis were calculated for all patients with malignancies over a 6-year period. Thus, information was made available to the attending physicians on the expected incidence for *P. carinii* pneumonitis for their patients. Without further guidelines each physician made the decision as to whether his patient would receive TMP-SMZ. Compliance was left to individual patient-physician relationships. The measure of success was based on the number of cases of *P. carinii* that occurred subsequently at this institution. Over the 3-year period TMP-SMZ was administered prophylactically to 786 patients. These had been selected out of a total group of about 1,000 patients/year at risk. During this time, 9 cases of *P. carinii* pneumonitis occurred, with none attributable to drug failure. All cases occurred in patients who either had not had the drug prescribed, were taking an inadequate dose or had had the drug discontinued prior to the onset of the pneumonia. Although the data are applicable to only one institution, the method for establishing the population at risk as an aid to the selection of patients who would be reasonable candidates for this prophylaxis could be adapted for other institutions.

Future Needs and Prospects

The mode of transmission and natural habitat of *P. carinii* are not known. Since *P. carinii* pneumonitis can be provoked with cortisone immunosuppression in nearly 100% of animals obtained from various suppliers, the organisms must be highly prevalent in the environment. When these aspects can be elucidated efforts can be directed to elimination and avoidance of the organism.

Although effective drugs are available the mortality rate remains at about 25% with treatment. A more effective drug is desirable. Especially intriguing is the high prevalence of serum antibody to *P. carinii* in otherwise healthy children. Clinical manifestations, if any, associated with infection in normal individuals need to be identified.

The definite diagnosis requires an invasive procedure which is associated with potential adverse effects to the patient. A more simple, noninvasive diagnostic test is urgently needed. Hopefully, methods for the identification and quantitation of circulating antigen can be developed and standardized. The antigen can be detected in serum of patients with *P. carinii* pneumonitis using counterimmunoelectrophoresis in gel. However, the antigen is also found in some immunosuppressed patients without any evidence of pneumonitis [28].

References

1 Carini, A.: Formas de eschizogonia do *Trypanosoma lewisi*. Comm. Soc. Med. Sao Paulo, 1910, p. 204.

2 Chagas, C.: Nova trypanomiazazia humana. Mem. Inst. Oswaldo Cruz *1:* 159–218 (1907).

3 Chusid, M. J.; Heyrman, K. A.: An outbreak of *Pneumocystis carinii* pneumonia at a pediatric hospital. Pediatrics *62:* 1031–1035 (1978).

4 Delanoe, P.; Delanoe, M.: De la rareté de *Pneumocystis carinii* chez les cobayes de la région de Paris; absence de kysts chez d'autres animaux, lapin, grenouille, trois anguilles. Bull. Soc. Path. exot. *7:* 271–275 (1914).

5 Delanoe, P.; Delanoe, M.: Sur les rapports des kysts de carinii du poumon des rats avec le *Trypanosoma lewisi*. C. r. hebd. Séanc. Acad. Sci., Paris *155:* 658–660 (1912).

6 Dutz, W.; Post, C.; Kohout, E., et al.: Cellular reaction to *Pneumocystis carinii.* Z. Kinderheilk. *140:* 1–11 (1973).

7 Farinas, E.; Quel, J. H.: Hypertension and duodenal ulcer associated with *Pneumocystis carinii* pneumonitis and dysgammaglobulinemia. Illinois med. J. *139:* 138–142 (1971).

8 Frenkel, J. K.; Good, J. T.; Schultz, J. A.: Latent pneumocystis infection in rats, relapse and chemotherapy. Lab. Invest. *15:* 1559–1577 (1966).

9 Geelhoed, G. W.; Levin, B. J.; Adkins, P. C., et al.: The diagnosis and management of *Pneumocystis carinii* pneumonia. Ann. thor. Surg. *14:* 335–346 (1972).

10 Harris, R. E.; McCallister, J. A.; Allen, S. A.: Prevention of *Pneumocystis carinii* pneumonia. Am. J. Dis. Child. *134:* 35–38 (1980).

11 Hughes, W. T.: Limited effect of trimethoprim-sulfamethoxazole prophylaxis on *Pneumocystis carinii.* Antimicrob. Agents Chemother. *16:* 333–335 (1979).

12 Hughes, W. T.; Feldman, S.; Aur, R. J. A., et al.: Intensity of immunosuppressive therapy and the incidence of *Pneumocystis carinii* pneumonitis. Cancer *36:* 2004–2009 (1975).

13 Hughes, W. T.; Feldman, S.; Chaudhary, S. C., et al.: Comparison of pentamidine isethionate and trimethoprim-sulfamethoxazole in the treatment of *Pneumocystis carinii* pneumonia. J. Pediat. *92:* 285–291 (1978).

14 Hughes, W. T.; Feldman, S.; Sanyal, S. K.: Treatment of *Pneumocystis carinii* pneumonitis with trimethoprim-sulfamethoxazole. Can. med. Ass. J. *112:* 47–50 (1975).

15 Hughes, W. T.; Kim, H. K.; Price, R. A., et al.: Attempts at prophylaxis for murine *Pneumocystis carinii* pneumonitis. Curr. ther. Res. *15:* 581–587 (1973).

16 Hughes, W. T.; Kuhn, S.; Chaudhary, S., et al.: Successful chemoprophylaxis for *Pneumocystis carinii* pneumonitis. New Engl. J. Med. *297:* 1419–1426 (1977).

17 Hughes, W. T.; McNabb, P. C.; Makres, T. D., et al.: Efficacy of trimethoprim and sulfamethoxazole in the prevention and treatment of *Pneumocystis carinii* pneumonitis. Antimicrob. Agents Chemother. *5:* 289–293 (1974).

18 Hughes, W. T.; Price, R.; Kim, H. K., et al.: *Pneumocystis carinii* pneumonitis in children with malignancies. J. Pediat. *82:* 404–415 (1973).

19 Ivady, G.; Paldy, L.: Ein neues Behandlungsverfahren der interstitiellen plasmazelligen Pneumonie Frühgeborener mit fünfwertigem Stibium und aromatischen Diamidinen. Mschr. Kinderheilk. *106:* 10–14 (1958).

20 Ivady, G.; Paldy, L.; Koltay, M., et al.: *Pneumocystis carinii* pneumonia. Lancet *i:* 616–617 (1967).

21 Kirby, H. B.; Kenamore, B.; Guckian, J. C.: *Pneumocystis carinii* pneumonia treated with pyrimethamine and sulfadiazine. Ann. intern. Med. *75:* 505–509 (1971).

22 Kluge, R. M.; Spaulding, D. M.; Spain, A. J.: Combination of pentamidine and trimethoprim-sulfamethoxazole in therapy of *Pneumocystis carinii* in rats. Antimicrob. Agents Chemother. *13:* 975–978 (1978).

23 Larter, W. E.; John, T. J.; Sieber, O. F., et al.: Trimethoprim-sulfamethoxazole treatment of *Pneumocystis carinii* pneumonitis. J. Pediat. *92:* 826–828 (1978).

24 Lau, W. K.; Young, L. S.: Trimethoprim-sulfamethoxazole treatment of *Pneumocystis carinii* pneumonia in adults. New Engl. J. Med. *295:* 716–718 (1976).

25 LeClair, R. A.: Descriptive epidemiology of interstitial pneumocystic pneu-

monia: an analysis of 107 cases from the United States. Annu. Rev. resp. Dis. *99:* 542–547 (1969).

26 Lipson, A.; Marshall, W. C.; Hayward, A. R.: Treatment of *Pneumocystis carinii* pneumonia in children. Archs Dis. Childh. *52:* 314–319 (1977).

27 Meuwissen, J. H. E. T.; Tauber, I.; Leeuwenberg, A. D. E. M., et al.: Parasitology and serologic observations of infection with *Pneumocystis* in humans. J. infect. Dis. *136:* 43–49 (1977).

28 Pifer, L. L.; Hughes, W. T.; Stagno, S., et al.: *Pneumocystis carinii* infection: evidence for high prevalence in normal and immunosuppressed children. Pediatrics *61:* 35–41 (1978).

29 Post, C.; Fakouhi, T.; Dutz, W., et al.: Prophylaxis of endemic infantile pneumocystosis with a 20:1 sulfadioxine plus pyrimethamine combination. Curr. ther. Res. *13:* 273–279 (1971).

30 Rifkind, D.; Faris, T. D.; Hill, R. B., Jr.: *Pneumocystis carinii* pneumonia. Studies on the diagnosis and treatment. Ann. intern. Med. *65:* 943–956 (1966).

31 Ruskin, J.; Remington, J. S.: The compromised host and infection. I. *Pneumocystis carinii* pneumonia. J. Am. med. Ass. *202:* 1070–1074 (1967).

32 Toth, G.; Balogh, E.; Belay, M.: Demonstration in tracheal secretion of the causative agent in interstitial plasma-cell pneumonia. Acta Paediat. Acad. Sci. hung. *7:* 25–30 (1966).

33 Van der Meer, G.; Brug, S. L.: Infection par Pneumocystis chez l'homme et chez les animaux. Annls Soc. belge Méd. trop. *22:* 301–307 (1942).

34 Varrek, J.: Atypical (interstitialni) pneumonie deti, vyvolaná *Pneumocystis carinii.* Cas. Lék. česk. *90:* 1121–1124 (1951).

35 Vanek, J.; Jirovec. O.: Parasitäre Pneumoniae. 'Interstitielle' Plasmazellen-Pneumonie der Frühgeborenen, verursacht durch *Pneumocystis carinii.* Zentbl. Bakt. *158:* 120–127 (1952).

36 Waalkes, T. P.; Makulu, D. R.: Pharmacologic aspects of pentamidine. Natn. Cancer Inst. Monogr. *43:* 171–176 (1976).

37 Walzer, P. D.; Perl, D. P.; Krogstad, D. J.: *Pneumocystis carinii* pneumonia in the United States. Ann. intern. Med. *80:* 83–93 (1974).

38 Western, K. A.; Perea, D. R.; Schultz, M. G.: Pentamidine isethionate in the treatment of *P. carinii* pneumonia. Ann. intern. Med. *73:* 695–702 (1970).

39 Wilber, R. B.; Feldman, S.; Malone, W. J., et al.: Chemoprophylaxis for *Pneumocystis carinii:* outcome of unstructured delivery. Am. J. Dis. Child. *134:* 643–648 (1980).

40 Winston, D. J.; Lau, W. K.; Gale, R. P., et al.: Trimethoprim-sulfamethoxazole for the treatment of *Pneumocystis carinii* pneumonia. Ann. intern. Med. *92:* 762–769 (1980).

41 Wolff, L. J.; Baehner, R. L.: Delayed development of *Pneumocystis carinii* pneumonia following administration of short-term high dose trimethoprim-sulfamethoxazole. Am. J. Dis. Child. *132:* 525–526 (1978).

42 Yoshida, Y.; Ikai, T.; Takeuchi, S.: Studies on *Pneumocystis carinii* and *Pneumocystis carinii* pneumonia. VII. Chemotherapy of 42 clinical cases. Jap. J. Parasit. *28:* 455–464 (1979).

43 Yoshida, Y.; Takeuchi, S.; Ogino, K., et al.: Studies on *Pneumocystis carinii* and *Pneumocystis carinii* pneumonia. III. Pyrimethamine plus sulfamonometh-

oxine and trimethoprim plus sulfamethoxazole. Jap. J. Parasit. *26:* 367–375 (1977).

44 Young, R. C.; DeVita, V. T.: Treatment of *Pneumocystis carinii* pneumonia: current status of the regimens of pentamidine isethionate and pyrimethamine-sulfadiazine. Symp. *Pneumocystis carinii* infection. Natn. Cancer Inst. Monogr. *43:* 193–200 (1976).

W. T. Hughes, MD, The Johns Hopkins University School of Medicine,
Baltimore, MD 21205 (USA)

Antibiotics Chemother., vol. 30, pp. 272–287 (Karger, Basel 1981)

African Trypanosomes

David A. Evans

Department of Medical Protozoology,
London School of Hygiene and Tropical Medicine, London, England

Introduction

The Parasites and Their Vectors

The organisms that cause African trypanosomiasis (sleeping sickness in man) are protozoa belonging to the genus *Trypanosoma* (subgenus *Trypanozoon*). It is usually considered that human sleeping sickness is caused by two species of trypanosome, *Trypanosoma gambiense* and *Trypanosoma rhodesiense,* the former causing the chronic West African form of the disease and the latter the acute East African form. These two trypanosome 'species' are, however, identical in morphological and many other respects, and many authorities consider them as either subspecies or even nosodemes (clinical races) of their presumed ancestral species *Trypanosoma brucei.* Thus, if we consider them as subspecies we have *T. brucei brucei* which is not infective to man, and the two man infective trypanosomes *T. b. gambiense* and *T. b. rhodesiense.*

The sleeping sickness trypanosomes are transmitted cyclically by dipteran flies of the genus *Glossina* (tsetse flies), and on rare occasions non-cyclically by a variety of biting flies. The life cycle of the trypanosomes in the tsetse fly is somewhat complex; trypanosomes imbibed by a tsetse fly feeding on an infected host undergo a series of complex morphological and biochemical changes in the gut of the fly. The initial development of the fly gut trypanosomes takes place in the midgut where they loose their mammalian infectivity and undergo extensive multiplication. The trypanosomes eventually invade the salivary glands of the fly where they undergo further transformations and regain their infectivity for mammals. The infective trypanosomes found in the salivary glands of the fly are known as metacyclic forms, and it is these that are responsible for the transmission of the infection when they are injected into a fresh mammalian host during the feeding process of the tsetse fly.

Historical

Human sleeping sickness has been known in West Africa for many centuries. It was more than 600 years ago when what is considered as the first recognisable description of the disease was recorded; this is in the writings of the fourteenth century Arab historian Al-Qaiqashandi who described the death of *Mari Djata,* Sultan of the Mandino people in 1373–4 from a lethargic disease, the symptoms of which are very like those of West African sleeping sickness [19, 24, 29].

It was not until 1902 that trypanosomes were first recognised as agents of human disease, when *Forde* demonstrated organisms (later recognised as trypanosomes by *Dutton*) in the blood of the captain of a steamboat which plied the River Gambia. These organisms were not immediately associated with sleeping sickness, but were thought to be responsible for *Trypanosoma* fever, a mild disease occurring both in the indigenous and European populations of tropical West Africa. The organisms were described and named *Trypanosoma gambiense* by *Dutton* [10]; sleeping sickness was thought at that time to be caused by a different organism, possibly a filarial worm. In 1903, *Castellani* [6] reported the finding of trypanosomes in the cerebrospinal fluid of 70 % of his sleeping sickness patients, and in the same year Colonel *David Bruce,* head of the Royal Society's Commission sent to Uganda to investigate a major sleeping sickness outbreak, and his colleagues confirmed that *T. b. gambiense* was the causative agent of the disease and that the tsetse fly *Glossina palpalis* was the vector.

It is generally accepted that the ancient foci of sleeping sickness were largely confined to the western coastal areas of tropical Africa, and that the rapid spread of the disease eastwards was due to the 'opening-up' of the country by European explorers and their porters travelling inland from the west and introducing human trypanosomiasis to new and completely susceptible populations. *Duggan* [9] describes in some detail the spread of West African sleeping sickness from an ancient focus extending some 100 miles inland on the banks of the Congo river. In 1885 the Congo Free State came into existance and soon after, steamers were brought into use on the river and many people including soldiers and labourers were transported to the upper regions of the river. About 10 years after these movements had begun, sleeping sickness was spreading into areas where it had been unknown, and by 1905 the endemic area at the mouth of the Congo river had expanded and the disease had reached the shores of Lake Tanganyika. It was estimated that some half a million people died of sleeping sickness in that area of Africa between 1896 and 1906.

Meanwhile a much more acute form of the disease was being encountered on the eastern side of the continent. An Englishman named *William Armstrong* developed this acute form of the disease in 1908 while travelling through the Luangwa Valley of the Zambesi river system; he was dead within 6 months. *Armstrong*'s companion *Beith* died of a similar infection soon afterwards. The trypanosome responsible for this acute form of the disease is considered by most authorities to be a separate subspecies – *T. b. rhodesiense* and to have evolved from the animal trypanosome *T. b. brucei;* others [32] have suggested that *T. b. rhodesiense* evolved from *T. b. gambiense* when the latter was introduced into the savannah area of south-east Africa. Origins aside, the acute Rhodesian (should we call it Zimbabwian now?) type disease became well established and spread northwestward reaching Tanzania in about 1910, southern Kenya in 1930 and the northern shore of Lake Victoria in about 1940 where an epidemic broke out in roughly the same area as the epidemic caused by *T. b. gambiense* half a century before [3]. Since then, the northern spread has continued into the southern areas of the Sudan and Ethiopia.

Epidemiology

Human trypanosomiasis in Africa occurs exclusively in the region bounded by the two tropics, and within this region to areas where the annual rainfall exceeds 500 mm [3]. The disease is not transmitted in the more arid areas of tropical Africa as the pupae of the tsetse fly vectors of the disease (*Glossina* spp.) are particularly susceptible to dessication.

As mentioned in the historical introduction, two distinct forms of human trypanosomiasis occur in Africa; on one hand we have the chronic Gambian type disease caused by *T. b. gambiense* which occurs mainly but not exclusively in the western part of the continent – it has occurred as far east as the northern shores of Lake Victoria. On the other hand we have the acute Rhodesian form of the disease caused by *T. b. rhodesiense* which is found in the east from the northern borders of South Africa northwards into Ethiopia. This is of course a gross over simplification and types of disease which fit neither the chronic nor acute categories exist. The epidemiology of trypanosomiasis in Africa is a vaste and complicated subject involving complex interactions between man, the parasite, the vector, mammalian hosts other than man, and of course the geophysical nature of the area where they coexist. To simplify the picture somewhat, I will confine myself to the two extremes of the disease condition (i) the chronic Gambian disease, and (ii) the acute Rhodesian disease.

The Gambian Disease. This form of human trypanosomiasis is characterised by a slow onset with low morbidity, only in the late stages of the disease do the classical sleeping symptoms appear, and 4 or more years may elapse between initial infection and death. At no time during the infection are large numbers of trypanosomes found; the level of parasitaemia found in the blood of an infected person is often as low or lower than 50 trypanosomes/ml of blood, indeed the concentration of trypanosomes is often higher in lymph and other tissue fluids than it is in blood. These low concentrations of trypanosomes in the blood cut down the likelihood of a tsetse fly taking a blood meal (tsetses feed exclusively on blood) containing sufficient trypanosomes to establish an infection. This taken in combination with the fact that only a very small percentage of tsetse flies will develop infections within their salivary glands capable of transmitting the infection (roughly 10% under laboratory conditions very much less in the wild), leads to the situation that only a very few flies will become infected. The fact that the disease exists at all may seem surprising, let alone that enormous epidemics arise from time to time. The explanations for the continuation of the disease must lie in the length of time an infected person remains active in the community as a mobile reservoir for the fly to feed upon – the longer an infected person is in circulation, the greater the chance the fly has of acquiring an infection from him.

The most important species of *Glossina* which transmit *T. b. gambiense* to man are the 'riverine' species belonging to the *palpalis* group – *G. palpalis, G. fuscipes* and *G. tachinoides*. These species, as their collective name implies, are found close to water, and it is in places close to water where people congregate, i. e. ferry crossings, fords, washing or watering places that are the classic sites for the acquisition of *T. b. gambiense* infections.

We come now to the vexed question as to whether or not there is an animal reservoir playing a part in the epidemiology of Gambian sleeping sickness. Certainly animals other than man can become infected with *T. b. gambiense,* usually though, the parasitaemias achieved in non-humans are even lower than those in man, and are often very short-lived, thus reducing the chances of tsetse infection from such a source even more. If animals were to be an important reservoir of infection then there would have to be close man-fly-animal contact, so we can exclude most of the wild ungulates from the reservoir role because of low levels of infection and lack of close man-fly-wild ungulate contact. Peridomestic animals such as cats, dogs, pigs and chickens could conceivably be implicated if they were susceptible to infection with *T. b. gambiense*. Pigs and dogs have recently been attracting increasing attention as possible reservoirs of Gambian sleeping sickness; they are found living close to man, *T. b. gambiense* has been isolated from domestic pigs in West Africa, and flies of the *palpalis* group like to feed on pigs. There is also at least one report of *T. b. gambiense* infections in chickens [33]. To be an important reservoir of the disease more than the odd individual needs to be infected, and the course of the infection should be long-running, and from the evidence collected so far, man is by far the most important reservoir of Gambian sleeping sickness.

The Rhodesian Disease. The epidemiology of Rhodesian sleeping sickness caused by *T. b. rhodesiense* is very different from that of the Gambian disease. The East African disease is essentially an acute disease with a rapid onset, high morbidity and almost 100% mortality in untreated cases. There are often high numbers of trypanosomes circulating in the bloodstream. Many wild mammals can support high parasitaemias of *T. b. rhodesiense* without apparent ill-effect. The main vectors of the Rhodesian type sleeping sickness are *Glossina* spp. of the *morsitans* group; these tsetse inhabit drier areas than the riverine *palpalis* group, and are to be found in the savannah country which extends from the forest edge to the desert or the sea. The three most important species as far as human disease is concerned are: *G. morsitans, G. pallidipes* and *G. longipalpis*. Rhodesian sleeping sickness is usually acquired by man when he enters areas where natural transmission of the infection between game animals and tsetse is occurring, so man, who is highly susceptible, enters the transmission cycle and becomes infected. Rhodesian sleeping sickness is therefore a zoonosis and can be thought of as an occupational disease, as except under epidemic conditions, man does not usually become infected in his peridomestic environment. Infections are acquired when man goes into the bush on activities such as hunting or honey gathering, just as the modern tourist gets his infection when he goes hunting with his camera in a wild life park. Man to man transmission is thought to be rare, as the disease is so debilitating that the individual is soon out of circulation and not in a situation where he is likely to be bitten by a tsetse fly. Under epidemic conditions man to man transmission certainly can occur and on occasions riverine tsetse such as *G. fuscipes* have been implicated in the transmission of the Rhodesian type disease.

Prevalence

African trypanosomiasis in humans remains important enough to warrant its inclusion as one of the major parasitic diseases in the UNDP/World Bank/WHO Special Programme for Research and Training in Tropical Diseases. The true prevalence of the disease today is very difficult to assess, as areas where it is thought to be on the increase are places of unrest such as Uganda, Southern Sudan, Ethiopia and Zambia, where it is reported that epidemics are occurring, but from where it is difficult to gather accurate statistics. Certainly the devastating epidemics of the early part of this century where up to one-third of the population of an area would die as a result of trypanosomiasis seem to be a thing of the past. Better medical care and tsetse control measures have certainly contributed to the control of the disease, but when medical and entomological control measures are abandoned, as in times of political termoil, the incidence of human infection rises. A good illustration of this is the situation that happened in Zaire. In 1972 Zaire had the highest sleeping sickness incidence in Africa. This high incidence followed a breakdown in the sleeping sickness control organisation during and after the disturbances of the civil war; the same is thought to be happening in Uganda today. World Health Organization statistics for 1978 show that human sleeping sickness was present in Angola, Benin, Chad, Congo, Gabon, Gambia, Guinea-Bissau, Mali, Mosambique, Uganda, United Republic of Cameroon, Upper Volta; and to this list one should almost certainly add Botswana, Ethiopia, Ivory Coast, Kenya, Sudan, Tanzania and Zambia.

Pathology

For detailed treatment of the pathology and pathogenesis of African trypanosomiasis in man see: *Mott* [27], *Van Bogaert* [31], *Ormerod* [28], *Connor* et al. [8] and *Boreham* [4].

Most of the known pathology of human sleeping sickness is based upon post-mortem appearance, and the central nervous system has received most of the attention. In patients that have died from African sleeping sickness the outward appearance of the brain may be normal, but in those with long-standing disease there can be obvious flattening of the surface convolutions due to dilation of the ventricles following atrophy of the subcortical white matter. The meninges are often thickened, and perivascular sheathing, hyperaemia and occasional ecchymoses are seen. Under the microscope the leptomeninges appear thickened and there is an infiltration of lymphocytes, plasma cells and histiocytes. The infiltrate involves the Virchow-Robin spaces and, sometimes, the vessel walls. Morula cells of Mott are seen in some cases (mainly Gambian-type disease); these cells are modified plasma cells up to 20 μm in diameter, they have the appearance of a raspberry, and are thought to secrete IgM. Trypanosomes are only very occasionally seen in tissue sections stained with haematoxylin and eosin, Giemsa staining will usually reveal some, but they are never easily recognised.

On examination of the CSF in advanced cases of trypanosomiasis the pressure is often raised as is the cell count. The cells that are seen are mainly lymphocytes and monocytes, with occasional morula cells (Gambian disease); cell counts of 15–500/mm^3 or more are achieved, and Giemsa staining often reveals the presence of trypanosomes. The CSF total proteins are very much increased and values of around 1 g/l (normal 0.2 g) are not uncommon; very high levels of IgM are also encountered.

The blood picture varies with the stage the disease has reached and also between the Rhodesian and Gambian forms, but in general, one finds hypoglycaemia, increased erythrocyte fragility, raised erythrocyte sedimentation rates, increase in serum potassium, microcytic anaemia, erythroblastic reaction in the bone marrow, increased numbers of lymphocytes, a fall in red cell count and haemoglobin due to increased cell breakdown, decreased serum albumin and increased serum globulin (the level of IgM reached is higher than with any other protozoal infection). Trypanosomes are usually present, but not necessarily in large numbers.

Lymphocytic tissue shows a general hyperplasia. The glands are soft and enlarged, and there is a great proliferation of lymphocytes. At first there is an increase in large mononuclear cells, lymphocytes and later fibroblasts. The glands are very vascular, and often early in the infection contain much higher concentrations of trypanosomes (Gambian especially) than the blood.

T. b. rhodesiense and less frequently *T. b. gambiense* may cause cardiac involvement with dilation, hypertrophy and pericarditis with effusion.

Endocardial thickening may also occur. Microscopical examination reveals infiltration of the endocardium, myocardium and epicardium by lymphocytes, plasma cells and histiocytes. The myocardium is oedematous, and there are lymphocytes and plasma cells in the interstices. Interstial fibrosis may follow. Pleural and pericardial effusions may contain trypanosomes, lymphocytes and mesothelial cells. The spleen may be enlarged and contain foci of histiocytic hyperplasia. Lymph nodes are enlarged and microscopically they have prominent germinal centres and occasional Russel bodies in the interstices.

Laboratory in vitro and in vivo Infections Models

In vitro

It is only within the last 3 years that is has been possible to cultivate the mammalian forms of *T. brucei* group trypanosomes in vitro. *Hirumi* et al. [18] were the first to achieve this; the secret of their method lying in the use of a feeder layer of bovine fibroblast-like cells, which presumbly help both with the nutrition of the trypanosomes and with the further metabolism of end products of trypanosome metabolism. The method involves daily changing of the rich culture medium (Hepes-buffered RPMI 1640 supplemented with 20% v/v fetal calf serum), and very careful adjustment of the ratio of trypanosome to fibroblast numbers. A highly successful modification of *Hirumi*'s original method has been pioneered in Switzerland [5]; this method again uses feeder cells (this time rabbit fibroblasts) but the medium in this case is based on MEM tissue culture medium again with Hepes but this time supplemented with extra glucose and pyruvate, non-essential amino acids and rabbit serum. The method works so well that bloodstream trypanosomes can be cloned, and also metacyclic forms taken from infected tsetse flies will develop into populations of infective 'bloodstream' forms. As far as I am aware no work has been published on the use of either of these culture systems in the assessment of chemotherapeutic agents.

Before the above methods were pioneered, the only trypanosome forms to survive and multiply in in vitro culture were the procyclic forms, forms equivalent to those which develop in the gut of the tsetse fly vector. These forms have a metabolism so different from the trypanosomes found in the mammalian host that their use as in vitro models of mammalian trypanosomiasis is highly questionable.

In vivo Models

The most widely used animal models are laboratory rodents (rats and mice). These animals are useful when one is dealing with *T. b. brucei* and *T. b. rhodesiense* infections, but both are fairly refractory to infection with *T. b. gambiense,* especially with freshly isolated stocks. With *T. b. gambiense* a variety of methods have been used in efforts to raise detectable parasitaemias in rats and mice; these include immunosuppression (chemical and physical) and the use of nursling animals. The Gambian pouched rat *(Cricetomys gambianus)* is supposedly more susceptible to *T. b. gambiense* infection, but the model is by no means well established, and very few of these animals have been imported into Europe.

The chief disadvantage of the rodent model for *T. b. rhodesiense* infections is that the animals often die from overwhelming bloodstream parasitaemias, usually before any central nervous system involvement is apparent. By careful choice of trypanosome stocks it is possible to find those which will cause chronic infections in laboratory rodents, and infection with such stocks will usually result in central nervous system involvement.

When using rodent models of African trypanosomiasis for the screening of potential trypanocides, it is of paramount importance to know what stage of infection the experimental animals have reached at the time one instigates treatment with the compound under test. Many compounds which are cureative in the very early stages of the infection often fail to cure when the infection is well established [14, 15, 21]. In most of the cases so far investigated this has been found to be due to the fact that as the infection progresses, the trypanosomes become established in extravascular sites, most importantly the brain, where effective concentrations of the potential drug are not reached; this has been shown to be the case for diminazine aceturate (Berenil), homidium bromide (Ethidium), pyrithidium bromide (Prothidium) and salicylhydroxamic acid/glycerol combination [14, 21].

Current Chemotherapy and Chemoprophylaxis

Suramin (Suraminum Natricum; Germanin; Bayer 205; Fourneau 309; Naganinum; Naganol)

The symmetrical 3″-urea of the sodium salt of 8-(3-benzamido-4-methylbenzamido)naphthalene-1,3,5-trisulphonic acid: $C_{51}H_{34}N_6O_{23}S_6$. Suramin is a dye-related compound brought into general use in the 1920s and remains the drug of choice in the early stages of sleeping sickness, especially when the infections are due to *T. b. rhodesiense* and before there is central nervous system involvement.

The mechanism of action of suramin is unknown, but the drug is known to inhibit numerous enzyme systems at low concentrations; among these is the glycerol-3-phosphate dehydrogenase system of *T. brucei* group trypanosomes [17]. Suramin forms firm complexes with proteins, and following intravenous administration the plasma concentration is high, but this falls rapidly in the first few hours, then more slowly for a few days, after which a low concentration is maintained for as long as 3 months. If trypanosomes are exposed to suramin in vitro and then washed, they loose their infectivity for animals, but remain active for over 24 h.

Suramin can cause severe side reactions in patients, especially in those who are malnourished; nausea, vomiting, shock and loss of conciousness are the most common reactions. The drug should be avoided in patients with kidney disease or adrenal insufficiency.

The drug is administered by intravenous injection; the usual adult dose is 5 g, given as an initial dose of 200 mg to test for tolerance to the drug, then 1 g after 24–48 h; the dose is repeated weekly until a total of 5 g have been administered. Suramin has been used prophylactically.

Pentamidine Isethionate (M & B 800; Lomidine)

This is the dimethanesulphonate salt of 1,5-bis(*p*-amidinophenoxy)-pentane-di-(2-hydroxyethane sulphonate): $C_{19}H_{24}N_4O_2$, $2C_2H_6O_4S$. As with suramin this drug is useful in the early stages of infection especially in cases caused by *T. b. gambiense.* It has a marked prophylactic activity, but again the mode of action is unknown. It is not of use once there is central nervous involvement. The usual prophylactic dose is 300 mg given intramuscularly every 3–6 months. Early trypanosome infections are treated with 150–300 mg i. m. daily for 7–15 days.

Pentamidine is absorbed fairly well from intramuscular injection sites, it is deposited in the tissues and only a small amount is detectable in the blood after a single injection. Experimental animals store the drug in the liver and kidney for months [23].

Diminazine Aceturate (Berenil)

p,p'-Diamidinodiazoaminobenzene diaceturate tetrahydrate: $C_{22}H_{29}N_9O_6$, $4H_2O$. This compound is in regular field use for cattle trypanosomiasis, and there are some reports of its successful use in the early stages of human sleeping sickness [20, 30]. In early human trials 3 doses of 5 mg kg^{-1} body weight at 2-day intervals were well tolerated; some relapse infections did, however, occur.

Melarsoprol (Melarsen Oxide-BAL; Mel B; RP 3845; Arsobal)

2-[*p*-(4,6-Diamino-1,3,5-triazin-2-ylamino)-phenyl]-4-hydroxymethyl-1,3,2-dithiarsolan: $C_{12}H_{15}AsN_6OS_2$. Melarsoprol is still the drug of choice in the meningoencephalitic stages of Gambian and Rhodesian sleeping sickness. Its precise mode of action remains unknown, but it probably works by interacting with SH groups essential for trypanosome metabolism. Certainly, melarsoprol has a profound inhibitory effect on one of the key glycolytic enzymes, pyruvate kinase; trypanosomal pyruvate kinase being more sensitive to the action of the drug than the corresponding mammalian enzyme [16].

The drug is administered by intravenous injection and the usual adult dose is 3.6 mg kg^{-1} body weight daily for 3 days. Children 1.8 mg kg^{-1} body weight daily for 3 days. The 3-day course is repeated after an interval of 10 days.

Side effects of melarsoprol can be severe range from an acute Herxheimer-type reaction due to the lytic action of the drug upon trypanosomes, to reactive encephalitis as a reaction to the arsenic moiety of the drug.

Melarsonyl Potassium (Melarsenoxide Potassium Dimercapto-succinate; Mel W; Pentylthiarsphenylmelamine; RP 9955)

Dipotassium 2-[*p*-(4,6-diamino-1,3,5-triazin-2-ylamino)-phenyl]1,3,2-dithiarsolan-4,5-dicarboxylate. $C_{13}H_{11}AsK_2N_6O_4S_2$. This is a water-soluble derivative of melarsoprol and may be administered by subcutaneous or intramuscular injection. The toxic effects are similar to those of melarsoprol, and it is considered as less effective than melarsoprol in the treatment of infections caused by *T. b. rhodesiense* where there is central nervous system involvement. It is used as an alternative to melarsoprol in the treatment of *T. b. gambiense* infections.

The usual dose is 2 mg kg^{-1} body weight, increasing to 4 mg kg^{-1} with a maximum of 200 mg total dose for an adult and 2 mg kg^{-1} for a child given s. c. or i. m. daily for 4 days. The 4-day course of 4 mg kg^{-1} daily may be repeated after an interval of 7–10 days.

Tryparsamide (Tryparsam; Tryparsamidium; Glyphenarsine;
Tryparsone)

Sodium *p*-carbamoylmethylaminophenylarsonate hemihydrate. $C_8H_{10}AsN_2NaO_4$, $^1/_2H_2O$. This arsenical compound is highly trypanocidal and able to penetrate the 'blood-brain barrier', thus it is of use in human sleeping sickness where there is central nervous system involvement. Its chief use has been in *T. b. gambiense* infections.

The major drawbacks to the use of tryparsamide are the fact that it has a severe toxic effect on the optic nerve and can cause blindness; there is also a problem of trypanosomes becoming resistant to the action of the drug. Because of the risk of blindness melarsoprol is now preferred, however, tryparsamide is still used, especially in conjunction with suramin in the late meningoencephalic stages of Gambian type disease where the general condition of the patient is extremely poor.

Tryparsamide is usually administered by intravenous injection; doses of 1–3 g are given once weekly for 6–8 weeks. In advanced *T. b. rhodesiense* infections with central nervous system involvement 30 mg kg^{-1} body weight of tryparsamide is given intravenously every 5–7 days for 10–12 doses together with suramin.

New Advances in Experimental Chemotherapy

The most exciting advances in this field have come from the 'logical approach' to chemotherapy, whereby differences in metabolism between parasite and host are researched, and inhibitors looked for that will act at specific points in the parasite's metabolism, and hopefully have little or no effect on the host. So a specific target in the parasite is chosen and inhibitors sought for that target, rather than the more usual giant screening procedures to look for drug activity that have been used in the past. The first such target that has been attacked in African sleeping sickness trypanosomes is their terminal respiration system; this is a cyanide-insensitive, cytochrome-independant, aerobic system that has glycerol-3-phosphate dehydrogenase and oxidase systems unique to the African salivarian trypanosomes. Many potential inhibitors were investigated until the discovery of a group of potent and specific inhibitors of the glycerol-3-phosphate oxidase component of the trypanosomes' terminal respiratory system; these were the aryl hydroxamic acids [11, 12]. At very low concentrations these acids give 100 % inhibition of the aerobic respiration of the trypanosomes, but the trypanosomes are able to survive this inhibition both in vivo and in vitro, and aryl hydroxamates on their own have been ineffective in curing trypanosome infections in laboratory rodents. The trypanosomes survive hydroxamate inhibition by using an anaerobic, hydroxamate-insensitive respiratory metabolism. *Clarkson and Brohn* [7] showed that by combining a commercially available hydroxamate, salicylhydroxamic acid (SHAM), with glycerol, a known inhibitor of the anaerobic respiration of glucose by sleeping sickness trypanosomes, that they were able to clear the bloodstream trypanosome infections of laboratory rodents. Very high doses of the drug combination were required, and the bloodstream parasitaemia always recrudesced within 7 days. *Evans and Holland* [13] showed that infections with the economically important cattle pathogen *Trypanosoma vivax* could be cured with a single but very high dose of SHAM and glycerol, and *Evans and Brightman* [14] showed that monomorphic trypanosomes belonging to the *T. brucei* group were curable with a single dose of SHAM and glycerol, but pleomorphic infections always recrudesced unless treatment was given very early on in the infection.

The enormously high doses of SHAM (500 mg kg^{-1}) and glycerol (4 g kg^{-1}) required to cure trypanosome infections, plus the problems encountered with recrudescence of the parasitaemia, make it unlikely that these compounds would ever be used as trypanocidal drugs, and as yet, no similarly acting compounds which are superior to SHAM and glycerol have been found. Salicylhydroxamic acid is excreted extremely rapidly, and this is probably the reason for the very high dosage required, and at these high doses the compound is certainly neurotoxic.

A more recent and most exciting advance in trypanosome chemotherapy has been the use of α-difluoromethylornithine (DFMO), an inhibitor of polyamine synthesis. Polyamines are low molecular weight compounds found in all cells, and are thought to participate in nucleic acid and protein synthesis, as well as acting to stabilize certain macromolecules. The role of polyamines in trypanosomatides has been under investigation for some time, and in these organisms as well as in all other cell types so far investigated, these compounds have an important role in cell replication. Recently, *Marcus* et al. [25] have demonstrated the presence of 2 forms of DNA polymerase activity in *T. b. brucei,* one of which is activated by polyamines, while *Lambros and Bacchi* [22] have shown that the vitally important NAD^+-linked glycerol phosphate dehydrogenase system in a related trypanosomatid, *Leptomonas* sp., requires polyamines for full activity. *Bacchi* et al. [1] have also shown that polyamines can negate the cureative action of several trypanocides.

The first step in polyamine biosynthesis is the formation of putrescine from ornithine, a reaction catalyzed by the enzyme ornithine decarboxylase. A specific and irreversible inhibitor of ornithine decarboxylase is α-difluoromethylornithine, and this compound has been used successfully by *Bacchi* et al. [2] to cure laboratory mice infected with *T. b. brucei*. *McCann* et al. [26] have reported similar cures of *T. b. rhodesiense* infected mice using DFMO. α-Difluoromethylornithine is apparently remarkably non-toxic and cures both *T. b. brucei* and *T. b. rhodesiense* infections in mice when 1–2 % of the inhibitor is added to the drinking water for 3–6 days. The outcome of further trials with DMFO as a trypanocide are eagerly awaited.

Future Needs

It seems unlikely that a vaccine for the protection of humans against infection with African trypanosomes will be forthcoming in the near future. Even the most enthusiastic tsetse fly irradicators do not foresee the elimination of the vector and consequently the disease, so chemotherapeutic and chemoprophylactic agents will have to be relied upon for the treatment and protection of people in areas of endemic trypanosomiasis. None of the present compounds available for human prophylaxis or treatment are satisfactory, all have side effects (often quite severe) of one form or another, and trypanosome resistance to the standard armoury of trypanocides is by no means uncommon. The most urgent need therefore is for a relatively non-toxic, cheap, easily administered drug, which will be capable of dealing with both early and advanced cases of African sleeping sickness. If such a compound were to have prophylactic action as well, then this would be as close to the ideal drug for combating African trypanosomiasis as it would be possible to imagine.

References

1 Bacchi, C. J.; Nathan, H. C.; Hutner, S. H.; Duch, D. S.; Nichol, C. A.: Negation of trypanocidal drug cures by polyamines; in Pollock, Current chemotherapy and infections disease. Proc. 18th Congr. Antimicrobiol. Agents and Chemotherapy, Boston 1979, pp. 1119–1121 (American Society of Microbiology, Washington 1980).

2 Bacchi, C. J.; Nathan, H. C.; Hutner, S. H.; McCann, P. P.; Sjoerdsma, A.: Polyamine metabolism. A potential therapeutic target in trypanosomes. Science *210:* 332–334 (1980).

3 Baker, J. R.: Epidemiology of African sleeping sickness; in Trypanosomiasis and Leishmaniasis with special reference to Chagas' disease. Ciba Foundation Symp. 20 (new series), pp. 29–43 (Associated Scientific Publishers, Amsterdam 1974).

4 Boreham, P. F. L.: The pathogenesis of African and American trypanosomiasis; in Levandowsky, Hutner, Biochemistry and physiology of protozoa, vol. 2; 2nd ed., pp. 429–457 (Academic Press, New York 1979).

5 Brun, R.; Jenni, L.; Tanner, M.; Schonenberger, M.; Schell, K.-F.: Cultivation of vertebrate infective forms derived from metacyclic forms of pleomorphic *Trypanosoma brucei* stocks. Acta trop. *36:* 387–390 (1979).

6 Castellani, A.: *Trypanosoma* in sleeping sickness. Br. med. J. *i:* 1218 (1903).

7 Clarkson, A.; Brohn, F.: Trypanosomiasis. An approach to chemotherapy by the inhibition of carbohydrate metabolism. Science *194:* 204–206 (1976).

8 Connor, D. H.; Neafie, R. C.; Dooley, J. R.: African trypanosomiasis; in Binford, Connor, Pathology of tropical and extraordinary diseases, vol. 1, pp. 252–257 (Armed Forces Institute of Pathology, Washington 1976).

9 Duggan, A. J.: A historical perspective; in Mulligan, The African trypanosomiases, pp. xli–lxxxviii (George Allen Unwin, London 1970).

10 Dutton, J. E.: Preliminary report upon a trypanosome occuring in the blood of man. Thomson Yates Lab. Rep. *4:* 455 (1902).

11 Evans, D. A.; Brown, R. C.: The inhibitory effects of aromatic hydroxamic acids on the cyanides insensitive terminal oxidase of *Trypanosoma brucei.* Trans. R. Soc. trop. Med. Hyg. *67:* 258 (1973).

12 Evans, D. A.; Brown, R. C.: *m*-Chlorobenzhydroxamic acid – an inhibitor of cyanide-insensitive respiration in *Trypanosoma brucei.* J. Protozool. *20:* 157–160 (1973).

13 Evans, D. A.; Holland, M. F.: Effective treatment of *Trypanosoma vivax* infections with salicylhydroxamic acid (SHAM). Trans. R. Soc. trop. Med. Hyg. *72:* 203–204 (1978).

14 Evans, D. A.; Brightman, C. A. J.: Pleomorphism and the problem of recrudescent parasitaemia following treatment with salicylhydroxamic acid (SHAM) in African trypanosomiasis. Trans. R. Soc. trop. Med. Hyg. *74:* 601–604 (1980).

15 Evans, D. A.; Brightman, C. J.; Holland, M. F.: Salicylhydroxamic acid/glycerol in experimental trypanosomiasis. Lancet *ii:* 769 (1977).

16 Flynn, I. W.; Bowman, I. B. R.: Further studies on the mode of action of arsenicals on trypanosome pyruvate kinase. Trans. R. Soc. trop. Med. Hyg. *63:* 121 (1969).

17 Fairlamb, A. H.; Bownman, I. B. R.: *Trypanosoma brucei.* Suramin and other trypanocidal compounds' effect on sn-glycerol-3-phosphate oxidase. Expl. Parasit. *43:* 353–361 (1977).

18 Hirumi, H.; Doyle, J. J.; Hirumi, K.: African trypanosomes. In vitro cultivation of animal-infective *Trypanosoma brucei.* Science *196:* 992–994 (1977).

19 Hoeppli, R.: Parasitic diseases in Africa and the Western hemisphere. Early documentation and transmission by the slave trade. Acta trop., suppl. 13 (1969).

20 Hutchinson, M. P.; Watson, H. J. C.: Berenil in the treatment of *Trypanosoma gambiense* infection in man. Trans. R. Soc. trop. Med. Hyg. *56:* 227–230 (1962).

21 Jennings, F. W.; Whitelaw, D. D.; Urquhart, G. M.: The relationship between duration of infection with *Trypanosoma brucei* in mice and the efficacy of chemotherapy. Parasitology *75:* 143–153 (1977).

22 Lambros, C.; Bacchi, C. J.: Properties of a purified, NAD-linked α-glycerophosphate dehydrogenase from *Leptomonas* sp; activation by polyamines. Biochem. biophys. Res. Commun. *68:* 658–667 (1976).

23 Launoy, L.; Guillot, M.; Jonchere, H.: Storage and Elimination of pentamidine in mice and white rats. Annls pharm. fr. *18:* 273–284, 424–439 (1960).

24 Lumsden, W. H. R.: Some episodes in the history of African trypanosomiasis. Proc. roy. Soc. Med. *67:* 789–796 (1974).

25 Marcus, S. L.; Lipschik, G.; Treuba, G.; Bacchi, C. J.: Chromatographic resolution of two DNA polymerase activities from bloodstream *Trypanosoma brucei*. Differential response to polyamine addition. Biochem. biophys. Res. Commun. *93:* 1027–1035 (1980).

26 McCann, P. P.; Bacchi, C. J.; Hanson, S. L.; Cain, G. D.; Nathan, H. C.; Hunter, S. H.; Sjoerdsma, A.: Effect on parasitic protozoa of α-difluoromethylornithine, an inhibitor of ornithine decarboxylase; in Advances in polyamine research (Raven Press, New York, in press, 1980).

27 Mott, F. W.: Histological observations on sleeping sickness and other trypanosome infections. Rep. Sleeping Sickness Commission Roy. Soc. *7:* 3 (1906).

28 Ormerod, W. E.: Pathogenesis and pathology of trypanosomiasis in man; in Mulligan, The African trypanosomiases, pp. 587–601 (George Allen & Unwin, London 1970).

29 Scott, H. H.: A history of tropical medicine (Edward Arnold, London 1939).

30 Temu, S. E.: Summary of cases of human early trypanosomiasis treated with berenil at EATRO. Trans. R. Soc. trop. Med. Hyg. *69:* 277–278 (1975).

31 Van Bogaert, L.: La trypanosomiase africaine; in Scholz, Spezielle pathologische Anatomie und Histologie, vol. 13, 2. Teil: Erkrankungen des zentralen Nervensystems II, pp. 1089–1099 (Springer, Berlin 1952).

32 Willett, K. C.: The problem of *Trypanosoma rhodesiense,* its history and distribution, and its relationship to *T. gambiense* and *T. brucei*. East Afr. med. J. *33:* 473–479 (1956).

33 Zillmann, U.; Mehlitz, D.: The natural occurrence of *Trypanozoon* in domestic chickens in the Ivory Coast. Tropenmed. Parasitol. *30:* 239–243 (1979).

D. A. Evans, PhD, Department of Medical Protozoology, London School of Hygiene and Tropical Medicine, Keppel Street, London WC1E 7HT (England)